INTENSIVE CORONARY CARE

A Manual for Nurses

INTENSIVE CORONARY CARE

A MANUAL FOR NURSES

Third Edition

LAWRENCE E. MELTZER, M.D.
Director, Section of Clinical Investigation
Presbyterian-University of Pennsylvania Medical Center
Philadelphia, Pennsylvania

ROSE PINNEO, R.N., M.S.
Associate Professor of Nursing
School of Nursing
University of Rochester
Rochester, New York

J. RODERICK KITCHELL, M.D.
Emeritus Chief of Cardiology
Abington Memorial Hospital
Abington, Pennsylvania

The Charles Press Publishers
Bowie, Maryland 20715

Intensive Coronary Care: A Manual for Nurses
Third Edition

Library of Congress Cataloging in Publication Data

Meltzer, Lawrence E.
    Intensive coronary care: a manual for nurses.

    Includes index.
    1. Coronary heart disease—Nursing.   2.   Coronary
care units.   I.   Pinneo, Rose, joint author.
II.   Kitchell, J. Roderick, 1906—   joint author.
III.   Title.
RC685.C6M44 1977   610.73′6   77-12120
ISBN 0-913486-79-5

Prentice-Hall International, Inc., London
Prentice-Hall of Australia, Pty., Ltd., Sydney
Prentice-Hall of India Private Limited, New Delhi
Prentice-Hall of Japan, Inc., Tokyo
Prentice-Hall of Southeast Asia (Pte.) Ltd., Singapore
Whitehall Books, Limited, Wellington, New Zealand

Printed in the United States of America

79 80 81 82   10 9 8 7 6 5 4

Contents

Preface

The system of intensive coronary care proposed in the original edition of this book (1965) is now a well established, standard method of hospital care throughout the world; indeed very few medical advances have been accepted as readily or with as much enthusiasm. It has been our premise from the outset that intensive coronary care is primarily and above all a system of specialized nursing care. The effectiveness of the plan in saving lives of patients with acute myocardial infarction depends finally on the ability of nurses to function as decision-making members of the coronary care team, capable of acting on their observations and judgment, particularly in emergency situations or whenever therapeutic decisions cannot be delayed. By demonstrating remarkable competence in this demanding role (and accepting the responsibilities that accompany it) coronary care nurses have broadened the horizons of clinical nursing, and have earned the sincere respect of their colleagues and patients.

We are extremely grateful for the extraordinary reception accorded the two previous editions of this book. *Intensive Coronary Care–A Manual for Nurses* has served as the standard textbook of coronary care nursing for the past 12 years; it has been translated into four languages, and more than 700,000 copies are in print.

In preparing this third edition we have attempted to increase the scope and depth of the presentation while preserving its simplicity and clarity. In effect, the style and format of the book remain unchanged but the text has been revised and expanded considerably. The revisions and additions are designed not only to present new concepts of coronary care that have evolved since the last edition but also equally important, to keep pace with the growing sophistication and quality of nursing education and nursing practice. To this end we have included detailed information about the pathophysiology of heart failure and cardiogenic shock, the pharmacology of antiarrhythmic drugs and diuretic agents, hemodynamic monitoring, coronary bypass surgery, and new concepts of the early management of acute myocardial infarction, among many other subjects involved in modern coronary care nursing.

We are indebted to Mrs. Elizabeth Meholick for her indispensable help in preparing this manuscript for publication.

Lawrence E. Meltzer, M.D.
Rose Pinneo, R.N., M.S.
J. Roderick Kitchell, M.D.

Philadelphia, Pennsylvania
September, 1977

INTENSIVE CORONARY CARE

A Manual for Nurses

1

Coronary Heart Disease

When the incredible complexity of the human system is considered along with the vast number of possible sources of illness and death, it seems incongruous that the life of so many depends finally on the health of two small arteries; but the fact is undeniable. Disease of the coronary arteries has become the single greatest threat to life in industrialized countries throughout the world. In the United States, for example, more than 600,000 deaths a year—or one-third of *all* deaths—are directly attributable to this one disease.

As the sole blood supply to the heart musculature (myocardium), the coronary arteries assume extreme importance. Any significant interference with blood flow through these vessels can impair the entire function of the myocardium, with dire consequences including sudden death. Before describing the clinical aspects of coronary disease it is pertinent first to consider the coronary arteries and the basic disease process that affects them.

THE CORONARY ARTERIES

The two coronary arteries, the left and right, arise from the aorta just above the aortic valve. The left coronary artery then divides into two large branches: the left anterior descending artery and the left circumflex artery. The relationship of these three arteries is shown in Figure 1.1.

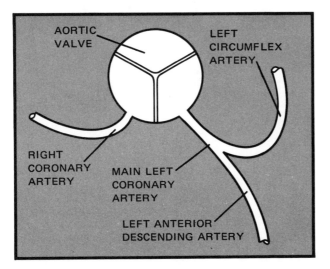

Figure 1.1. The coronary arteries as viewed from above (looking down at the aortic valve).

Each artery supplies a different area of the heart. Briefly, the left anterior descending artery supplies most of the anterior wall of the left ventricle, the anterior portion of the interventricular septum, as well as the anterior wall of the right ventricle. The left circumflex artery supplies the lateral aspect of the left ventricle and the left atrium. The right coronary artery supplies the right atrium and the right ventricle along with the posterior portions of the left ventricle and interventricular septum. The arteries lie on the outer surface of the ventricles and give off numerous branches that penetrate all parts of the heart (Fig. 1.2). The terminal branches of the arteries have many interconnections, forming an extensive vascular network throughout the myocardium.

The function of the coronary arteries is to bring oxygen-carrying blood to the myocardium, oxygen being an essential ingredient in producing the energy the heart requires to contract. As a pump that works incessantly (contracting more than 100,000 times a day), the myocardium has very great oxygen needs. This constant demand can be met only by an adequate coronary blood flow. Indeed, 250 cc of blood per minute—or 36,000 liters per day—pass through the coronary arteries to oxygenate the myocardium.

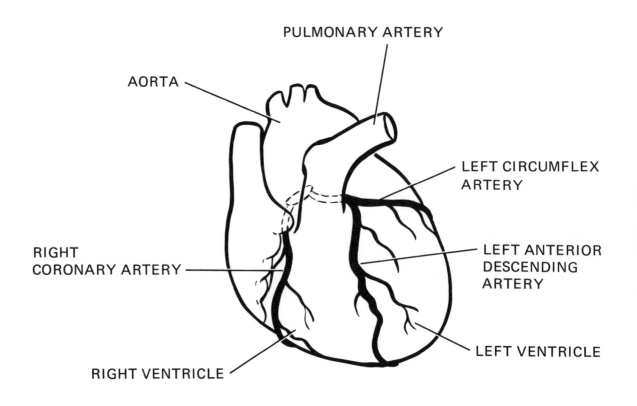

Figure 1.2. Coronary circulation.

CORONARY ATHEROSCLEROSIS

The primary disease affecting the coronary arteries is atherosclerosis, a process in which fatty substances (particularly cholesterol) deposit as plaques along the inner lining of the vessels and narrow the passages. If the narrowing reaches a stage where the blood flow through the arteries is insufficient to meet the oxygen demands of the myocardium, then coronary heart disease (CHD) is said to exist.

Coronary atherosclerosis usually develops gradually over a period of years. However, the process begins at an early age so that by adulthood most men (and women, to a lesser degree) have some evidence of atherosclerosis in the coronary arteries. Autopsy studies have shown, for example, that among young American soldiers (average age of 22 years) killed in action during the Korean war nearly 80% had definite signs of coronary atherosclerosis. It is essential to realize, however, that the critical determinant of coronary heart disease is not the mere presence of atherosclerosis but rather the extent of arterial narrowing and the reduction in blood flow the lesions produce. Atherosclerosis can be categorized into four grades according to the degree of arterial obstruction. Grade 1 atherosclerosis indicates that the diameter (lumen) of the artery is reduced by no more than 25%; grade 2 represents a 50% reduction, grade 3 a 75% reduction, and grade 4 complete (100%) obstruction of the vessel (Fig. 1.3). It is believed that an obstruction of at least 75% is necessary to produce a significant reduction in coronary blood flow; lesser degrees of narrowing can usually be tolerated without affecting myocardial function. Obstruction may occur in any (or all) of the coronary arteries, but involvement of the left anterior descending artery is particularly dangerous. This vessel supplies a much larger portion of the total myocardial mass than the right coronary and left circumflex arteries and therefore has the greatest blood flow.

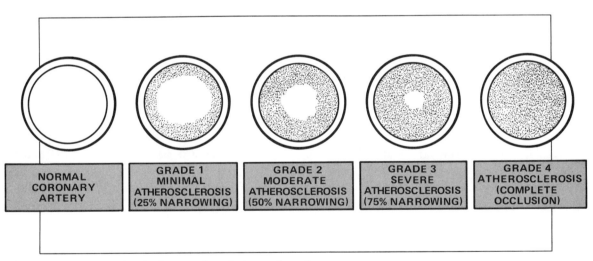

Figure 1.3. Criteria for the four grades of atherosclerosis.

Until recent years there was no way (except at autopsy) to determine the degree of arterial obstruction or the vessels involved. With the introduction of coronary arteriography, a technique which permits the arteries to be visualized by x rays, it is now possible to identify the site and extent of atherosclerotic lesions with reasonable accuracy. The procedure involves the insertion of a catheter into the aorta (by way of a peripheral artery) and the injection of a radiopaque dye through the openings (ostia) of the two main coronary arteries. As the dye is being injected a rapid series of x-ray films are taken to outline the arterial tree; advanced lesions can be readily detected in this way. Figure 1.4 compares a normal coronary artery with one that has a 90% obstruction in one segment.

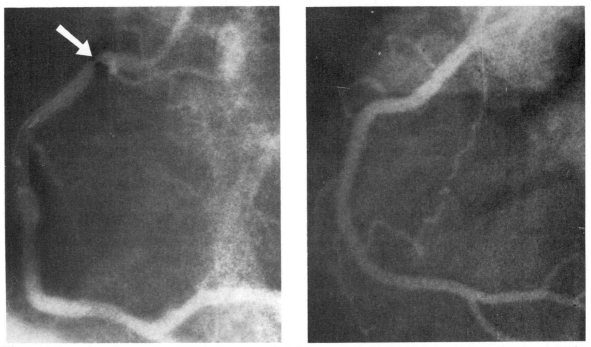

Figure 1.4.   Arteriograms comparing a normal right coronary artery (right) with one that has a 90% obstruction (left).

CAUSES OF CORONARY HEART DISEASE

An unrelenting search has been in progress for more than 50 years attempting to ascertain why and how the coronary arteries are affected by atherosclerosis. The question has never been answered, and the cause of coronary atherosclerosis remains unknown. However, one fundamental fact has emerged: combination of several factors is undoubtedly involved in the development of CHD; no single mechanism can be held responsible in its own right. According to this concept, all of the following factors (called risk factors) may contribute to the formation and progression of coronary atherosclerosis.

Sex and Age

CHD is distinctly more prevalent in men than in women. Indeed, during the childbearing years women are seemingly protected from CHD unless they have many other risk factors (e.g., hypertension and diabetes). After the menopause, however, the incidence of CHD in females rises rapidly and equals the male rate thereafter. In contrast, symptomatic CHD may occur in men as young as 30 years (or even younger). This sex–age discrepancy suggests that hormonal influences may be important in the disease.

The incidence of CHD increases greatly with age in both sexes. For example, a man in his fifties has four times the risk of a heart attack as a man in his thirties. The fact that young persons may develop CHD makes it clear, however, that coronary atherosclerosis is not simply a disease of aging.

Diet and Cholesterol

Several epidemiologic studies have demonstrated that the incidence of premature CHD (i.e., coronary disease occurring before the age of 60) can be correlated with the different dietary patterns of various societies. Specifically, in affluent countries (as the United States), where animal fats constitute a large percentage of the total diet, the frequency of CHD is very high; and in poorer countries, where animal fat intake is much less, the incidence of the disease is low. The gross disparity in the amount of animal fat eaten (e.g., eggs, butter, cream, milk, and fatty meats) in different parts of the world is believed to account for the fact that "normal" serum cholesterol levels in the United States may be 200–240 mg%, whereas in those countries in which CHD is uncommon the comparable levels are only 100–120 mg%. Further evidence in support of the danger of high-fat diets is the reported decrease in the number of deaths from CHD during World War II in those countries where animal fats became scarce, followed by a prompt increase in the death rate after the war ended when the economy improved and fats again became available. From data of this type many researchers have concluded that overeating of animal fats (also called saturated fats) is a prime factor in the etiology of CHD.

More specific information about the danger of high serum cholesterol levels has been obtained from the Framingham Heart Study. In this study more than 5000 men and women in the town of Framingham, Massachusetts, have been examined at regular intervals for 25 years to determine which factors contribute to the development of CHD. The results indicate that the risk of a heart attack is at least three times greater in men with serum cholesterol levels of more than 240 mg% than it is in those with levels of less than 200 mg%.

Hypertension

High blood pressure is thought to predispose to CHD by accelerating the rate of atherosclerosis and by increasing the oxygen demands of the myocardium. In the Framingham Heart Study it was observed that blood pressures in excess of 160/95 were associated with a fivefold increase in the incidence of CHD compared with normal pressures. Thus from a statistical standpoint hypertension appears to be one of the most serious risk factors.

Heredity

A familial pattern of CHD has long been recognized, but the degree of risk is still uncertain (because family histories are unreliable in many instances). However, our own experience suggests that heredity ranks among the highest risk factors, particularly when CHD occurs during the fourth or fifth decade of life. In these latter cases it is commonly found that a man's father, grandfather, and brothers often developed CHD at about the same age. It has been postulated (but not proved) that the physical structure of the coronary arteries and the rate of atherosclerosis may be genetically determined.

Diabetes

CHD develops more frequently and at an earlier age among diabetic patients than among nondiabetics. Even when diabetes is mild or well controlled the risk of CHD remains substantially greater. These facts along with data indicating that other metabolic diseases (e.g., gout) are associated with a high incidence of CHD suggest that a biochemical disturbance may be central to the underlying disease process.

Cigarette Smoking

There is statistical evidence to indicate that heavy cigarette smokers have a higher incidence of CHD than nonsmokers. In the Framingham study the risk of a heart attack was nearly twice as great in cigarette smokers. However, the risk is associated primarily with middle-aged men and is much less impressive in older men and in women. Curiously, cigar and pipe smokers are at no greater risk than nonsmokers, presumably because they do not inhale. The manner in which cigarette smoking affects the coronary arteries is not understood. The suggestion that nicotine may cause sufficient constriction of the arteries to reduce coronary blood flow has not been confirmed. On the other hand, nicotine increases the work of the heart (by increasing the heart rate and blood pressure) and could produce a relative oxygen deficiency. Moreover, cigarette smoking is associated with elevated carbon monoxide levels in the blood, which may also interfere with myocardial oxygenation.

Sedentary Life

Lack of physical activity has been incriminated as a risk factor in CHD, but the evidence for this belief is still inconclusive. Several studies have revealed, for example, that CHD occurs more frequently in sedentary workers (e.g., postal clerks) than in those whose occupations demand substantial physical activity (e.g., mail carriers); yet many observers have questioned the significance of these findings, noting that there were so many other variables between the two groups that physical inactivity should not be singled out as a risk factor in its own right. Although there is good reason to believe that exercise may benefit the myocardium, it remains to be seen if physical activity (or inactivity) affects coronary arteries and influences atherosclerosis.

Obesity

Insurance company statistics suggest that obesity predisposes to fatal CHD, but (as with physical inactivity) the issue is by no means settled. In fact in the Framingham study moderate obesity by itself was not associated with an increased incidence of CHD. However, overweight persons are especially prone to hypertension, diabetes, and elevated cholesterol levels, and it may be that the risk of obesity lies with these secondary effects. In any case obesity is classified as a risk factor even though its mechanism of action is uncertain.

Emotional Stress

Epidemiologic studies have consistently shown a markedly higher incidence of CHD in industrialized (civilized) countries than in primitive, less-demanding societies. Many believe that this gross disparity is a reflection or a direct result of emotional stress imposed by modern, fast-paced styles of life. For this reason CHD is considered by some to be a disease of "overcivilization." According to this theory civilized man has developed chronic anxiety in attempting to cope with rapidly changing socioeconomic and sociocultural forces, and this tension in some way promotes atherosclerosis. In principle, this is an attractive concept, since it has been demonstrated that anxiety is often accompanied by a distinct rise in serum cholesterol, which could favor the development of atherosclerotic plaques. Moreover, stress is known to accelerate blood coagulation, allowing small clots to form within the coronary arteries. Nevertheless, the relationship between emotional stress and CHD has been difficult to prove, particularly since there are no available methods to actually measure degrees of stress. Some research studies in fact have cast doubt on the importance of stress as a risk factor. For example, one large investigation involving telephone company employees showed that the incidence of CHD was actually less common among high-level executives (who presumably function under great stress) than it was among workers who installed or repaired equipment. Further facts will be needed to determine the significance of emotional stress as a risk factor.

Behavioral Patterns

Attempts have been made to correlate CHD with certain personality traits and behavioral patterns. The coronary-prone person—called a type A personality—is said to be one who is aggressive, ambitious, highly competitive, and most of all possessed with a profound sense of the urgency of time. Those with this type behavioral pattern reportedly have significantly higher cholesterol levels and an increased incidence of CHD than their counterparts (type B personalities), in whom these particular characteristics are not as apparent. This interesting observation requires confirmation, but many now accept type A behavior as a distinct risk factor.

Summary of Risk Factors

It is essential to point out that there is no definite evidence that any of the risk factors just described actually *cause* CHD. All that can be said is that individuals with multiple risk factors are high-risk candidates for CHD; conversely, the absence of these factors predicts little likelihood of developing the disease. For example, a man with hypertension and high serum cholesterol levels who is a heavy cigarette smoker may have ten times the risk of sustaining a heart attack than a person with none of these factors. In other words, there is a statistical association between risk factors and CHD but, on the other hand, no proof that these risk factors in themselves are the direct cause of coronary atherosclerosis.

THE CLINICAL SPECTRUM OF CORONARY ATHEROSCLEROSIS

Asymptomatic Coronary Atherosclerosis

If the degree of arterial obstruction is moderate and does not significantly reduce the blood supply to the myocardium, the disease may never be suspected by the patient or his physician. Results of autopsy studies among persons dying of other causes indicate that this is a common situation. In fact, practically all men in the United States have evidence of coronary atherosclerosis by age 50; it is only the degree of involvement that varies.

Even if the coronary arteries are grossly narrowed by intimal plaques, it still does not follow that the disease will be clinically evident or produce symptoms. This paradox can be explained by the fact that as the coronary arteries gradually narrow small branches of these vessels may enlarge or new branches may form in order to bring more blood to the myocardium. This additional blood supply, called *collateral circulation*, is of great importance in determining the clinical effects of coronary atherosclerosis since this network of vessels is often substantial enough to maintain an adequate blood supply to portions of the myocardium despite the presence of advanced atherosclerosis in a major vessel. It is the *total* blood supply to the myocardium rather than the state of the main coronary arteries that determines whether the disease will be symptomatic. In effect, any impairment of myocardial function produced by athero-sclerotic lesions depends finally on the rate of narrowing of the main arteries compared to the rate of widening and formation of collateral vessels.

Asymptomatic coronary atherosclerosis is sometimes referred to as coronary *artery* disease (CAD), in distinction to coronary *heart* disease (CHD), in which symptoms oc-cur because the total blood supply is insufficient to meet the demands of the myocar-dium.

Symptomatic Coronary Atherosclerosis

Coronary heart disease, by definition, implies that the myocardium is affected by inadequate coronary blood flow. The symptoms of CHD are due to myocardial oxygen deprivation and are manifested by progressive order of severity by three main clinical patterns: angina pectoris, the intermediate coronary syndrome, and acute myocardial infarction. Each of these syndromes is described separately in the following pages.

1. Angina Pectoris

The classic indication of impaired circulation to the myocardium is a distinctive type of chest pain called *angina pectoris*. As the result of the compromised blood supply the amount of oxygen available to the myocardium is reduced; it is this insufficient oxygen-ation (described as *ischemia*) that causes angina pectoris. In other words, angina pec-toris represents a warning signal from the heart, indicating that the myocardium does not have a sufficient amount of oxygen to meet its demands at the moment. Coronary arteriograms usually show at least 75% narrowing of one or more coronary arteries; most often two or three vessels are involved. Because this one symptom is often the key to the diagnosis of CHD it is important that the clinical pattern of angina be under-stood fully.

Site of Pain.   The pain reflecting myocardial ischemia is located most often directly under the breastbone. The pain may radiate from this substernal location to either the left or right arm, the neck, the jaw, the teeth, or the upper back. In some instances the pain occurs only at these latter sites without a substernal component; this pattern, how-ever, is much less common than pure substernal pain. The discomfort is usually de-scribed as a pressure, tightness, or constriction within the chest. Some patients place a clenched fist against the sternum in attempting to characterize the constricting nature of the sensation. Although angina pectoris generally lasts for only a few minutes (as described below), the pain is steady and is not influenced by breathing, breath-hold-ing, or change in body position. This constancy of substernal pain is the most charac-teristic aspect of angina and is more significant than other descriptive qualities (e.g., pressure, indigestion, or burning).

Occurrence of Pain.   Any condition that increases the myocardial demand for oxy-gen is capable of producing angina. In general, oxygen demand is related to the amount of work the heart performs. As would be anticipated on this basis, the pain is usually brought on by physical effort which increases the heart rate and work and, in turn, the myocardial oxygen requirements. Conversely, angina is relieved by rest. When physical activity stops, the oxygen demand falls promptly, and as a consequence the pain subsides. This relationship (activity → pain, rest → disappearance of pain) is typical of myocardial ischemia and distinguishes angina from other, nonischemic causes of chest pain in which this pattern does not appear. In addition to physical exer-tion, sudden emotional stress (e.g., anger, fear, or even the excitement of watching a football game) may precipitate an anginal attack. In these situations the work of the heart is transiently increased beyond the ability of the coronary circulation to satisfy the oxygen needs. In fact, any physical or emotional situation that suddenly increases the heart rate may cause angina. Although angina classically occurs with effort, it may develop during sleep (nocturnal angina) or at rest (angina decubitus); this paradoxical occurrence is not fully understood.

Duration of Pain. Angina is characteristically of *short* duration, lasting only seconds to a minute or two before abating with rest. Occasionally the pain may persist for longer periods (5–10 minutes), particularly if the stimulus for the attack is intense. The cessation of pain indicates that the myocardial demand for oxygen has been met, and that the oxygen deficit was only transient and not destructive to the myocardium. If the pain does not subside within minutes after rest, myocardial damage must be suspected.

Relief of Pain. Another distinctive feature of angina is the prompt relief of pain that follows the use of nitroglycerin. Failure of nitroglycerin, administered sublingually, to terminate ischemic chest pain is unusual and is cause for suspicion that the attack is not anginal in origin. Nitroglycerin (and other nitrites) act by dilating the coronary vessels, thus increasing the blood flow and oxygen supply to the myocardium.

Stable and Unstable Angina. As noted, in most instances angina pectoris behaves in a predictable manner: it occurs with certain types of physical effort or emotional stress and is relieved promptly by rest or nitrogylcerin. This pattern is described as *stable* angina. In contrast, if the pain pattern suddenly worsens and becomes unpredictable, occurring spontaneously or at rest, and is no longer controlled consistently by nitroglycerin, the condition is termed *unstable* angina. Unstable angina generally indicates progression of coronary disease and is more ominous than stable angina.

2. Intermediate Coronary Syndrome

Some patients with CHD develop chest pain that is more severe and longer lasting than angina pectoris but less severe and of shorter duration than the unrelenting pain of acute myocardial infarction. Because the pain pattern is between these two extremes, it is appropriately described as the intermediate coronary syndrome. An equally popular (but less descriptive) term for this ischemic pain is acute coronary insufficiency.

The intermediate coronary syndrome may occur as the initial symptom of CHD or as a sudden worsening of preexisting angina (unstable angina). This intermediate-type pain is more serious than stable angina, since frequently it is an immediate forerunner of acute myocardial infarction; in fact, this sequence occurs commonly enough that the pain pattern is often called *preinfarction* angina.

Theoretically the intermediate coronary syndrome implies that, although the myocardium was deprived of a sufficient oxygen supply for many minutes, adequate oxygenation was finally restored before myocardial destruction actually occurred. From a clinical standpoint, however, it is often very difficult to rule out the possibility that small areas of the myocardium were injured or destroyed during the prolonged period of ischemia. For this reason patients with the intermediate coronary syndrome are usually hospitalized until the diagnosis of acute myocardial infarction has been excluded (as described in the next chapter.)

3.   Acute Myocardial Infarction

If there is profound and sustained ischemia to a portion of the myocardium, the cells deprived of oxygen cannot survive, and local death of tissue (necrosis) develops in the involved area. This destructive process is termed *acute myocardial infarction*. The event that produces this irreversible tissue damage (infarction) is often called a coronary thrombosis, a coronary occlusion, a coronary, or a heart attack. These latter terms are used synonymously in clinical practice to describe what properly should be designated acute myocardial infarction.

Nearly all instances of acute myocardial infarction are the result of severe atherosclerosis of the coronary arteries. (Very rarely the arteries are narrowed or blocked by other processes, including collagen diseases, syphilis, or fragments of clots from other sites.) This final insult of progressive coronary atherosclerosis usually occurs when a main coronary artery or its branches become occluded; in most cases this obstruction takes place suddenly. The exact reason that a coronary vessel blocks off at a certain moment is not completely understood, but three different causes have been incriminated: 1) a blood clot may develop on the roughened surface of an atherosclerotic plaque and occlude the lumen of the artery (coronary thrombosis), 2) the atherosclerotic lesions may irritate the underlying arterial wall and cause bleeding beneath the plaque; this subintimal hemorrhage dislodges the plaque, which then obstructs the vessel, and 3) a piece of a large plaque may break off and block a smaller artery. Although these mechanisms offer a logical explanation for this sudden event, it is now clear that neither clot formation nor plaque disruption can account for *all* myocardial infarctions. Autopsy studies have shown that myocardial infarction may develop even though the coronary arteries are not completely closed. In these latter instances it is presumed that at a particular moment the heart may have an enormous demand for oxygen (e.g., during sudden vigorous physical exertion, as shoveling snow) which cannot be met by the available blood supply. In effect, even though the arteries are not completely obstructed, the myocardial demand for oxygen simply overwhelms its supply, and tissue necrosis occurs because of this relative oxygen deprivation. A similar situation may result from

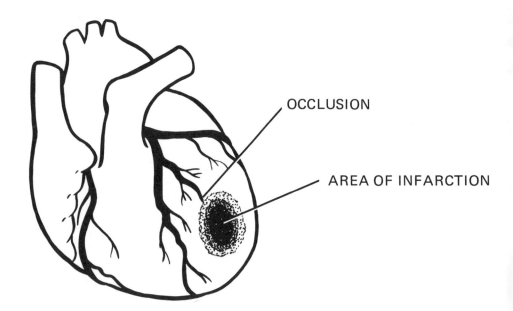

Figure 1.5.   Anterior myocardial infarction.

sudden, profound anemia (e.g., gastrointestinal hemorrhage) where oxygen available to the myocardium is grossly reduced, and infarction can develop in the presence of patent arteries.

The site of an infarction depends fundamentally on which coronary artery (or arteries) is blocked. When the left coronary artery or its branches are occluded, the infarction involves primarily the interior wall of the left ventricle and is called an *anterior infarction* (Fig. 1.5). Occlusion of the right coronary artery results in infarction of the inferior (diaphragmatic) wall of the left ventricle—an *inferior infarction* (Fig. 1.6). Very often more than one area of the left ventricle is damaged by the ischemic process; in these cases more specific terms are used to describe the location of the infarct. For example, if the infarction involves both the anterior and lateral walls of the left ventricle, it is termed an *anterolateral infarction*. Similarly, damage to the anterior wall of the left ventricle and to the interventricular septum is called an *anteroseptal infarction*. Infarction of the right ventricle is rare because this chamber receives a relatively greater proportion of blood for its muscle mass than the left ventricle and also has lesser energy (oxygen) requirements.

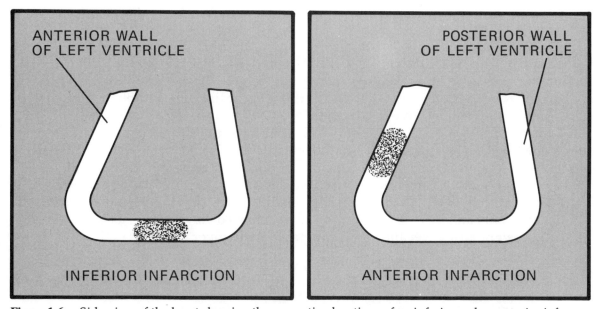

Figure 1.6. Side view of the heart showing the respective locations of an inferior and an anterior infarction. Because the inferior surface of the left ventricle faces the diaphragm, inferior infarctions are also called diaphragmatic infarctions.

The extent of an infarction is determined first by the size of the vessel obstructed and second by the capacity of the collateral circulation to bring blood to the oxygen-deprived areas. If there is widespread myocardial necrosis extending through and through the entire ventricular wall (from the endocardium to the pericardium), the infarction is termed *transmural* (Fig. 1.7). Lesser degrees of damage which do not involve the full thickness of the ventricular wall are categorized as *nontransmural* infarctions. Other descriptive terms for nontransmural infarctions are intramural and subendocardial infarctions.

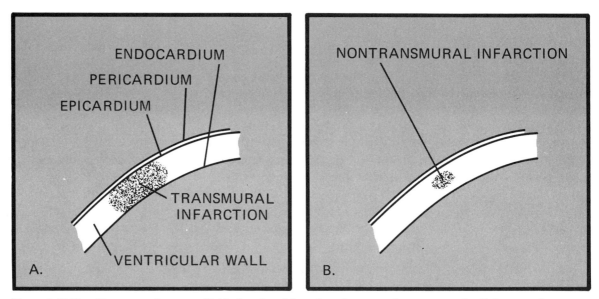

Figure 1.7(A).   Transmural myocardial infarction. Note that the necrotic area extends all the way through the ventricular wall from the endocardium to the pericardium.   **(B).** With a nontransmural infarction the damage is less extensive, involving only a portion of the ventricular wall.

In the early stages of acute myocardial infarction there are three zones of tissue damage (Fig. 1.8). The first zone consists of necrotic myocardial tissue that has been irreversibly destroyed by prolonged deprivation of oxygen. Surrounding this dead tissue is a second zone (zone of injury) in which the myocardial cells, although injured and jeopardized, may still survive if adequate circulation to the area is restored. Zone 3, called the zone of ischemia, represents cells that have not received adequate oxygen but can be expected to recover unless the ischemic process worsens. In effect, the ultimate size of an infarction depends on the fate of the injury zone and the ischemic zone.

Once the coronary circulation is interrupted and a myocardial infarction occurs, a series of events follow which place life and death in balance. This book concerns itself with these events and describes a concept of specialized care, known as *intensive coronary care*, designed to lower the death rate from acute myocardial infarction.

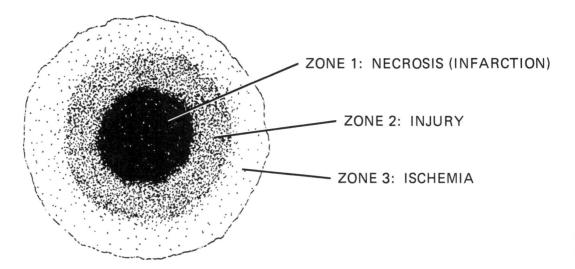

Figure 1.8.   Three zones of tissue damage associated with acute myocardial infarction. Zone 1 is irreversibly damaged, but zones 2 and 3 may recover if adequate circulation to these areas is restored by collateral circulation.

2

Acute Myocardial Infarction

THE ONSET OF THE ATTACK

Most patients with acute myocardial infarction seek medical assistance because of *chest pain*. The pain is usually quite distinctive; it occurs suddenly and is of severe, crushing quality. It is more intense than the pain of angina or the intermediate coronary syndrome and may be unlike any sensation the patient has experienced previously. Typically, the pain is concentrated directly beneath the sternum, but it frequently radiates across the chest or to the arms and neck. Patients commonly describe the pain as a heavy weight or pressure, or a knot in the chest. Unlike angina, the pain does not necessarily occur with exertion; in fact, it frequently begins during sleep. Its occurrence after eating explains why many patients interpret the pain as indigestion. The chest pain is continuous and is not relieved by change in body position, breath-holding, or by home remedies (e.g., bicarbonate) the patient may try. Nitroglycerin seldom influences the duration or severity of the pain. Shortly after the onset of the substernal pain drenching perspiration usually begins, and nausea and vomiting often occur at this time. Fear and apprehension are usual, and most patients sense that a catastrophe has happened. Within minutes, many patients are aware of dyspnea and marked weakness. This symptom complex of substernal pain, sweating, nausea, and vomiting along with dyspnea and weakness can be considered the typical history of acute myocardial infarction.

Not all patients, however, present such typical histories, and there are many variants of the story. Sometimes the major pain is not in the chest but, as with angina, is located in the neck, the arms, or the jaws. Sweating, nausea, vomiting, and dyspnea may not accompany this referred pain.

Acute myocardial infarction may also develop during surgery. In this situation the symptoms are masked by anesthesia, and the diagnosis of infarction is considered because of an unexplained drop in blood pressure or the development of shock during a surgical procedure.

Perhaps 10% of patients sustain acute myocardial infarction presumably without any chest pain or other symptoms. This diagnosis is surmised when there is evidence of an old infarction on a routine electrocardiogram and yet the patient denies any previous symptoms; these are called *silent* infarctions.

Some patients develop serious or fatal complications of acute myocardial infarction immediately after the attack, and in these cases it is the complication itself (e.g., sudden pulmonary edema or an arrhythmia) that arouses suspicion that an infarction has occurred.

THE CLINICAL COURSE IMMEDIATELY AFTER INFARCTION

It is apparent that the heart may respond in several different ways to the abrupt interruption of its blood supply. Some patients develop serious or lethal complications almost instantly, whereas others never experience any difficulties. It is not known with certainty which factors actually influence the heart's behavior once coronary occlusion has occurred. It has been presumed that the size of the infarction is the most important determinant of the subsequent clinical course. In general, if a main artery is occluded and there is extensive myocardial damage (transmural infarction), the course and prognosis are thought to be much poorer than if a branch vessel is blocked and the resultant injury is small. This relationship is not constant, however, and patients with limited areas of tissue destruction can develop serious complications. Because of this disparity it is evident that other factors play a role in determining the outcome of the illness. Considered to be of particular importance in this regard is the degree of collateral blood supply that can be diverted instantly to the deprived (ischemic) area of the myocardium. If the collateral supply is extensive, the area of myocardial damage may be minimal; conversely, if the collateral circulation is poor, widespread destruction may result since tissue oxygenation cannot be enhanced. Because of these variants (along with probably other influences which are not well understood) several possible clinical pictures may occur immediately after acute myocardial infarction:

1. If the infarcted area is limited in size and enough blood is diverted to the site by collateral channels, the myocardium may continue to function quite normally. The heart's pumping action may not be affected, and the rate and rhythm of the heart are not necessarily disturbed. The pain gradually subsides in these instances, and the patient appears in no distress.

2. When the involved area is larger and if there is only trivial collateral assistance, the myocardium may become sufficiently embarrassed that its function is impaired. This may be manifested by signs of decreased pumping action of the heart (heart failure) or by disturbances in the rate and rhythm of the heartbeat (arrhythmias). The degree of impairment may vary greatly; some patients have only mild shortness of breath and minor arrhythmias, whereas others are critically ill with marked dyspnea, pulmonary edema, and life-threatening arrhythmias.

3. If the pumping action of the heart is grossly reduced as a result of extensive structural damage to the myocardium, the left ventricle is simply unable to pump sufficient blood throughout the body to sustain circulation to the vital organs. Accordingly, the blood pressure falls, the heart rate increases, the urinary output decreases, and the skin becomes cold and clammy. This state is called *cardiogenic shock*; most patients with this complication die within hours.

4. In some patients death occurs almost instantly after interruption of coronary blood flow. These *sudden* deaths are almost always the result of lethal arrhythmias resulting from extraordinary changes in the electrical activity of the heart. In these instances the heart either stops abruptly (ventricular standstill) or beats ineffectively in a mere quivering fashion (ventricular fibrillation). There is no clear relationship between the size of an infarction and the occurrence of sudden arrhythmic deaths. Studies have shown that probably 50% of *all* deaths from acute myocardial infarction occur within the first hour after the attack as the result of arrhythmias.

Because of these different possibilities it can be appreciated that some patients admitted to the hospital with acute myocardial infarction have no pain by the time they arrive and are not in distress, whereas others are near death from cardiogenic shock or acute heart failure when first seen. The ultimate clinical course is related to a large degree, but certainly not entirely, to the clinical picture on admission. However, *complications can develop at any time in any patient!*

THE COMPLICATIONS OF ACUTE MYOCARDIAL INFARCTION

There are five major complications that threaten life after acute myocardial infarction. Each of these complications is considered in detail in subsequent chapters. They are mentioned here to provide an overview of the clinical course of the illness.

1. Arrhythmias

Disturbances in the cardiac rate or rhythm (arrhythmias) are the most common complication of acute myocardial infarction. At least 90% of patients with acute infarction develop some form of arrhythmia during the acute phase of the illness. Arrhythmias pose two serious threats: They may reduce the pumping efficiency of the heart, precipitating acute heart failure; and above all, they may produce *sudden death*. Although not all disorders of rate and rhythm are life-threatening, the critical fact is that *death-producing arrhythmias can occur at any time*.

2. Acute Left Ventricular Failure

The contractile ability of the myocardium is reduced after infarction, often causing the heart to fail as a pumping system. Such failure can occur suddenly, resulting in acute pulmonary edema, or gradually (if the ventricle recovers from the original ischemia but falters subsequently). Clinical signs of heart failure are observed in about 60% of patients; the degree of this pumping deficit varies considerably.

3. Cardiogenic Shock

The most advanced form of left ventricular failure is described as cardiogenic shock. It results when the heart is unable to sustain the circulation and provide adequate oxygen to the vital organs and tissues. Cardiogenic shock is an extremely serious complication. Despite all present forms of treatment the mortality is at least 80%. Although cardiogenic shock develops most often during the first 12 hours after the attack, it can occur several days later.

4. Thromboembolism

There is a propensity for blood to clot on the inner wall of the injured left ventricle. These clots may break loose and leave the heart (as emboli) to block the arterial supply to the brain, abdomen, or extremities. Emboli may also arise from the deep veins of the legs (presumably due to stasis of blood), and eventually find their way to the lungs and produce pulmonary infarction. Embolic phenomena, from either the left ventricle or the leg veins, can produce sudden death, but this complication is not common and accounts for a small percentage of deaths after infarction.

5. Rupture of the Left Ventricle

When there is extensive damage to the ventricular wall the necrotic area may weaken, leading to rupture of the left ventricle. When this catastrophe occurs blood from the ventricle instantly fills the surrounding pericardial sac and causes compression of the heart (cardiac tamponade). Death occurs usually within minutes. Ventricular rupture may develop at any time during hospitalization, but the highest incidence is within the first 7–10 days. Less than 5% of the total mortality from acute myocardial infarction is due to ventricular rupture.

THE DIAGNOSIS OF ACUTE MYOCARDIAL INFARCTION

The diagnosis of acute myocardial infarction is made essentially in three steps: the patient's history, the electrocardiogram, and enzyme studies.

The Patient's History

In many ways the patient's story of his illness is the prime factor in reaching the diagnosis of acute myocardial infarction. It is because of the history that the physician *suspects* the diagnosis and admits the patient to the hospital. The development of severe, substernal pain associated with nausea, sweating, and the other features already mentioned is often so distinctive the physician can safely anticipate subsequent confirmation of his diagnosis by the electrocardiogram and enzyme studies. However, the history, regardless of how typical it may be, is not diagnostic in its own right, and other steps must be taken to prove that acute infarction has actually occurred.

The Electrocardiogram

The diagnosis of acute myocardial infarction can be made *definitively* only by electrocardiographic means. When injury and local death (infarction) of myocardial tissue occurs, characteristic findings reflecting these changes are found in the electrocardiographic tracing. On many occasions the initial diagnostic (12-lead) electrocardiogram fails to show specific evidence of an infarction, and additional (serial) tracings must be obtained over the next several days until definite electrocardiographic proof has evolved. The diagnosis of acute infarction cannot and should not be made unless characteristic electrocardiographic changes are finally demonstrated. It is important to realize that the electrocardiogram does not show the actual extent of damage and by itself is not a true index of the seriousness of the attack.

Enzyme Studies

In some instances patients may give an impressive history suggesting acute myocardial infarction, but the electrocardiograms show equivocal (rather than definite) changes. In these cases other studies are necessary to verify the diagnosis. The most important of these laboratory determinations involves the measurement of certain enzymes in the blood. The basis of these tests is as follows: Several enzymes are normally present within the cells comprising the myocardium. When the myocardium is injured these enzymes escape into the bloodstream where they can be detected and measured. Thus after acute myocardial infarction a characteristic elevation of these enzymes in the serum is to be expected. The three most frequently used enzyme studies to confirm the diagnosis of acute myocardial infarction are creatine phosphokinase (CPK), serum glutamic oxaloacetic transaminase (SGOT), and lactic dehydrogenase (LDH).

Creatine Phosphokinase (CPK)

CPK is the first enzyme to increase after myocardial infarction, and elevated levels can be detected within 2–6 hours after the attack. The peak level usually is reached during the first 24 hours. After 2–3 days the CPK levels generally return to normal (Fig. 2.1). Accordingly, CPK levels should be measured at the time of admission, 24 hours later, and then at the end of the second and third days. Unfortunately, creatine phosphokinase is not only a myocardial enzyme but is produced also by the brain and the skeletal muscles. Therefore elevated CPK levels may be noted after brain damage (e.g., strokes) or with various muscle diseases or injuries. Even an intramuscular injection may cause a rise in serum CPK. (For this reason it may be wise, when possible, to draw a blood sample for CPK determination before any intramuscular injections are administered.)*

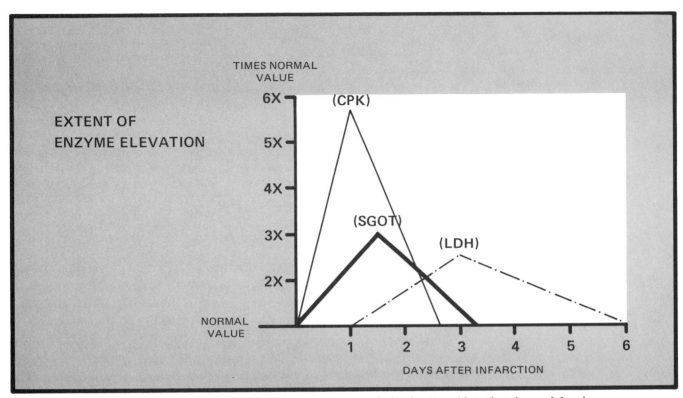

Figure 2.1. Typical enzyme elevation patterns after acute myocardial infarction. Note that the peak levels occur on different days; also that the extent of increase (i.e., two times, three times, or four times the normal value) is not the same for each enzyme. The normal values for the enzymes depend on the particular laboratory method used and therefore may vary from hospital to hospital. (It is important to ascertain the normal values at your own hospital in order to interpret the results of enzyme studies.)

Serum Glutamic Oxaloacetic Transaminase (SGOT)

SGOT levels rise less rapidly than CPK after myocardial infarction. Although minor increases in SGOT may be detected after 8 hours, the peak level does not occur until 24–48 hours have elapsed. The levels usually return to normal after 3–4 days. Therefore the concentration of this enzyme should be measured at 24, 48, and 72 hours after the attack. While SGOT levels are generally reliable in confirming myocardial damage, other diseases may also produce elevations of this enzyme. High SGOT levels are especially common in liver disease (hepatocellular damage) and, to a lesser degree, in congestive heart failure and after muscle injury.

Lactic Dehydrogenase (LDH)

Serum levels of LDH increase after infarction at a slower rate than CPK or SGOT. Peak concentrations do not occur usually until the second or third day, after which the levels return to normal on about the fifth or sixth day. This laboratory determination should therefore be performed on days 3, 4, and 5, but only if CPK and SGOT levels have not already confirmed the diagnosis. As with CPK and SGOT, LDH levels may increase from causes other than acute myocardial infarction. Elevations of LDH are known to occur with pulmonary, renal, and skeletal muscle diseases.

---

*It has been shown recently that total CPK consists of three separate components (isoenzymes), one of which, CPK-MB, is specific for myocardial necrosis. Thus by measuring CPK-MB it is now possible to determine if an elevated CPK level is due to acute myocardial infarction or another cause. However, the separation and assay of CPK isoenzymes is time-consuming and costly, and therefore only a limited number of hospitals are now prepared to perform this test routinely.

Although the degree of serum enzyme elevation cannot be correlated precisely with the size or severity of myocardial infarction, the levels do provide a general indication of the extent of tissue destruction. Markedly increased serum enzyme levels appearing promptly after infarction and remaining elevated longer than anticipated usually suggest an extensive myocardial infarction.

Because none of these enzymes are specific for myocardial damage (with the exception of CPK-MB), the diagnosis of acute myocardial infarction should never be made solely on the basis of elevated enzyme levels; the value of these tests is only supplemental. Conversely, negative results of enzyme studies should not be grounds to abandon the diagnosis of acute myocardial infarction in the presence of a typical history and characteristic electrocardiographic findings.

PHYSICAL EXAMINATION

In examining a patient with acute myocardial infarction the fundamental objective is to ascertain whether complications of the infarction have developed. Myocardial infarction in its own right does not produce abnormal physical findings; it is only the complications that can be detected by clinical examination.

As described in later chapters, each complication is associated with characteristic physical signs. For example, left ventricular failure is manifested by rales at the bases of the lungs and a gallop rhythm (among other findings). Hypotension, a rapid pulse rate, decreased urinary output, mental confusion, and cold clammy skin are found with cardiogenic shock. Arrhythmic disturbances are characterized by changes in the rate and rhythm of the heart.

It is understandable that the physical examination may be normal in patients who have not developed complications. Furthermore, it should be realized that acute myocardial infarction cannot be distinguished from other forms of heart disease solely on the basis of physical examination since circulatory failure and arrhythmias also occur with many different cardiac disorders.

THE ACUTE PHASE OF MYOCARDIAL INFARCTION

In general, the clinical course after infarction can be considered in two phases: the *acute* phase, which usually involves the first 5 days following the attack, and the *subacute* phase, which concerns the remaining period of hospitalization. During the acute phase patients are treated in a coronary care unit.

Clinical Course

The most characteristic aspect of the acute phase of myocardial infarction is its uncertainty; there is no typical course. The variation in the clinical picture is quite remarkable, but three broad patterns can be described.

1. There are some patients whose clinical course is truly uncomplicated. They show no evidence of cardiogenic shock, acute left ventricular failure, arrhythmias, or other major problems during this critical period of the illness. Most of these patients make uneventful recoveries regardless of the type of treatment employed. As will be shown in the next chapter, such uncomplicated courses are much less frequent than those associated with complications.

2. In other patients the illness appears benign at the time of admission, but suddenly major complications develop. These complications account for nearly all deaths, and it is the unpredictability of these catastrophes that makes myocardial infarction such a lethal disease. The concept of intensive coronary care is based on the prevention

or the immediate detection and treatment of life-threatening complications. By its ability to prevent sudden unexpected death in this group of patients, the system of intensive coronary care has made its greatest contribution.

3. When serious complications already exist at the time of admission, the clinical course is usually hectic and the prognosis becomes extremely poor. For example, if shock is present when the patient is admitted, there is more than a 90% likelihood that the patient will die within the next 48 hours. If acute heart failure is evident on admission, the mortality may be as high as 50%. Therefore the original clinical picture is very important in determining the ultimate course of the attack; but an uncomplicated picture on admission should not lead to a false sense of security for reasons stated in the preceding paragraphs.

That acute myocardial infarction may have such widely divergent courses explains why the death rate may be 90% at one extreme and 0%–5% at the other. Probably no other disease behaves in this unpredictable fashion. The final outcome of the illness depends on the presence or absence of complications.

Other Aspects of the Acute Phase

In addition to major complications, many other problems may develop during the acute phase. Some of these effects represent natural responses to tissue damage, whereas others can be considered actual complications.

Fever

Most patients with acute myocardial infarction develop temperature elevations during the acute phase of the illness. Typically, the body temperature rises after the first 24 hours of the attack to levels of 100°–101° F (or more) and remains elevated for 2–3 days before declining gradually. By the fifth day the temperature has usually returned to normal (Fig. 2.2). It is thought that this febrile pattern reflects local death of myocardial tissue. (The white blood cell count and the erythrocyte sedimentation rate also increase during this period for the same reason.) Thus the presence of fever is an anticipated finding and ordinarily does not indicate an infectious process in patients with acute infarction. However, if the fever is prolonged, excessively high, or develops after the first few days, the possibility of pneumonia, thrombophlebitis, or other systemic infection must be considered.

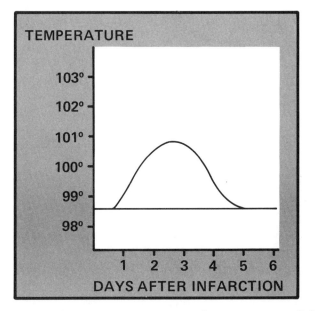

Figure 2.2.   Characteristic temperature pattern after acute myocardial infarction.

Pericarditis

Myocardial infarctions frequently extend to the epicardial surface of the heart and produce inflammation of the overlying pericardium. In most cases the pericardial reaction (pericarditis) is confined to the area over the infarction, but occasionally diffuse pericardial irritation may develop, probably from oozing of blood from the myocardium into the pericardial sac. Patients with pericarditis secondary to acute myocardial infarction usually experience chest pain which is often increased by deep breathing or changes in body position. The characteristic physical finding of pericarditis is a pericardial friction rub—a grating sound occurring each time the heart beats. A transient friction rub can be detected in nearly 50% of patients with acute myocardial infarction. Pericarditis usually disappears spontaneously within a few days and seldom causes serious problems.

Recurrent Chest Pain

Some patients develop additional episodes of ischemic chest pain during the acute phase of myocardial infarction. This pain may represent angina pectoris or, worse, an extension of the original infarction. (The possibility that the pain is caused by pericarditis must also be considered.) Recurrent ischemic pain generally indicates that the acute process has not stabilized and that further damage may occur. Serial electrocardiograms and enzyme studies should be performed after any significant chest pain episode.

Emotional Disturbances

Profound emotional reactions are frequently noted among patients with acute myocardial infarction during the period of intensive coronary care. The basis of this response can be readily appreciated: the abrupt interruption of normal life, the fear of death, and the possibility of permanent invalidism are powerful psychological threats. Because the patient's response to this stress is influenced by numerous factors inherent in his personality, the spectrum of reactions is very wide. The most common emotional problems associated with acute myocardial infarction are discussed in Chapter 6.

THE SUBACUTE PHASE OF MYOCARDIAL INFARCTION

The overall incidence of complications lessens markedly after the first 5 days, and for this reason patients are usually transferred from the coronary care unit (CCU) to other facilities within the hospital at that time.

During the remaining period of hospitalization (the subacute phase), while the infarcted area is healing, the main objective is to observe the clinical course carefully, focusing on the prevention of complications. At the same time it is important to prepare the patient for discharge by instructing and counseling him about his illness.

In the absence of serious complications the total hospital stay is generally 3 weeks in duration (including the period of intensive coronary care). Although some studies suggest that stays as short as 2 weeks or less are adequate for patients with uncomplicated courses, the more conservative approach is still followed in most institutions. During the subacute phase the patient's physical activity is restricted in order to limit the work of the heart as it heals. However, complete bed rest is no longer considered necessary, and it is now customary to allow patients to sit in armchairs and to walk to the bathroom. The use of chair rest rather than bed rest is beneficial not only for the emotional support derived from being out of bed but also because the sitting position may actually be more effective in terms of circulatory efficiency. Full ambulation should be started a few days before hospital discharge.

The hospital course of patients who develop complications varies with the nature of the problem and the response to treatment. Understandably, the basic program of care just described must be adapted according to the clinical picture.

Although the subacute phase is undoubtedly less hazardous than the acute phase, there is substantial evidence indicating that the period after transfer from the CCU is by no means without danger. *Indeed complications may develop at any time during the hospital stay.*

In an effort to reduce mortality during the subacute phase some institutions have established special care facilities for the postcoronary care unit period. These units, designated variously as intermediate coronary care units (ICCU), step-down units, or after-care wards, allow careful observation to be continued for a week or two after transfer from the CCU in a less-intensive but nonetheless prepared setting. The actual value of this intermediate care concept is still a subject of debate, particularly from the standpoint of the number of lives saved compared to the cost and effort involved.

CONVALESCENCE AFTER ACUTE MYOCARDIAL INFARCTION

Following discharge from the hospital it is customary for patients to remain at home on a limited-activity regimen until the infarction has healed. As a general rule, necrotic areas of the myocardium heal within 6–8 weeks after the attack. Thus if a patient was hospitalized for 3–4 weeks the period of convalescence at home would be an additional 3–4 weeks. The duration of convalescence depends on many factors, probably the most important of which are the patient's age and the functional capacity of the heart after the attack.

Physical activity is increased gradually during the convalescent phase. Excessive rest is unnecessary, but stair-climbing or household chores should be minimized. At the end of the healing phase a deliberate program of increasing physical activity is started in order to promote the development of collateral circulation to the myocardium. Although it is difficult to prove that the growth of collateral blood vessels is directly related to physical activity, the consensus is that regulated exercise is distinctly beneficial for this purpose. In concept, exercise may help to create what is in effect a new blood supply to the myocardium, taking over the role of the previously occluded artery. Walking is considered to be the most sensible and effective exercise to achieve this goal and should be encouraged, with the distance being increased daily. In addition to its helpful effect on the heart and circulation, physical activity at this stage of the illness is of great value in combating the weakness and fatigue that are so common after myocardial infarction. These symptoms, resulting mostly from disuse of the skeletal muscles during the period of hospitalization, are usually alleviated soon after a regular walking program is instituted.

Most patients, especially those without serious complications, are able to resume their customary lives and return to work about 3 months after the original attack. This time schedule must be flexible and adjusted according to the patient's age, general health, and cardiac status. It has become increasingly clear that the resumption of normal activity is highly desirable, and every effort should be made to fulfill this objective.

There is no reason to believe that deliberate inactivity or retirement from work after a myocardial infarction is conducive to longevity; in fact, the evidence is strictly to the contrary.

The resumption of a normal, useful life after a heart attack depends not only on physical recovery but also on emotional recovery. Some patients, despite excellent physical recoveries, develop such profound psychological reactions to their illness that they in fact become invalids. Emotionally-induced cardiac invalidism is a common problem and produces no less functional impairment than true physical invalidism. The clinical features of this distressing problem are inability to tolerate physical activity, weakness and fatigue (which are often overwhelming), and an intense awareness and concern about any discomfort or pain occurring anywhere above the waist.

3

The System of Intensive Coronary Care

THE PROBLEM OF CORONARY HEART DISEASE

A means to halt the ever mounting death toll from coronary heart disease (CHD) is desperately needed. Consider the magnitude of the problem in the United States alone: nearly 2000 persons a day—more than 600,000 a year—die from this one disease. The enormity of this mortality is brought into perspective by noting that all forms of cancer together—the second leading cause of death—take less than half this number of lives per year. Understandably, CHD has been described as the greatest epidemic modern man has ever faced. It is not only its awesome death rate that makes CHD such an overwhelming problem, but also the fact that the disease disables millions of other people, many of whom are in the most productive years of life. Current estimates indicate that at least 5 million Americans now suffer from CHD, with 1 million new cases being added annually.

What can possibly be done about such a devastating disease? Certainly the main attack should be directed toward the prevention of coronary atherosclerosis. Indeed, for more than a half century a relentless search has been in progress attempting to identify the cause of atherosclerosis with the underlying hope that once the mechanism was uncovered it would prove to be preventable or at least reversible. Unfortunately this search has not been fruitful thus far, and it has become increasingly clear that a usable method for inhibiting or controlling coronary atherosclerosis will not be forthcoming in the near future. Although certain risk factors associated with CHD have been identified (e.g., high serum cholesterol levels, smoking, and hypertension, among many others) there is still no proof (as explained in Chapter 1) that any of these factors specifically *cause* coronary atherosclerosis, or, even more significantly, that by reducing these risks CHD can in fact be prevented. Present indications are that it will take many more years to unravel this complex, multifactorial process and reach a point where coronary atherosclerosis can possibly be averted. (Those who believe that CHD is an effect of "overcivilization" or the emotional stresses of our times might have an even more pessimistic outlook since the likelihood of slowing the pace of present-day life seems difficult to envision.) On the positive side it should be pointed out that there is still hope that CHD may ultimately yield to *primary* prevention. This means that deliberate efforts will have to be made to control risk factors beginning in childhood and continuing throughout life. Specifically, forthcoming generations would have to recognize the danger of overeating, smoking, emotional stress, and other potential risk factors, and avoid these threats from an early age. This approach differs from the current plan of *secondary* prevention, which attempts to correct these habits (risk factors) after they have already become established. It remains to be seen if future generations will heed this advice and if primary prevention is in fact more effective than secondary prevention.

If we must accept the conclusion that there is no definite means at present to prevent or reverse coronary atherosclerosis, what other measures can be used to reduce the death rate from CHD?

The Surgical Approach to the Problem

One possibility for lowering mortality from CHD involves the use of surgical techniques to increase the blood supply to the myocardium after the coronary arteries have become critically narrowed. Many surgical methods have been attempted during the past 30 years in an effort to provide the heart with additional blood, but it was not until 1970, with the introduction of a new operation called the *coronary artery bypass graft* (CABG), that the surgical approach to CHD achieved widespread popularity. The procedure consists of suturing a segment of a vein (taken from the saphenous vein of the patient's leg) to a small opening made in the aorta at one end and to a coronary artery at the other. This vein graft bypasses the obstructed portion of a diseased artery and permits blood to pass from the aorta to the myocardium (Fig. 3.1). For the operation to succeed in its purpose, the distal end of the vein graft must be attached to a portion of the coronary artery that is relatively free of advanced atherosclerotic disease (as determined preoperatively by coronary arteriography). If the disease process is diffuse and extends throughout the entire length of the artery, the bypass will not be effective. Fortunately, atherosclerotic narrowing is most likely to occur near the point of origin of the artery, thus permitting vein grafts to be applied in many patients with CHD.

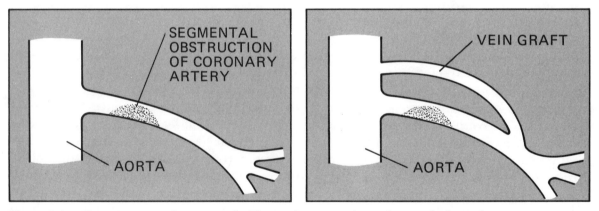

Figure 3.1. Coronary artery bypass graft. The saphenous vein graft extends from the aorta to a point distal to the obstructed segment of the coronary artery.

The operation was designed originally as a means of treating severe, disabling angina that could not be controlled by medical management; but now it is also being used in an effort to avert impending myocardial infarction. In principle the bypass graft brings an adequate oxygen supply to deprived areas of the myocardium and in this way controls angina pectoris and possibly prevents acute myocardial infarction. Many reports from various surgical centers have confirmed the fact that a very high percentage (about 80%) of patients with angina pectoris are relieved of their symptoms after CABG surgery. Much less certain at present is whether the operation is effective in preventing acute infarction. Above all, it is still not known if bypass surgery actually prolongs life. In other words, it is clear that the operation produces improvement of symptoms (and the quality of life), but it is still uncertain if patients undergoing this surgery actually live longer than those in whom surgery was not performed. This of course is the critical question, and until it is answered the true value of the surgical approach to CHD must remain a matter of speculation. Carefully designed studies sponsored by the National Institues of Health are now underway in several centers in the United States to determine the precise benefits (and risks) of CABG surgery, but the final results of this investigation will not be available until 1980 or later.

If coronary bypass surgery ultimately proves effective in prolonging life, it will certainly represent a major advance in the treatment of CHD in selected patients. However, it should be recognized that this (or any other) surgical method can have only limited application in terms of the overall problem of CHD throughout the world. It is not only that relatively few hospitals have facilities for open-heart surgery, but also the cost of surgery is so high that economic considerations would soon preclude this approach on a wide-scale basis. For example, the cost of CABG surgery in this country now averages $10,000 to $15,000 per patient. At its present rate of growth (currently 50,000 operations per year) the total cost for this single operation in the United States will soon exceed $1 billion a year!

Prevention of Clots

Another possibility for combating CHD concerns the prevention of clot formation within the coronary arteries. Recognizing that extensive atherosclerosis may be present for years without ever producing CHD (and its lethal complications), it can be postulated that unless a clot developed on an atherosclerotic plaque, acute myocardial infarction might never occur in many instances. The basic question is what causes a clot (thrombus) to form in the coronary arteries and why does it develop on one particular day rather than, for example, 2 months earlier or a year later. Research studies indicate that clot formation within arteries (in contrast to clots within veins) is the result of increased adhesiveness of blood platelets. Because of this unusual "stickiness," platelets tend to clump together and form the framework for a larger blood clot. There is reason to believe that platelet adhesiveness is influenced by the secretion of certain hormones (catecholamines) from the adrenal gland. Thus any outpouring of catecholamines (as occurs, for example, during stress) may increase platelet adhesiveness and lead to clot formation. If this theory is correct it may be possible to prevent clot formation in the coronary arteries by blocking catecholamine secretion with drug therapy. Along this same line, it has been shown that aspirin has antithrombotic qualities, and studies are now in progress to determine if daily administration of this simple drug will reduce the incidence of acute myocardial infarction. Much remains to be learned about this interesting and potentially useful concept.

THE CONCEPT OF INTENSIVE CORONARY CARE

Of the several methods proposed to reduce the extraordinary death rate from CHD, only one thus far has proved to be feasible, practical, and of unquestionable benefit. The plan is called *intensive coronary care*. It is based on the premise that until CHD can be prevented the main hope for reducing mortality is to provide optimal care after acute myocardial infarction has occurred and to salvage lives in this way. Admittedly, this after-the-fact approach to the overall problem of CHD is less meaningful than attempting to avert acute myocardial infarction, but the value of this concept has become clearly evident. Before the introduction of intensive coronary care in 1962, *at least 30% of all patients admitted to hospitals with acute myocardial infarction died during the period of hospitalization*. Thus of approximately 800,000 patients with acute myocardial infarction who were admitted each year to hospitals in the United States, more than 250,000 died before discharge. Since that time, as a direct result of the coronary care system, the death rate from acute myocardial infarction in hospitals has fallen to about 15%, or one-half the previous mortality. This means that if all hospitals in this country were now adequately prepared to provide intensive coronary care as many as 125,000 lives could possibly be saved each year. (Unfortunately a substantial number—perhaps 30%—of American hospitals do not have coronary care facilities because of their rural locations, small size, or lack of trained personnel; therefore the maximal reduction in mortality cannot be achieved at present.) Because of its proven effectiveness, intensive coronary care has become the strongest and most dependable weapon available for attacking the overall problem of CHD, and it promises to remain so in the foreseeable future.

THE DEVELOPMENT OF INTENSIVE CORONARY CARE

The concept of intensive coronary care was conceived in 1962 when two parallel avenues of research were finally brought together as a functional system of care. One area of research concerned the manner and mechanisms by which acute myocardial infarction causes death; the other involves new techniques of cardiac resuscitation.

It had been known for many years that death from acute myocardial infarction was always the result of *complications* of the attack, not occlusion of a coronary artery itself. However, the relative frequency in which the five main complications of acute myocardial infarction (as described in Chapter 2) produce death was uncertain. In 1961 Meltzer and Kitchell answered this question by studying the mechanisms of death in 171 patients who died of acute myocardial infarction. On the basis of their investigation they concluded that death was attributable to the following causes:

Arrhythmias	47%
Left ventricular failure	28% ⎤
Cardiogenic shock	15% ⎦ 43%
Emboli	8%
Rupture of ventricle	2%

These findings were extremely important in pointing out a way toward improving the survival rate after acute myocardial infarction. It was evident that rupture of the ventricle and embolism, the two complications that rarely can be treated successfully, were not common causes of death, comprising only 2% and 8%, respectively, of the total mortality. Left ventricular failure and cardiogenic shock, representing failure of the heart to pump effectively, collectively produced 43% of the deaths. *By far the most important observation was the unusually high percentage (47%) of deaths due to arrhythmias.* Although sudden and unanticipated deaths resulting from electrical disturbances in the heart were not unfamiliar events, the actual incidence of this lethal complication had been grossly underestimated in the past. (Indeed until this study the impression existed that arrhythmic deaths were relatively uncommon.) The fact that nearly one-half of all deaths from acute myocardial infarction resulted from arrhythmias became the cornerstone for the concept of intensive coronary care since it was known that *arrhythmic deaths were preventable!*

In fact, it had been shown more than 50 years previously that *ventricular fibrillation*, the arrhythmia responsible for at least 80% of all sudden deaths, could be terminated and the life saved if a powerful electric shock was delivered to the heart immediately after the onset of the arrhythmia. It was believed originally that the electrodes (which delivered the electric shock) had to be applied directly to the surface of the ventricles. Because this procedure required the chest to be opened (thoracotomy) to expose the heart, application of this lifesaving measure was confined primarily to the prepared setting of operating rooms. For this reason the technique of open-chest cardiac resuscitation never became a practical method for preventing death from acute myocardial infarction.

In 1956 this particular problem was solved when Dr. Paul Zoll and his colleagues demonstrated that ventricular fibrillation could be terminated by means of an electric shock delivered *externally* through the intact chest wall, thus eliminating the need for thoracotomy. Even this major medical advance had limited practical application until the development of the coronary care concept because of the extraordinarily short interval between the onset of ventricular fibrillation and irreversible death. *Normally only 1–2 minutes are available to stop ventricular fibrillation and restore an effective heartbeat.* The chance of accomplishing this maneuver (defibrillation) within this very brief period is understandably remote under ordinary hospital circumstances. Specifically, successful defibrillation in the precoronary care era required that a physician be in attendance when the death-producing arrhythmia began, that an electrocardiographic (ECG) machine (to identify the arrhythmia) and a defibrillator be brought to the bedside, and that an electric shock be delivered to the heart—*all within two precious minutes or less!* From the results of the study previously described in which nearly half of all deaths from acute myocardial infarction were due to arrhythmias, it is clearly apparent that these fortuitous circumstances rarely prevailed even though the hospitals involved had highly trained personnel and the necessary equipment to perform defibrillation.

Results of resuscitation from *ventricular standstill*—the second of the arrhythmias that cause sudden death—were equally poor. There was good evidence that if the heartbeat stopped (asystole) it could be reactivated under certain conditions by rhythmic electric stimuli delivered to the myocardium by a device called a pacemaker. However, again, although pacing techniques had been known for more than a dozen years, very few lives were ever saved with this ingenious method because of the same time limitation: restoration of the heartbeat after ventricular standstill can be accomplished only if the pacemaker is used within seconds after the onset of the arrhythmia.

Thus as late as 1960, despite the availability of methods and equipment to prevent arrhythmic deaths, little headway had actually been made in decreasing mortality from acute myocardial infarction. The fault was readily apparent: insufficient time to permit corrective action to be taken once a lethal arrhythmia developed. Attacking this critical problem, Kouwenhoven and co-workers at Johns Hopkins Hospital in 1960 devised a simple procedure to sustain the circulation until defibrillation or cardiac pacing could be performed. The method, now known as cardiopulmonary resuscitation (CPR), involves rhythmic compression of the lower sternum (to massage the heart) and mouth-to-mouth ventilation (to supply oxygen). With this technique the circulation can be adequately supported for many minutes (or longer), thus providing additional time to terminate the arrhythmia. Although CPR was instrumental in saving the lives of many patients who would have died otherwise, it soon became evident that this resuscitative method could not be expected to reduce substantially the total number of arrhythmic deaths. The reason was that most patients who died of lethal arrhythmias were unattended at the moment of the catastrophe, and by the time the event was recognized it was too late to initiate CPR because death was already irreversible.

Finally in 1962 Day, at Bethany Hospital in Kansas City, Kansas, and Meltzer and Kitchell, at the Presbyterian–University of Pennsylvania Medical Center in Philadelphia, independently conceived a plan by which arrhythmic deaths among patients hospitalized with acute myocardial infarction might be prevented in nearly all instances. Both research teams reasoned that, if patients were kept under constant surveillance in a special unit where the cardiac rhythm could be observed continuously and where resuscitative equipment was always ready for immediate use, it would be possible to detect and terminate lethal arrhythmias the instant they occurred. In this way sudden, unexpected death from arrhythmias could be avoided. *Were this scheme successful, the in-hospital mortality rate from acute myocardial infarction might be reduced by nearly 50%.*

The development of monitoring equipment which permitted the cardiac rate and rhythm to be viewed constantly brought the plan closer to reality. One last step had to be accomplished before intensive coronary care could be implemented: to train personnel to assess the patient's clinical course, to identify and interpret arrhythmias, and, above all, to act on their own if necessary in terminating lethal arrhythmias. But who would assume this demanding role? It seemed at first that only physicians could possibly undertake the responsibility, but then research studies at the Presbyterian–University of Pennsylvania Medical Center revealed that specially trained nurses were fully capable of serving in this critical position. It was with this background that the original system of intensive care was finally designed and tested.

THE BASIC SYSTEM OF INTENSIVE CORONARY CARE

Intensive coronary care is a *system* of care designed primarily to prevent death from the complications of acute myocardial infarction. As with any effective system, optimal function depends on the interrelationship of its various components; individually the components are not self-sufficient and cannot achieve the desired result. The interrelationship of the components of the system of coronary care is shown in the following diagram.

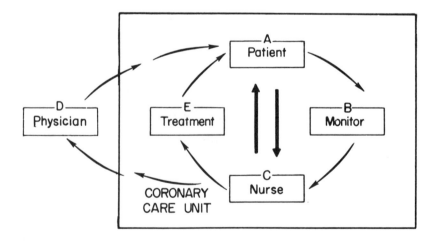

The patient (A) with suspected or confirmed acute myocardial infarction is admitted directly to the coronary care unit (CCU), a fully equipped facility within which all materials necessary for the detection and treatment of the complications of acute myocardial infarction are centralized. (The design of the unit and its equipment are described in Chapter 4.)

Monitoring equipment (B), attached to the patient, provides a continuous display of the electrocardiogram on an oscilloscopic screen. In this way the rate and rhythm of the heart is apparent at all times, and the onset of any arrhythmia can be detected immediately. Cardiac monitors also include rate meters which indicate the minute-to-minute heart rate, as well as alarm systems which alert personnel to significant changes in the heart rate. Thus if the rate of the heart exceeds or falls below preset limits, an alarm is triggered. (The details of cardiac monitoring are described in Chapter 8.) In addition to electrocardiographic monitors, other monitoring equipment to assess circulatory (hemodynamic) function is available for diagnostic purposes.

The nurse (C), who has been specifically trained for this specialized role, remains in constant attendance within the unit. Of the multiple nursing duties and responsibilities, one of the most essential is to interpret the electrocardiographic findings displayed on the oscilloscope and to recognize the significance of changes in cardiac rate or rhythm. In addition the nurse must repeatedly assess the clinical condition of the patient at the bedside by planned careful observation and physical examination in order to detect signs of other complications of myocardial infarction. In the event of any change in the patient's status, either clinically or electrocardiographically, the nurse must decide upon a course of action which may involve either further observation, notifying a physician, or acting immediately on her own in emergency situations. (The nursing role is described in detail in Chapter 6.)

The physician (D), unlike the nurse, is not in constant attendance. He relies fundamentally on the observations made by the nurse members of the team who advise him of their assessments, particularly when there is a change in the clinical course. That the physician delegates unusual authority to the nurse members of the physician–nurse team is one of the most distinguishing characteristics of the system of intensive coronary care.

The treatment program (E) is designed to prevent lethal complications. The plan of therapy is directed by the physician but carried out, for the most part, by the nurse. In emergency situations—especially when lethal arrhythmias develop—the nurse must perform lifesaving measures (e.g., defibrillation) in the absence of the physician.

From the foregoing description of the coronary care system it is readily apparent that *the nurse is the key to the success of the entire system of coronary care*. This is not to say that nursing practice alone determines the effectiveness of intensive coronary care, but it does indeed mean that without specially trained, highly skilled nurses the system can never achieve full effectiveness. In fact, without specialized nursing practice intensive coronary care is no more than a token gesture. This advanced concept of nursing care implies much more than simply having a nurse stationed in a CCU to observe the cardiac monitor and to call a physician when an alarm sounds or another problem arises. For the intensive care program to fulfill its objectives the nurse must be able to anticipate complications, assess each problem as it arises, and, above all, assume a *decision-making* role. Unless nurses are delegated authority to make and carry out therapeutic decisions based on their own observations and judgment, the coronary care system is weakened seriously. This point was demonstrated decisively by the initial experience with intensive coronary care at New York Hospital–Cornell Medical Center. When the coronary care unit began operation, the nursing staff was *not* empowered to act on its own in emergency situations and had to call a house officer to defibrillate patients. With this restrictive policy the mortality at the end of the first year among patients treated in the CCU was the same (31%) as that noted on the general medical wards. As soon as nurses were granted authority to defibrillate patients in the absence of a physician, the mortality in the unit fell promptly.

It should also be emphasized that monitoring equipment alone, regardless of its sophistication or elegance, must not be construed as intensive coronary care. Monitoring is only one component of the total system and can never be self-sufficient. In the absence of a skilled nursing staff monitoring equipment by itself does not warrant its expense.

AGGRESSIVE MANAGEMENT OF ARRHYTHMIAS

When the system of intensive coronary care was first tested at the Presbyterian–University of Pennsylvania Medical Center and the Bethany Hospital it proved effective immediately and a significant decrease in mortality from acute myocardial infarction was observed in both hospitals. At each institution the death rate fell from more than 30% to 20%—a relative reduction of 33%. On the basis of these impressive results the concept of coronary care was accepted readily and enthusiastically, and within a few years hundreds and then thousands of CCUs were established in hospitals throughout the world.

As would be anticipated from its background, the original plan of coronary care focused primarily on resuscitation from lethal arrhythmias. The fundamental objective was to terminate ventricular fibrillation and ventricular standstill the moment they occurred. That this system was capable of preventing sudden arrhythmic deaths was clearly evident: the 33% reduction in mortality was achieved almost entirely by successful defibrillation and (to a much lesser extent) by cardiac pacing.

While observing the clinical course of patients who developed death-producing arrhythmias it became apparent that ventricular fibrillation and ventricular standstill seldom occurred spontaneously; in practically all instances the catastrophes were preceded by lesser (warning) arrhythmias. When it was demonstrated that warning arrhythmias could be controlled by antiarrhythmic drugs or transvenous pacing, the theme and emphasis of coronary care switched abruptly from resuscitation to the *prevention* of lethal arrhythmias. This step marked the beginning of the second stage of development of the coronary care system—the aggressive management of warning arrhythmias.

According to this new concept, vigorous treatment of warning arrhythmias would prevent ventricular fibrillation and ventricular standstill, relegating resuscitation to a role of lesser importance (at least in principle). The value of this plan was confirmed promptly. For example, Lown, at the Peter Bent Brigham Hospital in Boston, reported a zero incidence of ventricular fibrillation among 130 consecutive patients in whom this preventive approach was used. Aggressive management of warning arrhythmias became, and remains, the byword of coronary care.

THE ATTACK AGAINST DEATH FROM PUMP FAILURE

With the ability to prevent arrhythmic deaths an accomplished fact, coronary care entered its third (and present) stage of development: an attempt to reduce the death rate from left ventricular failure and cardiogenic shock (pump failure).

By 1970 (when many major medical centers had reported their experience with intensive coronary care) it was clear that the reduction in hospital mortality had already reached a plateau (at about 18%–20%, as noted in Table 3.1), and that no further de-

Table 3.1. Mortality from Acute Myocardial Infarction at Major Medical Centers

Series	Place	No. of patients	Hospital mortality (%)
Day and Averill	Kansas City	280	20.0
Meltzer and Kitchell	Philadelphia	500	18.0
Lown et al.	Boston	300	17.7
Julian and Oliver	Scotland	552	19.2
Killip and Kimball	New York	300+	21.0
Sloman et al.	Australia	350	18.0

crease in the death rate could be anticipated with the existing program of care. The reason for this limitation was readily apparent: the system of care was capable of preventing nearly all sudden arrhythmic deaths, but it was not effective in saving lives from the other complications of acute myocardial infarction. In particular, the mortality from pump failure showed no improvement compared to the results obtained without coronary care. The inability to combat death from cardiogenic shock and advanced left ventricular failure made pump failure the most common cause of death among patients treated in CCUs. In fact more than 90% of the total mortality from acute myocardial infarction is now due to pump failure. The change in the relative incidence of death-producing complications before and (8 years) after the introduction of the coronary care system at the Presbyterian–University of Pennsylvania Medical Center is shown in Table 3.2.

Table 3.2. Incidence of Death-Producing Complications Before and After Introduction of Coronary Care

Complication	Complication rate (%)	
	Before CCU	After CCU
Arrhythmias	47	2
Pump failure (left ventricular failure and cardiogenic shock)	43	91
Emboli	8	4
Ventricular rupture	2	3

Little headway could be made in the battle against pump failure until simple and safe methods were devised (during the early 1970s) actually to measure the heart's pumping performance during the acute phase of myocardial infarction. With these measurements treatment can now at least be structured in a rational, deliberate way according to the particular hemodynamic disturbance.

Of the many different approaches now being used to control pump failure, four methods seem to hold the greatest promise: 1) detecting heart failure at its earliest stages so prompt treatment can be initiated in an attempt to prevent progression; 2) improving pumping efficiency by correcting adverse hemodynamic effects (e.g., by lowering elevated blood pressure) with drug therapy; 3) increasing left ventricular function (particularly in cardiogenic shock) by means of mechanical circulatory assist devices (aortic balloon pumping); and 4) attempting to limit the size and extent of a myocardial infarction with various drugs, thus reducing structural damage and preserving left ventricular pumping action. (These methods are described in Chapter 7.) Although the ultimate effectiveness of this multipronged attack must still be determined, it is fair to say that the possibility of reducing the mortality from pump failure is brighter than before.

BASIC PRACTICES OF INTENSIVE CORONARY CARE

Selection of Patients

The criteria for admission to a CCU are distinctly different from those used to determine the need for other forms of intensive care. Usually admission to an intensive care unit is based primarily on the level of patient care required rather than on a specific clinical disorder, but this is not the case with acute myocardial infarction and intensive coronary care. Every patient with acute myocardial infarction, regardless of the severity of the attack, should be admitted directly to a CCU. Admittedly, patients who show evidence of complications on arrival at the hospital have a far greater chance of developing additional problems than those who are free of complications initially; therefore it might be argued that intensive coronary care (being as comprehensive and expensive as it is) should be reserved for patients who are acutely ill when first seen. This reasoning is fallacious, however, because the clinical course during the acute phase of myocardial infarction is by no means predictable. *Many patients who appear perfectly stable on admission may be candidates for sudden death.* The fact is that arrhythmias and other complications can develop at any time. For example, in studying the clinical course of 100 patients *without* complications at the time of admission to the CCU at the Presbyterian–University of Pennsylvania Medical Center, we found that 38% of the group subsequently developed serious arrhythmias, 22% left ventricular failure, and 4% cardiogenic shock. The mortality among these so-called "good risk" patients was 9%. In other words, it is foolhardy to attempt to predict the outcome of acute myocardial infarction according to the clinical picture on admission: good risk patients can be identified only *in retrospect*, and therefore all patients with acute myocardial infarction should be treated in a CCU.

This cautious policy also involves the admission of patients with *suspected* myocardial infarction. Very often patients arrive at a hospital with chest pain or other symptoms suspicious of acute myocardial infarction, but a positive diagnosis cannot be established at the time because the ECG fails to reveal characteristic findings of an acute infarction. Should these patients be admitted to a CCU to "rule out acute myocardial infarction" or should they be observed elsewhere in the hospital until a definitive diagnosis is made? The answer is clear: any patient whose *history* suggests the possibility of acute myocardial infarction should be admitted to a CCU and treated as if an infarction had in fact occurred. That the initial ECG does not show evidence of myocardial ischemia, injury, or necrosis is unimportant since these findings may take many hours or days to develop. If this practice is followed, the diagnosis of acute myocardial infarction will not be confirmed in approximately one of every three patients admitted to the unit (usually because the problem is ultimately classified as angina or the intermediate coronary syndrome rather than acute infarction). Although this conservative approach may seem wasteful in terms of personnel, bed usage, and cost, it is nevertheless a sound principle to adopt, particularly since lethal arrhythmias may develop with bewildering speed in the presence of myocardial ischemia. Any compromise with this admission policy is a flirtation with danger.

The Duration of Intensive Coronary Care

Under ordinary circumstances patients with acute myocardial infarction usually remain in the CCU for 5 days. The reason for this particular duration of stay is that the majority of complications and hospital deaths from acute myocardial infarction occur within this period. As shown in Figure 3.2, approximately 40% of all deaths take place during the first day of hospitalization, and by the end of the fifth day 65% of the total mortality has already occurred. Because the fatality rate decreases sharply after the third day many hospitals prefer to limit the stay in the unit to 3 rather than 4 or 5 days. Our experience, however, suggests that 5 days of intensive coronary care is a safer compromise.

Since complications are not predictable and can develop at any time after infarction, it might seem sensible to provide intensive coronary care throughout the entire hospital period. This is not a feasible approach to the problem for several reasons. First, the unit would have to be inordinately large to accommodate all patients with acute myocardial infarction for this length of time. (Surveys have shown that about 8% of a hospi-

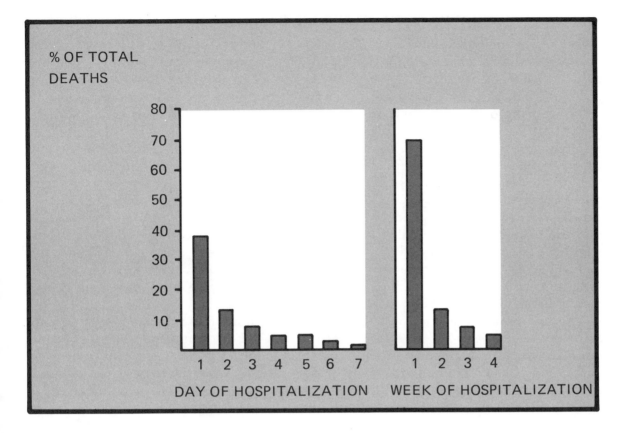

% OF TOTAL
DEATHS

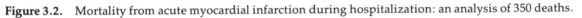

Figure 3.2.   Mortality from acute myocardial infarction during hospitalization: an analysis of 350 deaths.

tal census on any given day is comprised of patients with acute myocardial infarction; thus in a 300-bed institution the coronary unit would require about 25 beds.) Second, intensive coronary care is prohibitively expensive, and the total cost for prolonged sojourns in the unit would create a tremendous economic burden for the patient. A final deterrent to extended coronary care is the adverse psychologic effects it produces among certain patients; abnormal behavior is frequently noted in this circumstance.

In an effort to prevent death after transfer from the CCU, some hospitals have established intermediate coronary care units. The plan for this subacute care involves a separate facility (usually contiguous with the CCU) to which patients are transferred after the period of intensive care. The subacute care unit permits additional surveillance of patients with myocardial infarction in a setting that is intermediate between intensive care and customary hospital care. As mentioned in Chapter 2, the actual benefit of this concept has not been clearly established.

Preventive Treatment

As explained previously, one of the main objectives of coronary care is to prevent arrhythmic deaths by recognizing and treating warning arrhythmias. Usually antiarrhythmic drugs are administered only after a warning arrhythmia is identified; however, some clinicians believe that prophylactic treatment should be used *routinely*, even before warning arrhythmias occur. This latter practice, although attractive in theory, carries the risk of producing undesirable side effects from the drug when in fact treatment may not be required. Although the concept of preventive treatment is wholly endorsed by all, the extent and aggressiveness of the practice varies to some degree among institutions.

Prompt Initiation of Coronary Care

One of the major weaknesses of the coronary care concept is its failure to combat death *before* hospitalization. Ordinarily intensive coronary care begins when the patient finally reaches a CCU (which may involve a delay of many hours after the onset of symptoms). This delay is a serious drawback since it has been shown that the majority of deaths (probably 60% or more) from acute myocardial infarction occur before the patient can be brought to a hospital and admitted to a CCU.

In an effort to reduce the *prehospital* mortality rate several communities have established mobile coronary care units. The primary purpose of these units is to prevent arrhythmic deaths at home or in transit to the hospital by initiating intensive coronary care outside the hospital as soon as possible. The mobile units are large vehicles (or ambulances) specially designed and equipped for handling acute cardiac emergencies; they are usually staffed by allied health personnel (Emergency Medical Technicians) who have been trained to defibrillate the patient, administer intravenous drugs, and perform other lifesaving measures. By shortening the period between the onset of symptoms and the start of medical care, mobile coronary care units have been instrumental in saving many lives.

A second problem interfering with the prompt initiation of intensive coronary care is the prolonged period of time patients often wait in busy emergency wards of hospitals before being examined and then transferred to the CCU. There are two basic ways of removing this weak link in the chain of hospital care. One is to bypass the emergency facility and admit patients as quickly as possible to the CCU. This plan functions in the following way. As soon as a patient whose history suggests acute myocardial infarction enters the receiving ward he is placed on a litter equipped with a battery-powered monitor and defibrillator, and cardiac monitoring is started immediately. The patient is then transported to the CCU accompanied by a nurse or physician. No attempt is made to confirm the diagnosis of acute myocardial infarction or to obtain customary hospital admission data.

An alternative approach to preventing death in the emergency ward is to equip and staff part of the facility as a separate CCU, where intensive care can be started instantly. Unfortunately only a few hospitals can afford to maintain and staff two CCUs; therefore this scheme is less feasible than rapid transfer to the CCU. *In any case, the sooner intensive coronary care can be initiated, the better is the survival rate.*

4

The Coronary Care Unit

A coronary care unit (CCU) is a specially designed and equipped facility staffed by highly skilled personnel to provide optimal care for patients with suspected or confirmed acute myocardial infarction. Many institutions have expanded the function of the CCU by admitting patients with other cardiac emergencies to the unit. Included in this latter group are patients with acute pulmonary edema, major arrhythmias (unrelated to myocardial infarction), and those requiring pacemakers.

The object of this chapter is to discuss the design, equipment, and staff of an effective CCU.

DESIGN OF THE CCU

Because most hospitals now have CCUs, little purpose would be served here by presenting a detailed description of the physical design of these specialized facilities. However, it is useful for nurses to understand some of the basic concepts and problems involved in planning a CCU. This knowledge is important particularly when the nursing staff is asked to participate in designing a new unit or remodeling an old one. Moreover, the physical layout of the unit influences patient care, and the nurse should appreciate this relationship. The following design factors are considered relevant.

1. Ideally the unit should consist of a series of individual private rooms. An open ward-type facility with curtains or partitions between beds is unsuitable for providing the peacefulness and serenity required in the overall treatment program. Furthermore it is important that patients be unaware of each other so they are not affected by emergencies occurring in adjacent areas. Seeing a crisis elsewhere in the unit can be a devastating emotional experience.

In the same vein, the unit should be designed in such a way that beds and litters can be moved to and from the individual rooms without the risk of disturbing other patients. This unobtrusive movement is particularly important when deaths occur.

2. All beds should be directly visible (through glass windows) from a central nursing station. Direct visual observation is an integral part of coronary care nursing, and it is thoroughly disadvantageous to rely on monitor surveillance as the prime means of patient assessment. Some hospitals have utilized closed circuit television from patient rooms to the nursing station when space limitation prevents direct observation. This technique is less than desirable and has proved to be an unfortunate compromise from the patient's standpoint. In very large units more than one nursing station may be required to provide close observation of all patients.

3. Patient's rooms should be at least 12 × 12 feet in size to allow adequate space for equipment and multiple personnel (particularly at the time of emergencies). Since many patients in the CCU are admitted because of suspected myocardial infarction and may not be desperately ill, it is important that the unit be attractively and cheerfully decorated with this fact in mind. A window should be present in each room; "inside" rooms are very depressing to patients. Provisions for noise control are essential, and acoustical materials for ceilings and floors should be used whenever possible. It is helpful to furnish rooms with clocks, calendars, a radio, and music so the patient does not become totally separated from his normal environment.

4. It is beneficial to locate the CCU at a site contiguous with (or nearby) the hospital's general intensive care facility. This arrangement allows for sharing of certain basic facilities and services (e.g., utility rooms, pantries, storage areas) that would otherwise require duplication. On the other hand, it is not wise to combine these two specialized units into one facility served by a single staff. Experience has shown that independent, full-time nursing staffs for the respective units are more effective than a joint staff (as would be expected with the advancement of specialization in nursing). Furthermore, the general intensive care unit is usually much too hectic a setting for patients with acute myocardial infarction.

Another important consideration in choosing the location of the CCU is to have the unit as close as possible to the emergency or receiving ward of the hospital. Tragically, many deaths occur during transit to the CCU. This threat can be reduced by minimizing the distance between the admission area and the unit.

5. In the design plan it is worthwhile to provide certain additional rooms for purposes other than patient care. Of special importance are the following areas:

a. A waiting room for families. Because of the abrupt and critical nature of cardiac emergencies it is understandable that families gather and remain near the patient for prolonged periods. Unless provisions are made to accommodate these visitors in a separate room outside the unit, disturbance and congestion at the nurses' station and patient care areas usually results. This family waiting room should have adequate telephone facilities.

b. A nurses' lounge. Since nursing personnel must be in continuous attendance within the unit it is important that a room be allocated within the unit for the nursing staff. This lounge should include bathroom facilities, lockers, and comfortable furniture.

c. A physicians' consultation room. Although certainly less essential than the two areas just described, a separate room for the use of physicians has proved very useful in many institutions. This space provides not only an office for the physicians but sleeping quarters as well when necessary.

6. Air conditioning and an efficient ventilatory system are mandatory not only for patient and nurse comfort but also for proper upkeep of the monitoring equipment. Many monitoring systems and other equipment are heat-sensitive, and proper room temperatures must be maintained to ensure satisfactory function.

7. Multiple, separately fused electrical outlets are absolutely essential and should be considered in the early stages of planning. Approximately eight grounded outlets are required for each bed. Electrical grounding within the unit must have unquestionable integrity. Unless true and effective grounding is provided, there is a potential danger of patient electrocution, particularly when several electrical devices are used simultaneously. Grounding that consists of no more than connecting a wire to a convenient water or heating pipe is wholly inadequate, and a three-pronged plug by itself is not a

real safety measure. No compromise can be made without a proper grounding circuit.

Because of increasing use of major electrical equipment within units (including portable x-ray machines), 220-volt lines should be included in the electrical system. An emergency power supply should also be available in the event of electrical failure of the primary circuit.

8. Effective communication and alarm systems are of great importance. The objective of the system should be to permit the nursing staff to summon help instantly and directly. The usual hospital communication network, which involves the circuitous chain of dialing the operator, paging physicians, and returning the call to the unit results in too much delay. A special alarm signal (or code) which bypasses the customary route is very desirable at each bedside.

9. In addition to the specialized equipment described in the following section, each room should be furnished with the following items:

a. Hydraulic bed. A manually operated hydraulic bed is preferable to an electric bed in a CCU. Electric beds pose the potential threat of electric shock to the patient. Also, changing the patient's position with an electric bed is too slow a process in times of emergency.

b. Toilet facilities. A "pullman" toilet or a bedside commode should be kept near each bedside. Bedpans are undesirable for patients with acute myocardial infarction because of the physical effort expended in their use. A portable toilet requires minimal space and can be brought directly to the bedside.

c. Blood pressure apparatus. A wall-mounted sphygmomanometer is required next to each bed. The ready accessibility of this instrument is advantageous because of the frequency with which blood pressures must be recorded.

d. Hangers for intravenous solutions. At least two metal rods with hooks should be suspended from the ceiling above each bed to hang intravenous solutions. These hangers are less cumbersome than floor standards and do not obstruct access to the patient.

EQUIPMENT FOR A CCU

To fulfill its objectives a CCU must contain equipment for detecting, assessing, and treating complications of acute myocardial infarction (and other cardiac emergencies). The type of equipment depends to a large degree on the role and function of the unit. For instance, a CCU that serves as a research or teaching facility or a referral center may be equipped with computerized systems and sophisticated instruments that are unnecessary in other settings. The following discussion focuses on the basic equipment considered necessary in an up-to-date CCU.

Equipment for Detection

Cardiac Monitoring System. The most important detection instrument in the CCU is the cardiac monitor used to identify arrhythmias on a continuous basis. A separate monitor, consisting of an oscilloscope, a rate meter, and an alarm mechanism, is required for each patient. (The specific details of cardiac monitoring are discussed in Chapter 8.) In some CCUs the monitors are placed at each bedside with "slave" oscilloscopes and alarm systems at the central nursing station; in others the monitors are situated in the nursing station with the "slave" attachments at the bedside. The second alternative is probably more effective; it combines the advantage of the patient being unaware of the business of monitoring with its inherent problems (e.g., false alarms) and at the same time allows those attending the patient to observe the electro-cardiographic pattern at the bedside without having to return to the central station. This latter benefit is important during emergency situations (e.g., defibrillation) and avoids the necessity of leaving the bedside to ascertain the effectiveness of treatment.

Electrocardiographic Machine. In addition to the monitoring system the unit requires one or more ECG machines for obtaining 12-lead ECGs for diagnostic purposes. The machine is also used to document arrhythmias seen on the oscilloscope when the monitoring equipment does not include a direct ECG writeout device.

X-Ray Equipment. A portable x-ray machine is very useful for detecting early heart failure and should be readily available for use in the CCU. (In many institutions this equipment is brought to the CCU from the radiology department each time an x ray is ordered.)

Equipment for Assessment

Hemodynamic Instruments. To assess the clinical status of patients with cardio-genic shock or left ventricular failure effectively it is often necessary to measure pressures directly in veins and arteries. Apparatus for this purpose should be on hand in the CCU. The equipment includes manometers, transducers, hemodynamic catheters, and appropriate tubing for determining central venous, intraarterial, and pulmonary artery pressures.

Blood Gas Determinations. Arterial blood gases (and to a lesser degree, venous blood gases) are used to assess tissue oxygenation and metabolism, particularly in the presence of circulatory failure. Needles, syringes, and collecting tubes for blood gas studies should be readily available in the CCU.

Equipment for Treatment and Resuscitation

Defibrillators. A defibrillator should be present at all times at *each* bedside. Although this number of defibrillators may seem redundant, the safety and assurance afforded by individual defibrillators certainly justify their cost. Operating the unit with a lesser number of defibrillators is not without risk.

Pacemakers. Battery-operated pacemakers for temporary cardiac pacing should be readily available in the CCU. Also required is an assortment of different-sized pacing catheters for transvenous insertion.

Respirators. Respiratory assistance equipment should be kept permanently in the unit. Of the many mechanical respirators now available, perhaps the most useful in a CCU is the pressure-cycled machine which inflates the patient's lungs until a preset pressure has been reached. In addition to mechanical respirators, manual breathing bags are essential.

Crash Cart. A mobile cart which contains all supplies, equipment, and drugs needed for cardiac emergencies and resuscitation attempts must be ready for use at all times in the CCU. This cart should be easily movable, constructed of heavy gauge stainless steel, and have a low center of gravity to prevent tipping. Preferably the cart should contain three or more shelves, the topmost of which serves as a work area. Separate drawers for drug storage are located between the first and second shelves. The equipment drugs and supplies customarily contained in a crash cart are noted in Table 4.1.

Oxygen Supply. A dependable oxygen supply piped in from a central source to each bedside is mandatory. Face masks and nasal cannulas for oxygen delivery should be available for immediate use.

Aspiration Equipment. An effective system for aspirating and suctioning nasotracheal secretions should be located in each patient area. A laryngoscope, nasotracheal tubes, and endotracheal tubes are also required.

Tourniquets. Part of the treatment program for acute left ventricular failure is to reduce the work of the heart by applying tourniquets to the extremities in order to diminish the amount of blood returning to the heart. Either plain rubber tubing or a rotating tourniquet machine can be used for this purpose.

Automatic Timing Device. Because it is critically important to know precisely how much time has elapsed after the onset of a lethal arrhythmia, it is useful to have an automatic timer in the CCU. The nurse activates the device at the bedside by pushing the alarm signal as soon as a death-producing arrhythmia is identified.

Bed Board. Either a board or a cafeteria tray should be kept at each bedside for use during cardiopulmonary resuscitation. Without firm support behind the patient's thorax, external cardiac massage may be ineffective.

Prepared Trays. Sterile packages (trays) for venous cutdown, urinary catheterization, tracheostomy, and other procedures should be kept in readiness.

DRUGS FOR THE CCU

Because medications usually have to be administered at a moment's notice in cardiac emergencies, all necessary drugs and fluids must be immediately available in the CCU. A specific list of drugs for the unit should be established, and an adequate supply of these preparations kept on hand at all times. The responsibility for checking the inventory and reordering drugs should be assigned to the head nurse or her designate.

It is essential that the drugs be stored in a precise, orderly way so every nurse in the unit knows exactly where to find a particular item without having to search for it. The importance of this theme cannot be overemphasized: every second counts in a life-threatening emergency.

Although physicians have individual preferences about the specific drugs that should be stocked in the CCU, the basic drug list does not vary greatly at different hospitals. The drugs and intravenous solutions stocked in the CCU at the Presbyterian–University of Pennsylvania Medical Center are given in Table 4.2.

THE STAFF OF THE CCU

It is absolutely essential that the care of patients in a coronary unit be delegated to a *team* of physicians and nurses. In fact, the team approach is the most distinguishing characteristic of the coronary care concept. Because all members of the team understand the aims of care and recognize their respective responsibilities and functions, the effectiveness of the system of care is markedly enhanced. Furthermore, a team effort develops clarity of communication and a mutual respect among the individual members. Unless the physicians and nurses in a CCU function as an organized team, the ultimate result of the entire program will prove very disappointing.

The ideal CCU team is composed of a director, attending physicians (and in some hospitals the intern and resident staff), and a group of nurses specially trained in the principles and practices of coronary care nursing.

Director of the Unit

As with any successful team effort, one person must be in charge and serve as its responsible member and representative. Ideally, the director is a cardiologist or an internist who has the knowledge, dedication, interest, and time to coordinate the whole program. The general duties and responsibilities of the director are to: 1) assume authority and responsibility for establishing basic policies of the unit regarding admission of patients, length of stay in unit, physicians' privileges, and other administrative decisions; 2) establish an overall plan of care for patients in the unit and delegate specific duties to the respective members of the team; 3) supervise and participate in the training program for nurses and other members who comprise the CCU team; 4) be responsible for the selection of equipment and supplies used in the unit; 5) serve as liaison between the attending staff, hospital administration, and members of the CCU team concerning problems that may arise; 6) assume command of patient care in critical situations if the attending physician is not immediately available; 7) evaluate periodically the effectiveness of the unit; and 8) serve as a consultant to the attending physician upon request.

In some hospitals the overall responsibility for the proper functioning of the CCU is shared by a committee comprised of the director of the unit and representatives from the nursing service, hospital administration, and medical staff. The advantage of this plan is that all parties participate in making decisions that may affect their respective departments.

Attending Physicians

It is generally agreed that the care of the patient in the CCU should be supervised by his own physician. The director of the unit and the other members of the team essentially assist the attending physician but do not displace him or assume his role. However, it is essential that the attending physician be willing to delegate some of his normal responsibility to the other team members. In particular, the attending physician must transfer certain authority to the nurse so she can assume a decision-making role on her own when the situation demands.

The delegation of authority from one physician to another in the CCU has broad implications, and the extent of this practice varies considerably among hospitals. In some institutions this delegation of authority involves no more than an agreement that any physician who happens to be present at the time of a catastrophe may assume command (e.g., defibrillate a patient of another physician). In other hospitals the director of the unit (or a committee of physicians) is empowered to act not only in the event of emergencies but also if the general treatment program prescribed by the attending physician fails to meet the care standards of the unit.

Attending physicians should participate in the ongoing training program for nurses (and house officers). Their presence at team conferences is especially important when the patients to be discussed are under their care.

The Intern and Resident Staff

In many hospitals interns and resident physicians become part of the coronary care team as delegates of the attending physician. It should be recognized that these house officers are in training and that their primary function is not to replace the attending physician in the direct care of patients; their assignment to the CCU is meant to be an educational experience.

It is customary practice for a house officer to be notified when the CCU nurse detects a change in the patient's clinical status or if a life-threatening problem develops. It is the decision the house officer makes at these times that often means the difference between life and death. In many instances the house officer has time to confer with the attending physician or the unit director before deciding on a course of action, but with catastrophic situations the resident physician alone makes the ultimate decision of treatment; therefore his role is vitally important to the success of the entire program. Certain aspects regarding house officers' responsibilities are worth considering, particularly as they relate to the team approach.

The unique role of the CCU nurse and her status on the team should be carefully explained to the house staff by the director of the unit. As might be anticipated, the traditional physician-nurse relationship is changed in this setting, where the nurse assumes duties and responsibilities far beyond those generally expected of nurses. Not infrequently, because of their constant exposure to the problems related to myocardial infarction, CCU nurses become extremely competent in the detection and management of arrhythmias and other complications, and the wise house officer will recognize the value of their judgment and experience.

An on-call schedule for the house staff should be posted daily in a conspicuous site so the nurse knows which physician to call for advice or for emergencies during each shift. Preferably two physicians should be listed for both day and night tours. This type of call system is more effective than having the nurse sound a general alarm in catastrophic situations which may be answered by any physician who happens to be nearby. General alarms tend to create confusion, with the sudden assemblage of several members of the house staff but without one person responsible for making decisions.

House officers and the nursing staff should make daily patient rounds in the unit jointly. In this way patient problems that may not be apparent to individual members of the team may be identified and solved. This form of communication is fundamental to effective care.

The Nurse Members of the Team

The success of the coronary care system depends above all on the competence of the nurse members of the CCU team. As noted, unless nurses are adequately trained for their role and are delegated authority to make and carry out therapeutic decisions based on their own observations and judgment, coronary care is merely a token gesture.

For optimum effectiveness a CCU should maintain a ratio of one professional nurse for every two or three patients at all times. Thus a four- or six-bed unit requires two nurses per shift—or a total nursing staff of at least 10 or 12 professional nurses for full coverage. This high quota of nurses may be unrealistic or unachievable in many hospitals. In this circumstance, licensed practical nurses can be employed to assume some of the lesser duties of the professional nurse. However, it is essential that at least one professional nurse be present in the CCU at all times; the responsibility of the unit must never be delegated to a licensed practical nurse, even for a few minutes. This is not to say that highly motivated practical nurses cannot provide valuable assistance in patient care, but it does mean that the duties and responsibilities of coronary care nursing are so encompassing that none but specially trained professional nurses should undertake them. When practical nurses are included as members of the CCU team, they should participate in the training program offered to professional nurses.

Because of its great importance, the role of the CCU nurse is considered separately in the two following chapters. Chapter 5 concerns the selection and preparation of the CCU nurse, and Chapter 6 presents an overview of the responsibilities and duties involved in coronary care nursing.

Table 4.1.   Equipment and Supplies for a Crash Cart

Top Shelf
  Defibrillator
  Electrode paste
  Syringes (3, 5, 10, and 50 cc)
  Needles (18, 20, 21, and 25 gauge)
  Intracardiac needles (3.5-inch spinal needle, 19 gauge)
  Alcohol sponges (one jar)
  Intravenous tubing and adaptors, including Solusets and a three-way stopcock
  Oral airway and padded tongue blades
  Drug tray containing

Atropine SO_4 (1 mg/ml)	1 ml ampule
Lidocaine 1% (10 mg/ml)	50 ml vial
Lidocaine 2% (20 mg/ml)	50 ml vial
Isuprel (0.2 mg/ml)	5 ml vial
Sodium bicarbonate (1 mEq/ml)	50 ml vial
Epinephrine (1:10,000)	10 ml vial
Sterile water for injection	30 ml vial
Sterile normal saline solution for injection	30 cc vial

Shelf 2
  Ambu bag and tubing
  Sterile gloves and drapes
  Endotracheal tray containing
    Endotracheal tube (No. 7) and guide
    Universal adaptors (2)
    T-tubes (2)
    Largyngoscope with three blades
    Batteries
    Lidocaine 4% (40 mg/ml) 50 ml, with atomizer
    Adhesive tape
    Lubricating jelly
    McGill forceps
    Hemostat, rubber-tipped
  Armboards (2)
  Tourniquets
  Venosets (3)
  Angiocaths (3)
  Intracaths (3)
  Scalp vein set
  Pacemaker and pacing catheters

Shelf 3
  Venous cutdown tray
  Tracheostomy set
  5% Dextrose in water—500 ml
  5% Sodium bicarbonate solution—500 ml
  Sterile (4 × 4) dressings

Table 4.1. Equipment and Supplies for a Crash Cart (continued)

Side of Cart
  Resuscitation Board

In Drawers

Sodium bicarbonate (1 mEq/ml)	50 ml ampules (5)
Digoxin (0.25 mg/ml)	2 ml ampules (2)
Levophed (0.2%)	4 ml ampules (4)
Aramine (10 mg/ml)	10 ml vials (2)
Wyamine sulfate (30 mg/ml)	10 ml ampules (1)
Aminophylline (0.5g/20 ml)	20 ml ampules (3)
Dilantin (100 mg/2 ml)	2 ml ampules (2)
Pronestyl (100 mg/ml)	10 ml vials (3)
Atropine sulfate (1 mg/ml)	1 ml ampules (3)
Lidocaine 2% (100 mg/5 ml)	Prepared syringes (2)
Lidocaine 4% (2000 mg/50 ml)	Prepared syringes (2)
Inderal (1 mg/ml)	1 ml ampules (2)
Valium (5 mg/ml)	10 ml ampules (2)
Lasix (10 mg/ml)	2 ml ampules (4)
Solu-Medrol (125 mg/vial)	Prepared vials (2)
Mannitol (12.5 g/50 ml)	50 ml vials (1)
Intropin (200 mg/5 ml)	5 cc ampules (2)
Calcium chloride (100 mg/ml)	10 ml ampules (5)

Table 4.2.   Drugs Stocked in the CCU at the Presbyterian–University of Pennsylvania Medical Center

Antiarrhythmic Agents
   Atropine sulfate
   Isoproterenol (Isuprel)
   Lidocaine
   Diphenylhydantoin (Dilantin)
   Potassium chloride
   Procainamide (Pronestyl)
   Propanolol HCl (Inderal)
   Quinidine sulfate

Anticoagulants
   Heparin
   Warfarin sodium (Coumadin)

Anticoagulant Antagonists
   Protamine sulfate
   Vitamin K_1 oxide (Mephyton)

Antiemetics
   Prochlorperazine (Compazine)
   Trimethobenzamide HCl (Tigan)

Antihypertensive Agents
   Aldomet
   Diazoxide (Hyperstat)
   Reserpine
   Sodium nitroprusside (Nipride)

Bronchodilators
   Aminophylline

Coronary Dilators
   Isosorbide dinitrate (Isordil)
   Nitroglycerin
   Nitroglycerin ointment (Nitrol ointment)

Digitalis Preparations
   Deslanoside (Cedilanid-D)
   Digoxin
   Ouabain

Diuretic Agents
   Furosemide (Lasix)
   Mannitol
   Spironolactone (Aldactone)
   Thiazides

Electrolyte Solutions
   Calcium gluconate
   Magnesium sulfate
   Potassium chloride
   Sodium bicarbonate
   Sodium chloride

Table 4.2. Drugs Stocked in the CCU at the Presbyterian–University of Pennsylvania Medical Center (*continued*)

Hypnotics and Sedatives
   Brevital
   Chloral hydrate
   Flurazepam HCl (Dalmane)
   Phenobarbital
   Amytal sodium

Intravenous Solutions
   Dextran 6%
   Dextran 10%
   Dextrose 5% in saline 0.9%
   Dextrose 5% in 1/4 strength saline
   Dextrose 5% in 1/2 strength saline
   Dextrose 5% in water
   Normal saline 0.9%

Narcotics
   Codeine sulfate
   Hydromorphone (Dilaudid)
   Meperidine HCl (Demerol)
   Morphine sulfate
   Pentazocine (Talwin)

Narcotic Antagonist
   Naloxone HCl (Narcan)

Steroids
   Hydrocortisone sodium succinate (Solu-Cortef)
   Methylprednisolone (Solu-Medrol)
   Prednisone

Tranquilizers
   Chlordiazepoxide HCl (Librium)
   Diazepam (Valium)
   Hydroxyzine pamoate (Vistaril)

Vasopressor Agents
   Dopamine HCl (Intropin)
   Epinephrine
   Levarterenol bitartrate (Levophed)
   Mephentermine sulfate (Wyamine)
   Metaraminol bitartrate (Aramine)
   Phenylephrine HCl (Neo-Synephrine)

5

The Selection and Preparation of CCU Nurses

Nursing in a coronary care unit (CCU) requires skills, knowledge, and judgment beyond that which can be acquired in a basic nursing school curriculum. Consequently, additional training is necessary to prepare nurses (even those with extensive general duty experience) for their specialized role in the CCU. Before describing the details of this instructional program, it is pertinent to consider some of the most important qualifications (personal and professional) for coronary care nursing.

SELECTION OF NURSES FOR THE CCU

Despite hospital staffing problems, CCU nurses must be deliberately selected for their role rather than accepted merely because of their availability or willingness to work in the unit; under no circumstances should nurses be forced or persuaded to work in a CCU against their desire. The underlying purpose of the selection process is to ensure that the members of the nursing staff are all well qualified and able to work together as a team in providing quality nursing care. In view of the time, effort, and cost involved in preparing CCU nurses and the responsibilities they will be asked to assume, it is important for prospective candidates to decide at the onset if they are qualified and suited for coronary care nursing. To this end, it is useful for the nursing director to establish a list of basic requirements for those who contemplate working in a CCU. This practice minimizes misconceptions about CCU nursing and reduces undue turnover; it also results in a stable, smoothly functioning unit. The following personal and professional qualifications should be included among the selection criteria for CCU nurses.

Personal Qualifications

Emotional Stability

It must be recognized that patients admitted to a CCU are usually seriously ill and that the death rate among them is substantially higher than in other divisions of a hospital. The prospective CCU nurse should evaluate her personal reactions to working in this potentially depressing setting and make certain that she can cope with it. Also to be considered is whether making decisions instantly and assuming serious responsibility—inherent elements in coronary care nursing—are likely to produce adverse emotional effects. To be weighed and balanced against these emotional challenges is the sense of accomplishment and satisfaction that CCU nurses derive from saving lives through their own efforts—an experience that is probably unique in the nursing profession.

Social Maturity

Because intensive coronary care is a team effort, an ability to work closely with others is an essential attribute for CCU nurses. It is understandable that in a small, confined area as a CCU, where team members are together constantly, frictions may develop easily, particularly during stressful situations. Unless mature interpersonal relationships are maintained, the team's effectiveness is greatly weakened and the quality of care diminishes.

In addition to working collaboratively with fellow nurses, CCU nurses must also maintain a secure interdependent relationship with the physician members of the team. Unfortunately, some physicians are still unaccustomed to delegating authority to nurses, and problems may arise because of this. It is not uncommon, for example, for CCU nurses to become more proficient in interpreting arrhythmias than some physicians, thus challenging the physician's status and judgment. It takes considerable discretion and a mature approach for nurses to handle these situations.

Motivation

Although usually an exciting experience, coronary care nursing can become dull and routine if the nurse lacks enthusiasm for her work and motivation to learn continually. The nurse should appreciate that nursing in a CCU is meant to be an ongoing learning experience—something to look forward to and enjoy. The degree of enthusiasm of the nursing staff correlates well with the quality of care offered. In fact, one of the most revealing characteristics of a superior CCU is a highly enthusiastic nursing staff.

Integrity

The importance of honesty in a CCU cannot be overemphasized. Errors are bound to occur at one time or another because actions often must be taken instantly and usual safeguards are bypassed. If the errors are recognized and reported immediately, corrective measures can be instituted. Thus total integrity on the part of all CCU personnel is mandatory. Those who cover up their mistakes or are fearful to admit them are ill-suited to work in a CCU.

Dependable Attendance

Nurses who are frequently ill or who are unable to comply regularly with the CCU time schedule for other reasons are poor candidates for coronary care nursing. Recognizing that the proper function of a CCU depends on an adequate nursing staff at all times, it is understandable that any absence or lateness can create a serious problem. This is particularly true in small coronary units where there are a limited number of nurses available as replacements.

Employment Commitment

In view of the time required to prepare CCU nurses (and for them to acquire enough experience to assume full responsibilities), it is only reasonable that candidates agree to remain employed for at least 1 year, unless some unforeseen circumstance arises. Lesser periods of employment weaken the stability of the CCU team and are defeating for all concerned.

Age

As a general rule, nurses who are relatively recent graduates of basic nursing programs are the most adaptable and make the best adjustment to the demands required of CCU nurses. On the other hand, older nurses with excellent qualifications need not be excluded from CCU nursing solely because of their age.

Professional Qualifications

Nursing School Record

All CCU nurses must be graduates of an accredited school of nursing, preferably a baccalaureate program. It is clear that a high ability to learn is an important requisite for nurses selected to work in a CCU. The specialized training program for CCU nurses includes many new concepts and skills which must be mastered quickly. Therefore nurses whose academic record in nursing school indicates a high level of intelligence and superior learning ability are apt to be the best candidates for coronary care nursing.

Dedication to Bedside Nursing

Because coronary care nursing is concerned almost entirely with direct patient care, it is essential that CCU nurses be dedicated to bedside nursing care and enjoy the nurse-patient relationship inherent in this role. Unless a nurse has a keen interest in direct patient care, working in a CCU is ill-advised.

Previous Nursing Experience

Nursing experience with acutely ill patients (as obtained, for example, in general intensive care units, recovery rooms, or emergency departments) is a valuable asset for the prospective CCU nurse. This background facilitates the transition to coronary care nursing, particularly since many of the required technical skills have already been acquired.

PREPARATION OF THE CCU NURSE

After being selected to work in a CCU (according to the criteria just described), nurses must receive sufficient preparation to provide the skills and knowledge necessary to assume responsibilities in the unit. As mentioned previously, a nurse cannot function in a CCU solely on the basis of undergraduate education, and specialized training is required.

Ideally each hospital should conduct its own coronary care training program. When this is not feasible, cooperative programs can be developed with other hospitals or nurses can be sent to nearby medical centers for primary training; the latter alternatives are less desirable.

Although there are many methods for preparing the nurse for her duties in the CCU, the overall educational program can be considered in two phases: the basic orientation program and the continuing educational program.

The Basic Orientation Program

The customary training program for coronary care nursing involves classroom instruction and clinical experience. The two methods should be integrated in order to reinforce both aspects of the learning experience, with classroom instruction preceding clinical instruction. The total program is usually given as a concentrated course of 3 or 4 weeks' duration.

Because the background and previous experience of the students may vary considerably, the design and objectives of the course should be tailored to meet the diverse needs of the class. This requires an evaluation of the nurses' knowledge and skills (usually determined by a preassessment test).

By the completion of the orientation program the nurse should be able to perform the following tasks:

1. Use monitoring devices and other equipment required for assessment and treatment.
2. Assess the patient's physical and psychological status by bedside observation and appropriate examinations.
3. Institute measures designed to prevent complications.
4. Detect and interpret early signs and symptoms of complications.
5. Provide effective nursing care which meets the patient's physiologic, psychologic, and social needs.
6. Initiate emergency therapy and assess its effects.
7. Evaluate the results (both desired and untoward) of various means of intervention.
8. Determine patients' needs for instruction about rehabilitation, and start a teaching plan early in the course of hospitalization.
9. Function as a member of the CCU team in planning, evaluating, and delivering patient care.

Classroom Instruction

Learning is facilitated when a student is an active participant in the program rather than a passive listener. Therefore it is desirable to minimize formal classroom lectures, which involve very little interaction between the instructor and the student, and to focus instead on conferences and demonstrations whenever possible. Several excellent teaching aids are available to complement the instructional program, including films, film strips, slides, audiotapes, videotapes, and programmed instructional books. A typical outline for classroom instruction is presented below.

Topics for Classroom Instruction and Discussion

1. *Introduction to the concept of intensive coronary care:* rationale; prevention of complications; physician-nurse team approach to care; tour of CCU
2. *Anatomy and physiology of the heart:* the coronary circulation; electrophysiology; hemodynamics
3. *Coronary heart disease:* the problem; risk factors; pathophysiology; approaches to combating the problem
4. *Acute myocardial infarction:* the patient's history; physical findings; diagnosis; enzyme and other laboratory studies; complications of the attack; clinical course
5. *Cardiac nursing care:* comprehensive care to meet the patient's changing needs; methods of clinical assessment; physical and psychological care; patient instruction and rehabilitation
6. *Electrocardiography:* basic principles; monitoring leads; ECG wave forms; the normal ECG
7. *Arrhythmias:* classification; identification; interpretation; relative dangers
8. *Drug treatment of arrhythmias:* specific drugs; anticipated effects; side effects; nursing role

9. *Electrical treatment of arrhythmias:* defibrillation; elective cardioversion; temporary cardiac pacing; permanent cardiac pacing
10. *Lethal arrhythmias:* emergency treatment program; cardiopulmonary resuscitation; emergency drugs; nursing role
11. *Left ventricular failure:* hemodynamics; clinical assessment; drug therapy; nurse's role in therapy
12. *Cardiogenic shock:* hemodynamic measurements; clinical assessment; intraaortic balloon pumping; the nurse's role
13. *Other complications of acute myocardial infarction:* ventricular rupture; thromboembolism; papillary muscle dysfunction; pericarditis
14. *Assisted respiration and oxygen therapy:* indications; methods; problems
15. *Fluid and electrolyte balance:* clinical signs; replacement therapy; use of diuretics
16. *Rehabilitation of the cardiac patient:* assessing needs; follow-up care; patient teaching

Clinical Experience

Clinical training in coronary care nursing is obtained for the most part at a nurse-to-nurse level, with an experienced CCU nurse serving as the preceptor. This plan involves much more than simply assigning the student to work in a CCU under the supervision and observation of the preceptor. Instead, the program should consist of a planned, orderly sequence of learning activities designed to prepare the nurse for specific duties and responsibilities (as described in the next chapter). These clinical activities should be scheduled to follow the classroom discussion of the particular subject. However, this is not always possible, and the clinical program must be flexible so each day's plan can be adjusted according to circumstances within the unit. For instance, if on the learner's third day in the unit, a patient requires a temporary pacemaker, it is logical to provide clinical experience with cardiac pacing then, rather than at a later, scheduled time.

Normally the clinical program covers a 3-week period but can be extended according to the needs of individual students. During the first 2 weeks, at least, the trainee should work side by side with the preceptor (who often is the head nurse). After this initial period the student obtains further experience by working with a staff nurse during the evening shift.

In addition to this direct form of clinical training, other practical experience can be obtained outside the CCU. The following methods are helpful in enabling the nurse to become skillful in some of the procedures used in a coronary unit.

Electrocardiographic Techniques.   To become adept at recording 12-lead ECGs, it is useful for the nurse to spend a day or two in the Heart (ECG) Station. By recording many ECGs here, the technique can be learned promptly. Particular attention should be given to the methods used to obtain high quality (distinct) ECGs.

Venipuncture and Intravenous Infusions.   Many nurses are not experienced in collecting blood samples (for laboratory studies) or in starting intravenous infusions, both of which are essential duties within the CCU. These skills can be acquired by having the nurse accompany laboratory technicians and the "IV team" as they make their rounds in the hospital.

Use of Respiratory Equipment.   By assigning nurses to the inhalation therapy department, valuable practical experience can be obtained in the use of positive-pressure machines, manual breathing bags, mechanical respirators, and in the use of various methods of administering oxygen. Since arterial blood gas studies are frequently performed in patients receiving inhalation therapy, the nurse can also learn the procedure for collecting arterial blood samples and preparing them for the laboratory.

The Technique of Precordial Shock.   Unquestionably the most unique experience for the beginning CCU nurse is the use of a defibrillator to terminate ventricular fibrillation. A machine that delivers 7000 volts of electricity has frightening implications. Because the same equipment is used in terminating other, nonfatal arrhythmias (e.g., atrial fibrillation) on an elective basis, it is extremely beneficial if nurses are allowed actually to give the precordial shock, under the supervision of a physician, in these nonemergency situations. In this way the nurse becomes familiar with the equipment she later will use on her own if death-producing arrhythmias occur.

Cardiopulmonary Resuscitation.   It is mandatory that each nurse be able to perform closed-chest compression and mouth-to-mouth ventilation in a wholly effective manner (according to the American Heart Association's standards). Practicing this life-saving procedure on life-sized manikins (e.g., Resusci-Anne or Recording Annie) is an excellent method for learning the technique of cardiopulmonary resuscitation. Also, nurses should attend and observe actual resuscitation attempts made in all areas of the hospital to get a view of how a team functions in practice.

Simulated Emergencies.   As a means of achieving optimal efficiency during emergency situations, simulated catastrophes ("fire drills") can be staged, using a manikin as a "patient" who has suddenly developed ventricular fibrillation. The nurse carries out the planned program of resuscitation while other members of the team fulfill their particular roles. The sequence of nursing actions and the time they take to accomplish are evaluated by the instructor or preceptor.

Continuing Educational Program

It is important to realize that the basic training plan just outlined is only an introduction to coronary care nursing, and that to achieve greater skill and competence nurses must continue to learn (and apply) new concepts and techniques. To this end, each hospital should develop a continuing educational program for the CCU nursing staff. By participating in this ongoing learning program, the nurse increases her knowledge, and the quality of nursing care in the unit improves steadily. Some of the methods used to conduct an effective ongoing educational program are described below.

Team Conferences

Team conferences, in which nurse and physician members of the coronary care unit team meet jointly, have proved to be useful and popular teaching exercises for the unit's staff. The meetings, which usually consist of case presentations or discussions of policies and practices within the unit, should be scheduled once a week with the unit director presiding. These conferences provide an opportunity for mutual learning in an informal setting and are extremely worthwhile.

The format we employ involves a case history presentation given by a house officer (or the attending physician), after which a nurse (assigned in rotation) describes her observations about the patient's clinical course. The treatment is reviewed and the group identifies special problems. The following is an excerpt from one of our team conferences.

RESIDENT PHYSICIAN: Mr. Scott is a 48-year-old man who was admitted to the unit yesterday afternoon following an episode of typical substernal pain along with vomiting and sweating. On admission the pulse was 120/minute, but there were no signs of left ventricular failure. Other than the chest pain, which by then had persisted for an hour, his condition was quite stable. He was given 75 mg Demerol after which the pain disappeared. The ECG showed marked elevation of the ST segments in the precordial leads typical of acute anterior wall infarction. Monitoring revealed sinus tachycardia but no other arrhythmias. The first CPK enzyme level was markedly elevated. There wasn't much question about the diagnosis. I haven't seen him since late last evening, but he was doing quite well then. I should add that the patient is a known diabetic who apparently has been reasonably well controlled with insulin.

DIRECTOR: Dr. Edwards, as the patient's physician, could you tell us a little more about his history? Did he have known coronary disease in the past?

ATTENDING PHYSICIAN: Although this man has never had angina and an ECG 6 months ago was normal, I am not really surprised that he had a coronary. He would really be considered a high risk candidate. In addition to the diabetes, he smoked two packs of cigarettes a day, had an elevated serum cholesterol, and was 20 pounds overweight. Unfortunately, I was unable to get him to change his ways. Furthermore, his father died of a coronary at age 51.

DIRECTOR: We would all agree this man was looking for trouble. Now, Jane, could you tell us about his course since admission?

NURSE: In general, his condition hasn't changed much during the night. He did have one other episode of chest pain about 8 PM, and he was given an additional injection of Demerol. He didn't sleep well, but he has not been dyspneic nor does he have any other complaints this morning. The night nurse, however, was concerned about his pulse rate. It remained between 100 and 120 since admission, and none of us is sure why this sinus tachycardia has persisted.

DIRECTOR: That is an important observation. We have a patient who seems stable but has a rapid heart rate. What do you make of this, John?

RESIDENT PHYSICIAN: Many patients have sinus tachycardia. It may be due to temperature elevation or anxiety, or it may reflect an early sign of impending heart failure.

DIRECTOR: Quite right. What do you think is causing this patient's tachycardia?

RESIDENT PHYSICIAN: If it persisted all night and he was restless, I would be suspicious that we may be seeing early left ventricular failure.

NURSE: That is what we guessed too.

DIRECTOR: Has a chest film been taken this morning?

SECOND NURSE: Yes, I called for the report just before the conference, and the interpretation was early left ventricular failure.

ATTENDING PHYSICIAN: I just examined his chest, and there were no rales present.

DIRECTOR: That would not be unusual. The x-ray findings and the persistent tachycardia often precede clinical failure.

Nursing Conferences

Nursing conferences, which represent a variation of nurse-to-nurse teaching, offer another means for providing continuing education. The main objective of these meetings is to allow the nursing staff as a group to identify and seek solutions to particular problems encountered in the unit. The success of this learning experience depends on an active exchange of ideas and opinions. Therefore the conferences should be scheduled at times that permit the largest attendance (without reducing nursing care in the unit). An excerpt from a nursing conference follows:

MODERATOR: Mr. Clark was admitted yesterday with an acute myocardial infarction. He has not had any chest pain since admission and his course has been uneventful—no problems at all. We've noticed, however, that he has become increasingly upset about having his vital signs checked every few hours, and I thought it might be worthwhile to discuss this situation.

NURSE ONE: He certainly does get upset. As I walked into the room to take his blood pressure, he sat up in bed and said, "You're going to take my blood pressure *again*? I feel all right. Why is it necessary to check me so often?"

NURSE TWO: What did you say?

NURSE ONE: I told him we routinely check the blood pressure of each patient every few hours as a means of preventing complications. I tried to reassure him that his condition was stable and that there were no complications.

NURSE TWO: Didn't that help?

NURSE ONE: I guess not because Mary had the same experience with him at 8 o'clock.

MODERATOR: Why do you think he reacts this way?

NURSE THREE: Perhaps he believes his condition is worsening and we aren't telling him about it.

MODERATOR: That's one explanation, but I wonder if there isn't more to the problem than that?

NURSE TWO: I've seen other patients who question everything the nurse does and seem to resent it. Usually these patients have great anxiety, and complaining to the nurse is their way of seeking further reassurance.

NURSE ONE: If that's the case, we should try to reassure him more often, not only after he complains about vital signs.

MODERATOR: I think that would be a good plan.

NURSE THREE: I hope you're right—since I'm just coming on duty.

Hospital Ward Rounds

Because nurses working in a CCU are involved in the care of patients with myocardial infarction for a period of only 4 or 5 days (the acute phase), they have little opportunity to observe the subsequent course of the illness. This is a disadvantage since patients in the CCU usually ask many questions about the remaining period of hospitalization and the program after discharge. In order to respond intelligently to these questions, it is important for CCU nurses to obtain a complete picture of the overall management of acute myocardial infarction. What medications are used during the subacute phase of hospitalization? What activities are permitted and when? Do the emotional responses noted initially (e.g., anxiety or depression) disappear after transfer from the CCU? What instructions does the physician give the patient at the time of hospital discharge? This type of information can be gained readily if CCU nurses make ward rounds throughout the hospital with the attending physician. A schedule should be established so that each nurse has the opportunity of participating in these rounds at regular intervals.

Physicians' Lectures

A lecture series given by physicians in different specialties is a valuable component of an ongoing educational program. The presentations should provide advanced, in-depth information; they should not review basic material already covered in the orientation program. It is desirable for the nursing staff to suggest and select the subjects to be discussed. Examples of various lecture topics (and speakers) for the series include the following.

Emotional Aspects of Myocardial Infarction—Psychiatrist

• Clinical assessment of the patient • Methods of coping • Intervention techniques • When is psychiatric consultation needed? • The nurses' own emotional responses • Emotionally induced cardiac invalidism

Electrocardiography—Cardiologist

• Interpretation of complex arrhythmias • Heart block and His bundle electrograms • The ECG diagnosis of myocardial infarction • Monitoring leads • Electrical axis of the heart

Diagnostic Methods—Cardiologist

• Echocardiography • Cardiac scanning • Other noninvasive techniques • Cardiac catheterization • Stress testing

Assisted Respiration—Anesthesiologist

• Mechanical respirator therapy • Complications of artificial respiration • Oxygen toxicity • Interpreting blood gas studies • Intermittent positive-pressure breathing

Pathology of the Heart—Pathologist

• Current concepts of atherosclerosis • Complications of myocardial infarction • Enzyme studies and size of infarction • Interpretation of laboratory studies • Papillary muscle dysfunction

Heart Surgery—Cardiac Surgeon

• Coronary artery bypass graft surgery • Ventricular aneurysm surgery • Permanent pacemaker implantation • Intraaortic balloon pumping in cardiogenic shock • Surgery for preinfarction angina

6

Coronary Care Nursing

In the final analysis intensive coronary care is a system of specialized nursing. Indeed, the number of lives saved in a coronary care unit (CCU) is directly related to the competence of the nursing staff; no other element of coronary care is as important.

To define this specialized nursing role clearly it is appropriate first to outline the overall duties and responsibilities of the CCU nurse and then to consider specific aspects of nursing care from the time of admission to discharge from the unit.

AN OUTLINE OF NURSING DUTIES AND RESPONSIBILITIES

The primary goals of coronary care are to preserve life, prevent complications, and restore the patient to his maximal functional capacity (physically and emotionally). To achieve these objectives the nurse members of the CCU team must assume the following responsibilities.

I. **Continuous Assessment of the Patient's Clinical Status**

A. **By Means of Electrocardiographic Monitoring**

Because arrhythmias are the most common cause of death after acute myocardial infarction, it is absolutely essential that the heart rate and rhythm be monitored continuously in all patients in the CCU. The nurse must be able to identify arrhythmic disorders, assess their relative danger, and decide what action to take when an arrhythmia develops. Much of the success of intensive coronary care depends on this nursing responsibility.

B. **By Direct Observation of the Patient**

Cardiac monitoring provides information only about the electrical activity of the heart; the remaining aspects of cardiac performance are assessed by other means. To evaluate the heart's function as a pump a series of planned observations at the bedside must be made. To this end, it is essential that the nurse examine the patient carefully at regular intervals to detect signs or symptoms of left ventricular failure and cardiogenic shock. In fact the detection of all complications except arrhythmias depends on direct observation of the patient. This nursing duty should not be overshadowed by cardiac monitoring.

C. **By Means of Hemodynamic Monitoring**

In patients with advanced left ventricular failure (or other circulatory complications) it is often necessary to measure venous and arterial pressures repeatedly in order to assess the severity of the problem and the effects of treatment. This type of monitoring—called hemodynamic monitoring—involves the insertion of long, indwelling intravenous or intraarterial catheters (by the physician) and the measurement and recording of the pressures at frequent intervals by the nurse. Hemodynamic monitoring requires technical skill; but far more important, the nurse must be able to interpret the findings so that the treatment program can be altered accordingly.

II. Anticipation and Prevention of Complications

A. Intravenous Infusions

Because of the unpredictable nature of acute myocardial infarction and the threat that a serious arrhythmia (or other complication) may develop suddenly, it is standard practice to establish and maintain a "keep open" intravenous line in every CCU patient. In this way intravenous drugs can be administered instantly in critical situations. It is the duty of the CCU nurse to start the intravenous infusion, verify the patency of the system, and control the rate of flow.

B. Oxygen Therapy

CCU nurses are permitted to start oxygen therapy at their own discretion. The need for oxygen is determined by the patient's clinical condition. In addition to its use in circulatory failure, oxygen is administered as a preventive measure (in the hope of improving myocardial oxygenation) when ischemic chest pain or arrhythmias develop.

C. Treatment of Warning Arrhythmias

One of the fundamental objectives of coronary care (as explained in Chapter 3) is to prevent ventricular fibrillation and ventricular standstill by treating warning arrhythmias. When a warning arrhythmia is recognized the nurse must anticipate the treatment program and prepare appropriate antiarrhythmic drugs for immediate use. In keeping with this preventive approach, CCU nurses are authorized to administer intravenous drugs (e.g., lidocaine or atropine) when necessary. Depending on the particular policies of a CCU (discussed subsequently) a specific order may be required in each instance, or, under coverage of a standing order, the nurse may administer the drug on the basis of her own clinical judgment when dangerous arrhythmias occur.

D. Cardiac Pacing

The prevention of ventricular standstill is based primarily on the insertion of a temporary transvenous pacemaker when advanced heart block exists. The pacing catheter is positioned by the physician with the assistance of a nurse. Thereafter the nurse must determine if the pacemaker is functioning properly at all times and, if necessary, identify sources of malfunction. These are important responsibilities because abrupt failure of a pacemaker (e.g., as the result of battery failure or a disconnected wire) can be disastrous.

III. Emergency and Resuscitative Treatment

A. Defibrillation

Although preventive measures certainly reduce the risk of ventricular fibrillation, the fact remains that this death-producing arrhythmia can develop at any time. The preservation of life after the onset of ventricular fibrillation depends in nearly all instances on the ability of the CCU nurse to recognize the arrhythmia and terminate it immediately by means of precordial shock (defibrillation). This nursing responsibility is of supreme importance.

B. Cardiopulmonary Resuscitation

When sudden death occurs because preventive treatment is ineffective or cannot be accomplished in time, the final hope for survival is cardiopulmonary resuscitation by means of external cardiac compression and mouth-to-mouth ventilation. This technique maintains the circulation, allowing corrective procedures to be attempted. Every nurse—indeed all personnel in the CCU—must be proficient in performing effective cardiopulmonary resuscitation.

C. Assisted Respiration

Mechanical respirators are sometimes required in the treatment of advanced circulatory failure to provide adequate tissue oxygenation. Although in most hospitals respiratory therapists operate and maintain this equipment, the CCU nurse must be familiar with the operation of mechanical respirators and must be able to recognize problems that occur during their use. Also necessary is the ability to use a manual breathing bag to assist respiration.

D. Rotating Tourniquets

Part of the treatment program for acute left ventricular failure (pulmonary edema) involves the application of tourniquets to the arms and legs to reduce venous return to the heart. The nurse applies these tourniquets and rotates them from limb to limb at set times. Included in this nursing responsibility is the prevention of arterial constriction from overly tight tourniquets.

IV. Diagnostic Procedures

A. Twelve-Lead Electrocardiograms

In other areas of the hospital electrocardiograms (ECGs) are recorded by technicians, but in the CCU the nurse usually assumes this duty. The reason for this is that ECGs must be taken frequently, and often at a moment's notice (e.g., during episodes of chest pain). Furthermore, the presence of many hospital personnel within the unit at one time is undesirable because it creates confusion and disturbs serenity.

B. Laboratory Studies

To minimize patient fears and at the same time to develop a close nurse-patient relationship it is beneficial for the CCU nurse, rather than a laboratory technician, to draw the many blood samples required each day for diagnostic purposes. Technical skill in venipuncture is a valuable asset for the nurse.

C. Arterial Blood Gases

To evaluate oxygen (and other gas) concentrations arterial blood samples are required. The arterial puncture and aspiration of blood is performed by a physician. Nursing duties include preparation of the syringe (with heparin), placing the blood sample in a container of ice, and sending the specimen immediately to the laboratory for blood gas analysis.

V. General Nursing Care

In addition to their specialized duties, CCU nurses are expected to provide high level general nursing care to patients in the unit. The nursing care plan for the coronary patient should be very flexible; establishing rigid routines for carrying out nursing procedures is ill-advised. The most practical approach is to develop a broad plan for each day which can be adjusted according to the patient's needs at a particular time. (Specific aspects of general nursing care are described in the following pages.)

VI. Emotional Support

High on the list of nursing responsibilities is the identification and management of anxiety, depression, and other emotional responses that may affect the patient's clinical course and ultimate rehabilitation. The nurse should be able to recognize verbal and nonverbal clues of emotional stress, and understand the basic mechanisms for helping the patient to cope with his problems. (Because of its special importance the subject of emotional support is considered separately in this chapter, after the sections on admission procedure and subsequent care of patients in the CCU.)

VII. Communication

As the member of the CCU team who constantly attends the patient, the nurse must communicate not only with the patient and his family but also with physicians, fellow nurses, and other hospital personnel involved in the care program. The specific duties involved in this communication are:

a. To explain to the patient the objectives of coronary care, as well as the reasons for various procedures and how they are accomplished; and, above all, to answer questions about the illness.

b. To apprise the family of the patient's clinical condition and progress, to allay their fears, and to enlist their cooperation.

c. To serve as a liaison between the physician, the patient, and the family.

d. To keep the physician advised of the patient's clinical status and to report any meaningful changes as soon as they occur.

e. To present succinct, comprehensive reports to the other members of the nursing staff about the condition of each patient so that the continuity of effective care will not be interrupted.

VIII. Collection and Recording of Data

A. Nursing History

A sometimes tedious but always important nursing duty is to obtain and record pertinent information about the patient's personal health habits, social history, and other factors that influence nursing care. A representative form for recording these facts is shown in Figure 6.1. Pertinent information from the nursing history should also be recorded on the Kardex for day-to-day nursing care plans.

B. Admission Summary

It is essential for the nurse to summarize the patient's clinical condition at the time of admission in order to establish a base line for comparison. These findings are usually reported on a separate admission note (Fig. 6.2); however, in some CCUs these data are included in the nursing history form described above.

C. Documentation of Arrhythmias

At hourly intervals, or whenever a significant arrhythmia appears on the monitor, the nurse should record an ECG strip—called a rhythm strip—to document the heart's rate and rhythm at the time. These serial tracings are extremely useful for detecting progressive changes.

D. Drug Therapy

The dosage, time of administration, and effects of all cardiac drugs must be noted specifically. This information is extremely important in assessing whether changes are necessary in the treatment program.

Nursing History

Patient's Name _____

Admitting Diagnosis _____

Date of Admission _____ Time_____

Attending Physician_____

    Notified by_____ Time_____

House Officer _____

    Notified by_____ Time_____

Mode of Arrival_____ Accompanied by _____

Responsible Family Member_____ Telephone _____

Informant Other than Patient _____ Telephone _____

Language Spoken _____

Medications Before Admission:

    Cardiac _____

    Other _____

    Last dose _____

Medications Removed from Patient's Bedside?_____

    Taken home by family _____

    Stored in nurse's station _____

Known Allergies? _____

Personal Information:

    Glasses_____ Contact lenses _____ Hearing aid _____

    Dentures_____: Upper _____ Lower _____ Partial _____

    Customary activity: Limited _____ Unlimited _____

    Diet: Unrestricted_____ Restricted _____ Type _____

    Sleep pattern: Hours at night _____

               Hours during day_____

               Requires sedatives? _____

               Number of pillows _____

    Bowel pattern: Frequency _____

               Laxatives? _____ Type_____

               Last B.M. _____

    Bladder pattern: Frequency _____

               Nocturia?_____

General Observations:

    Patient's level of understanding _____

    Reliability of information _____

    Hygiene _____

    Skin: Integrity _____ Rashes? _____

          Pressure sores? _____ Ulcers? _____

    Deformities or abnormalities _____

    _____

    _____

    _____

Other Pertinent Information _____

_____

_____

Nursing History Obtained by _____

Figure 6.1. Nursing history.

Nurse's Admission Summary

Name _____ Age _____ Sex _____

Date of Admission _____ Time_____

Diagnosis _____

Past History:

    Known angina _____ Previous infarction _____

    Hypertension _____ Diabetes _____ Respiratory_____

    Other diseases _____

    Previous hospitalizations _____ Here _____ Other _____

Emergency Drugs Before Admission to CCU and Time Administered _____
_____

Condition on Admission:

    Chest pain _____

    Dyspnea_____

    Diaphoresis_____ Skin color _____

    Mental status _____

    BP _____ Pulse _____ Respirations_____ Temperature _____

Cardiac Rhythm _____

    (*Attach rhythm strip to back of this sheet*)

Summary of Clinical Condition _____
_____

Laboratory Studies

	Ordered	Performed	Nursing Comments
CBC			
Urinalysis			
BUN			
Blood sugar (__hours p.p.)			
CPK			
SGOT			
LDH			
Sedimentation			
Electrolyte panel			
Prothrombin time			
ATPP			
Other			
ECG (12-lead)			
Chest x ray			

Figure 6.2. Nurse's admission summary.

E. **Nursing Notes**

The emphasis of nursing notes in the CCU should be on changes in the patient's clinical status that occur during a particular shift. Observations regarding symptoms, signs, and emotional responses are especially relevant.

IX. **Student Teaching**

The experienced CCU nurse is expected to serve as a preceptor for new nurses joining the coronary care team. Moreover, each nurse in the unit can benefit from the wisdom of colleagues.

X. **Patient Teaching**

Although detailed teaching of patients is not usually attempted during the acute phase of the illness, CCU nurses nevertheless have a responsibility to at least begin a teaching plan on an informal basis. This can be accomplished by responding to patient's questions (or cues) in a simple but informative manner. The subjects discussed with the patient should be recorded so that the teaching plan is consistent and can be continued after transfer from the unit.

ADMISSION OF PATIENTS TO CCU

Admitting a patient to the CCU involves a sequence of steps, the final order of which is determined by the nurse. Certain procedures are of overriding importance and demand immediate action; others, although essential, have a lower priority. The critical factor in establishing priorities is the patient's clinical condition (and needs) at the time of admission.

For patients who are not in acute distress on arrival, the primary goal of the admission process is to institute as quickly as possible a program for preventing complications while at the same time attempting to allay the patient's fears. In contrast, when complications already have developed and patients are in acute distress on admission, initial efforts must be channeled toward combating the existing problem (e.g., acute left ventricular failure, cardiogenic shock, or major arrhythmias) and preventing further complications. The admission procedure for patients in both of these categories is described in the following paragraphs.

Patients Not in Acute Distress

1. Initiate cardiac monitoring. The first step in the admission of any patient with suspected acute myocardial infarction is to attach electrodes to the chest and begin cardiac monitoring. Death-producing arrhythmias can develop at any time (especially during the immediate hours after the attack), and therefore it is essential that ECG monitoring be instituted immediately, regardless of the patient's clinical condition. (The procedure for cardiac monitoring is described in detail in Chapter 8.)

2. Explain the monitoring system to the patient and outline the general program of coronary care. Being admitted to a CCU is a frightening experience for most patients, and the nurse must attempt to allay these anticipated fears from the onset. As discussed later in this chapter, one of the most useful ways of helping the patient is to explain every step to be undertaken. While applying the electrodes the nurse should briefly describe the purpose of cardiac monitoring and demonstrate how it is accomplished. The main point to emphasize is that cardiac monitoring is used to prevent complications and that by observing the monitor the nurse is able to detect any minor change in the heart rate or rhythm, which can then be corrected immediately, before a problem arises. So that the patient will not become awed by the importance of the machine, the nurse should make it clear at once that cardiac monitoring is only one aspect of coronary care, not the entire program. Because the patient is unlikely to remember detailed descriptions given during the stressful period of admission, it is wise to provide simple explanations at first and elaborate later.

*3. **Record an ECG-strip from the monitor.*** An ECG recording of the heart's rate and rhythm (as detected by the monitor) should be obtained soon after admission. This rhythm strip documents the ECG pattern seen on the monitor screen and serves as a base line for future comparison. After the cardiac rhythm has been identified the rhythm strip is attached to the nurse's admission notes.

*4. **Inquire about the presence of chest pain.*** A basic rule of therapy in acute myocardial infarction is to control chest pain promptly. Ischemic pain is usually a source of great apprehension to the patient, and relief of this distressing symptom must be accomplished without delay. If the patient indicates that he has chest pain, the nurse should administer a narcotic as ordered by the physician.

*5. **Start an intravenous infusion.*** As an early step in the admission procedure, the nurse should insert an indwelling venous catheter and start an infusion of 5% glucose in water. The intravenous line is kept in place all during the patient's stay in the CCU. To prevent overloading of the vascular system, the rate of fluid administration must be carefully regulated (using a microdrip technique). The usual flow rate is 15–60 microdrops per minute.

*6. **Evaluate the patient's clinical condition.*** Even though a patient appears comfortable and is not in acute distress, early signs or symptoms of complications may nevertheless be present. One of the main objectives of the initial evaluation is to determine if there is any evidence of a beginning complication (particularly early left ventricular failure or cardiogenic shock). This is accomplished by questioning the patient about symptoms and by physical examination (as described in Chapter 7). In addition, information must be obtained about the patient's past medical history (including preexisting diseases, medications, and allergies) which may influence the treatment program. These facts should be recorded carefully on the admission summary sheet (Fig. 6.2).

*7. **Notify the physician.*** After high priority procedures have been completed, the nurse should communicate with the physician responsible for the patient's immediate care (i.e., the attending physician or a house officer) and describe all pertinent findings on admission. The nurse's description of the patient's status is extremely important because it influences the physician's decision about initial treatment.

*8. **Record a 12-lead ECG.*** This tracing, the first of a series that will be taken during the period of hospitalization, is required to confirm the diagnosis of acute myocardial infarction. This initial recording is compared with subsequent ECGs to identify sequential changes associated with myocardial injury and necrosis. The full (12-lead) ECG also provides information about certain arrhythmic disturbances that cannot be identified specifically from a monitor rhythm strip. If a 12-lead tracing has been recorded in the receiving ward or the physician's office just before admission to the unit it is not necessary to repeat the ECG at this time. In the event a patient develops recurrent chest pain after admission the nurse should record a 12-lead ECG during the pain episode if possible; diagnostic changes are most likely to appear in the presence of ischemic pain.

*9. **Collect blood and urine specimens for laboratory studies.*** In most CCUs a routine series of laboratory studies are ordered for all patients admitted to the unit. The tests usually include a complete blood count (CBC), urinalysis, serum enzymes, erythrocyte sedimentation rate, and a screening profile (glucose, urea nitrogen, uric acid, cholesterol). Potassium and sodium are measured in patients who have been receiving diuretics. When anticoagulant therapy is used, a prothrombin time or an activated partial thromboplastin time (APTT) is ordered.

10. Assist the physician in the physical examination of the patient. The nurse's presence at the bedside during the examination is very helpful for all concerned. While assisting both the physician and the patient, the nurse is also able to compare her original findings and impressions with those of the physician. Changes in the blood pressure, pulse rate, cardiac rhythm, or other clinical parameters since the time of admission are extremely important in planning the treatment program.

11. Begin the treatment program as ordered by the physician. The proposed management of the patient must be discussed in detail with the physician so that the nursing staff has a clear picture of the aims of therapy and of any problems that may be anticipated. Drug therapy should be started promptly, and the time of administration carefully recorded.

12. Arrange for other studies. The physician may order several other studies for purposes of diagnosis or clinical assessment. These may include chest x rays, arterial blood gases, and hemodynamic measurements. The nurse should arrange for the procedures ordered and assist in performing them.

13. Explain the situation to the family. The great concern of a family for a patient with acute myocardial infarction and the worry of the patient about his family must always be recognized. The patient is one of the family and cannot be set apart simply because he is in a hospital. With this in mind the nurse should provide a general description of the purpose of the unit to family visitors and explain the type of care the patient will receive. In many CCUs families are given prepared brochures which describe the monitoring system, visiting hours, and other pertinent information regarding the patient's stay in the unit. It is a mistake to view the family as burdensome; indeed every effort should be made to enlist their cooperation. Reassuring the family is often every bit as important as reassuring the patient.

Patients in Acute Distress

1. Connect the monitor. Although the clinical picture of patients in acute distress is usually dominated by signs of acute left ventricular failure or cardiogenic shock, it is critically important that cardiac monitoring be started before attempting to control the obvious complications. Because most deaths that occur within the first 30 minutes after admission are due to lethal arrhythmias, preparation for the detection and treatment of these sudden catastrophes should precede other therapy.

2. Notify the physician immediately. That a patient is admitted in acute distress indicates that a serious complication of acute myocardial infarction has already developed and that therapy must be started as soon as possible. The sooner treatment is initiated in these critical circumstances, the better the chance for survival. For this reason the nurse should advise the physician at once of the patient's status.

3. Start oxygen therapy. Oxygen should be administered without delay to all patients in acute distress. The most effective method for delivering oxygen in this situation is by means of a tight-fitting face mask with an oxygen flow rate of 8–10 liters of oxygen per minute. An oxygen concentration of at least 60% can be achieved with this method. (In contrast, a two-pronged nasal cannula with an oxygen flow rate of 6–8 liters per minute usually provides a concentration of only 30–40%).

4. Start an intravenous infusion. Because intravenous drugs will be used in the immediate treatment program, an intravenous conduit must be established as soon as practicable. A long, indwelling venous catheter is preferable in this situation in that it can also be used in measuring central venous pressure.

5. Evaluate the patient's clinical status. The clinical condition of patients admitted in acute distress can change very rapidly, and therefore it is essential to promptly obtain base line levels for comparison. The blood pressure, pulse rate, cardiac rhythm, number and quality of respirations, skin color, presence or absence of sweating, mental status, and urinary output should be determined and recorded.

6. Assist the physician in performing assessment procedures. Physical examination alone often fails to provide sufficient information about the severity of a complication or the manner in which it should be treated. In these instances arterial blood gases and direct hemodynamic measurements may be required. The assistance of a nurse is required in performing these procedures.

7. Prepare for emergency treatment program. Anticipating that various equipment and drugs will be required in the management of complications, the nurse can save precious time by bringing all necessary items to the bedside and preparing them for immediate use.

8. Start the treatment program as ordered by the physician or in accordance with the standing orders of the CCU. Having identified the underlying complication, the CCU team must institute a planned treatment program. The nursing role in the treatment of each major complication is described in the following chapters.

SUBSEQUENT CARE OF PATIENTS IN THE CCU

The preventive regimen started at the time of admission is continued throughout the patient's stay in the CCU. The main objective of nursing care during this period is to *anticipate* problems. Included in this anticipatory care are the following measures.

Cardiac Monitoring

Constant vigilance is essential if warning arrhythmias are to be detected and lethal arrhythmias prevented. This does not imply that it is necessary to watch the monitor incessantly, but it does mean that the nurse must always be aware of the heart rate and rhythm. So that sudden changes in the heart rate can be recognized instantly, the alarm system of the monitor should be utilized to its fullest advantage (as explained in Chapter 8). Although death-producing arrhythmias are most likely to develop within the early hours after myocardial infarction, it can never be assumed that the risk period has in fact passed, even though the cardiac rhythm appears stable.

Clinical Evaluation

The use of monitors and elaborate equipment is meant to complement direct nursing care, not replace it. Careful evaluation of the patient's clinical condition at regular intervals is mandatory. Basically the assessment consists of eliciting symptoms, measuring vital signs, and examining the patient for signs of heart failure. As a general rule the evaluation is conducted every 2 hours during the first 8 hours after admission (or until the patient's condition is stable), and then every 4 hours thereafter.

Chest Pain

As part of the assessment process the nurse should specifically inquire about the recurrence of chest pain. Also, the patient should be instructed to notify the nurse promptly whenever chest pain develops. Depending on the intensity and duration of the pain (along with clinical findings) the nurse must decide whether to administer nitroglycerin or an analgesic. One helpful method of judging the severity of chest pain is to ask the patient to rank the discomfort on a scale of 1 to 10. This ranking provides some guide for comparison of the intensity of pain episodes.

Preparation for Emergencies

Despite every effort at prevention, unexpected catastrophes can and do occur in patients with acute myocardial infarction. In these circumstances survival hinges on split-second decisions and actions. Not only must the nursing staff itself be prepared for these emergencies, but it is absolutely essential that all resuscitative equipment and supplies are always ready for instant use. Machines—particularly defibrillators—should be tested regularly to verify that they are functioning properly.

Intake and Output

Maintaining fluid balance is highly important in the care of coronary patients. Over-hydration or underhydration pose serious threats to circulatory efficiency, particularly in the presence of left ventricular failure or cardiogenic shock. Moreover, the effectiveness of diuretic therapy is determined primarily by the urinary output volume. In order to assess fluid balance wholly accurate records of fluid intake and output must be maintained at all times. This essential nursing duty should not be minimized by delegating it to untrained personnel.

Bed Rest

One of the mainstays of the treatment program for acute myocardial infarction is to reduce the workload of the heart until the injured myocardium has healed. Bed rest is the least stressful activity for the heart, and for this reason patients are confined to bed during the CCU period. While at bed rest the patient should be positioned in a way that assures his comfort. Usually a semi-Fowler's position is the most comfortable; it also allows for full lung expansion by lowering the diaphragm. If the patient's condition is stable, arm chair rest may be permitted after the third or fourth day. (The energy expenditure involved in sitting is only slightly greater than with bed rest.)

Activity

Although limitation of physical activity is important, complete restriction of all activity is seldom necessary. Certainly the patient should not be led to believe that he must be rigidly in bed for fear that any movement may overburden his heart. Immobility not only causes weakness and loss of muscle tone, but it is also a source of emotional depression. Unless the patient's clinical state dictates otherwise, the following activities are usually permissible, particularly after the first few days: washing hands and face, brushing teeth, combing hair, self-feeding, and passive motion of the lower extremities. On the other hand, activities that demand sustained muscle tension (e.g., straining at stool) must be avoided since isometric muscle contraction substantially increases cardiac work. The heart rate and ECG should be monitored during and after physical activity to determine if the exercise produces any deleterious effects. Also, if the patient describes angina or dyspnea with exertion, the degree of activity must be curtailed.

Maintaining a Serene Atmosphere

Physical and emotional rest can be achieved only in a setting conducive to these needs. Ideally the CCU is the quietest place in the hospital. The nursing staff must make every effort to maintain a calm, serene atmosphere by providing care in an efficient, unhurried manner and, second, by controlling noise, avoiding commotion, and reducing traffic in the unit. Scheduling visiting hours to meet the needs of the patient and his family and limiting the number of visitors in a room to one or two at a time are helpful measures. In addition, it is worthwhile as part of the nursing plan to include deliberate rest periods for the patient in which he can relax without interruption. During these periods the room should be darkened to minimize distractions.

Elimination

Patients should be allowed to use a bedside commode (or pullman toilet) for urination and defecation. Indeed the physical effort involved in using these facilities is much less than that expended with a bedpan. Male patients may stand at the bedside to void. Bedpans are required only if patients are desperately ill and cannot get out of bed. Stool-softening drugs and mild cathartics are useful in facilitating bowel movements and preventing straining. Enemas should be avoided because rectal stimulation may induce undesirable cardiovascular reflexes.

Diet

Because many patients experience nausea and vomiting during the first day (particularly if narcotics have been administered), a liquid diet is usually ordered initially. After the gastrointestinal symptoms have subsided and the patient's appetite has returned, the choice of diet depends to a large degree on the philosophy of the individual physician about the need for sodium (and cholesterol) restriction at this stage of the illness. Some physicians believe that all patients should receive a low-sodium diet for at least 4 or 5 days as a preventive measure; others restrict sodium intake only if there are signs of heart failure. Many patients find low-sodium diets unpalatable and therefore do not eat their meals. The nurse should assess the adequacy of the patient's nutrition and assist him in selecting foods he will enjoy. Low-sodium diets can be made tastier by using flavors such as lemon, thyme, vinegar, and sodium-free spices. Coffee, tea, and other caffeine-containing beverages are generally excluded from the diet during the CCU period. Also to be avoided is iced water (or any iced drink); it is believed that the chilling effect of these drinks may affect the cardiac rate and rhythm through reflex mechanisms.

Prevention of Thromboembolism

Venous stasis predisposes to clot formation in the lower extremities, and therefore measures designed to prevent pooling of venous blood in the legs are important, particularly in elderly patients and those with heart failure in whom the risk of thrombosis is greatest. Antiembolic stockings are helpful in this respect and should be used in all high-risk patients. Also, patients must be instructed not to cross their legs at the calves because external pressure in this area may compress venous channels and promote stasis of blood. Another useful nursing measure is to place a foot board at the end of the bed against which the patient can extend his feet; this exercise promotes the return of venous blood. (Further details of the nursing role in preventing thromboembolism are described in Chapter 7.)

Passive Exercises

Muscles weaken rapidly during bed rest, and an effort must be made to combat this deconditioning. Active exercise is undesirable because of the work imposed on the heart, but passive exercise can be tolerated without difficulty. Several times a day the nurse should move the patient's extremities through their full range of motion.

Medications

The nurse must carefully observe the clinical response to all medications administered. Has the drug achieved its desired effect? Are there any side effects? These observations strongly influence subsequent decisions about treatment, and therefore repeated assessment is essential. (The actions and side effects of cardiac drugs are described in Chapter 18.)

TRANSFER FROM CCU

In the absence of serious complications patients are transferred from the CCU to regular hospital quarters usually after the fourth or fifth day. Leaving the protective setting of a CCU is often a disquieting experience for the patient. The source of this apprehension is readily understandable: no longer will the patient be under constant surveillance and protected from sudden death. Furthermore the abrupt interruption of the close relationships between the patient and the CCU team may lead to a sense of loss and abandonment. There are several ways to help the patient adjust to this transition.

1. A day or two before transfer the nurse should advise the patient his condition has improved to a point that intensive care will no longer be needed. Being moved from the unit is an indication that the clinical course has been satisfactory and that the acute phase of the illness has passed. Repeated reassurance along these lines is often necessary to convince the patient of the safety and desirability of the change.

2. It is also wise to tell the patient that apprehension on his part about being transferred is a normal reaction, one that most patients experience. Allowing the patient to express his feelings and to ask questions is a very helpful approach.

3. Introducing the patient to the head nurse of the floor to which he is being transferred is a valuable method of demonstrating continuity of care. The introduction should be made while the patient is still in the CCU, not on arrival in the new ward.

4. After transfer is accomplished, a nurse from the CCU should visit the patient in his new quarters. The psychological effects of transfer often do not become apparent until after the patient is situated in his new surroundings, and therefore seeing a familiar face offers a sense of security.

5. To avoid the problems associated with the sudden termination of coronary care, some hospitals utilize intermediate (step-down) units, to bridge the gap between intensive and regular nursing care. These units serve as halfway houses; a patient is kept under surveillance but not with the same intenseness as the CCU. As an alternative, cardiac monitoring can be continued after transfer from the CCU by means of telemetry. This permits the patient to be assigned to an ordinary hospital room and to be ambulatory while still being monitored in the coronary unit.

6. A concerted effort should be made to maintain continuity of patient teaching plans after transfer from the unit. In some institutions CCU nurses make follow-up visits for this purpose; in others, staff nurses assume this responsibility. In either case it is important to establish a check list for nurses to note which subjects they have discussed with the patient.

EMOTIONAL SUPPORT OF THE PATIENT

An extraordinarily important part of coronary care nursing is to help the patient manage (and cope with) the profound emotional stress that accompanies acute myocardial infarction. This intervention is essential not only for compassionate reasons (inherent in all nursing care), but also because emotional stress can adversely affect the clinical course and eventual outcome of the illness. For example, severe anxiety during the early days after acute myocardial infarction is a serious threat since it results in a rapid heart rate, a rise in blood pressure, and an increase in the oxygen demands of the myocardium. These emotionally induced cardiac effects (mediated through the sympathetic nervous system) may lead to life-threatening complications including heart failure, pulmonary edema, lethal arrhythmias, and extension of the size of the original infarction (as explained in Chapter 7). Furthermore it has been reported that the patient's emotional adjustment during the coronary care period significantly influences rehabilitation and long-term survival. Some studies indicate that patients who adjust poorly while in the coronary unit are less likely to return to work and more prone to develop another myocardial infarction than those who make good adjustments during the early stages of hospitalization. In light of these facts it is understandable that the management of emotional problems is a major nursing responsibility in a coronary care unit. Although professional nurses are well prepared to identify and resolve emotional reactions to illness (indeed very few health disciplines emphasize these principles as strongly), the psychological effects of acute myocardial infarction are unique in many ways and demand special attention. Before describing the basic elements of the nursing role, it is pertinent to mention some of the factors that contribute to the severe stress the patient with acute myocardial infarction encounters initially, and to consider the most common emotional responses observed in the coronary care unit.

Sources of Emotional Stress

Experiencing a myocardial infarction is a terrifying feeling from the very onset. The realization that death may be imminent, the unrelenting chest pain, the dependence on others to provide help, the rush to a hospital (usually by ambulance), and the looks of anguish on the faces of relatives or friends are just a few of the many fears that immediately confront the patient; but this is only the beginning of his ordeal. As soon as the patient reaches the coronary care unit (or while still in the emergency ward) he encounters other unexpected threats and his burden of fear mounts. Monitoring electrodes are attached to his chest, an intravenous infusion is started, oxygen is administered, injections are given, blood samples are drawn, and unfamiliar nurses, physicians, and technicians hurriedly enter and leave his room. The thought, "Am I dying," runs through the patient's mind. The coronary unit itself contributes to his terror: the room is small; strange machines encircle him; he sees bottles, syringes, tubes, and needles; he hears the sounds of the equipment and the voices of the staff. Thus from the moment of the attack the patient is subjected to an enormous *sensory overload*, both internal and external, over which he has no control.

Adding to the already formidable problem is the fact that the patient is inadequately prepared, if at all, for this sudden sensory overload. Unlike many illnesses in which the patient can anticipate some of the fears and frights he will experience, acute myocardial infarction occurs suddenly and unexpectedly, and therefore precludes adequate preparation. Because of this lack of preparation, the patient's fears are intensified greatly.

Another factor that contributes to the profound psychological stress of acute myocardial infarction is that the patient does not have the opportunity, at least at first, to mobilize his emotional resources and attempt to resolve ("work through" as psychiatrists say) the stressful situation. He is preoccupied with more crucial thoughts, particularly survival, and consequently other problems are of much less importance.

The combination of marked sensory overload, inadequate preparation for this stress, and inadequate opportunity to mobilize emotional resources to reduce the stress represent the three characteristic features of an overwhelming emotional experience. It is readily understandable that patients with acute myocardial infarction face great difficulty in maintaining emotional equilibrium, particularly during the acute phase of the illness.

Emotional Responses To Acute Myocardial Infarction

The severe stress associated with acute myocardial infarction provokes a wide variety of emotional responses. Fundamentally, patients attempt to cope with the stress by relying on defense mechanisms that have served them in the past with other crises. Because each person responds according to his own psychological makeup, the behavioral pattern among patients in a coronary care unit is by no means constant. Nevertheless there are certain predictable emotional responses, the most common of which are described below.

Anxiety

The emotional response observed most often during the coronary care period is anxiety (which for practical purposes is synonymous with fear). The degree of anxiety is influenced by many psychosocial factors and varies considerably among patients. Psychological studies suggest that the main source of anxiety is the prospect of sudden death. Consequently, signs of anxiety are most likely to be noted during the early days of hospitalization, when recurrent symptoms develop (e.g., chest pain or shortness of breath), or when special procedures are required (e.g., insertion of a temporary pacemaker or cardioversion). Curiously, perhaps there is no definite relationship between anxiety and the seriousness of the illness. It appears that anxiety depends more on how the patient perceives the threat to his life rather than on the severity of infarction itself.

Anxiety is often difficult to identify in patients with acute myocardial infarction because many of them attempt to hide or deny the fact that they are anxious (as explained below). Objective evidence of anxiety is probably a more reliable clue to the problem. Patients who are anxious usually appear tense, apprehensive, fidgety, restless, and seem unable to relax. Sweating is frequently apparent on the palms of the hands and the axillae. Particularly important from a nursing standpoint is that patients with anxiety repeatedly seek reassurance in one way or other. For example, they may ask the nurse time and again about coronary disease, monitoring, laboratory tests, and methods of treatment—all in an effort to be reassured. What may appear to be intellectual curiosity is usually a sign of anxiety.

Denial

Many patients attempt to cope with emotional stress by means of denial. There are two principal forms of denial: denial of fact and denial of meaning. Denial of fact means that the patient does not acknowledge that he has actually had a heart attack. He attempts to pass off or minimize the event by saying, for example, "I am sure it's not a heart attack, nobody in my family had heart disease," or "we are going on vacation next week." Denial of meaning, probably the more common mechanism, is defined as a conscious or subconscious effort to deny the emotional feelings (e.g., anxiety or depression) associated with acute myocardial infarction and hospitalization. The patient does not admit his fears and, in fact, often displays an optimistic attitude. Both forms of denial are a reaction against reality posed by the illness.

Denial usually can be recognized by statements the patient makes in conjunction with the way he acts. For instance, the patient may tell the nurse that he feels well and is not upset, yet it is evident that he is sweating and has a look of fear in his eyes. Threatening to sign out of the hospital against advice is a manifestation of severe denial.

Depression

It is understandable that patients generally become despondent when they begin to consider the implications of a heart attack. They realize that their activities, earning capacity, and way of life may be affected drastically. This is a normal response and is of concern only when the depression is prolonged or severe.

Patients often deny depression just as they do anxiety; therefore the problem may not be readily apparent. However, moderate or severe depression has characteristic signs: disinterest in the surroundings, a sad look, slow speech, listless behavior, loss of appetite, insomnia, and crying.

Anger

Patients who have hostile personality traits may react to emotional stress by displaying anger. The anger may be self-directed or aimed at the family or CCU staff. Self-anger is expressed in questions such as "Why me?" or "Why did this happen now?" Anger directed at the staff is usually manifested by repeated complaints about the quality of care or the manner of treatment. In effect, nothing pleases the patient and he is hostile or angry about everything.

Nursing Intervention

Explanation and Clarification

One of the most useful methods of helping the patient adjust to the emotional stress of acute myocardial infarction is to explain his illness to him. The main object is to dispel common misconceptions about heart disease and its consequences. The patient's concept of a heart attack is usually grossly distorted and therefore many of his fears are unrealistic and unwarranted. For example, patients commonly believe that even if they recover from a heart attack they will have to take medication for the rest of their lives or that sexual activity is no longer permissible. To combat these fears the nurse should offer repeated explanations about various aspects of myocardial infarction, always attempting to identify and clarify any misconceptions the patient may have. It is important to answer the patient's questions in a forthright manner. By avoiding a question or simply saying, "You will have to ask the doctor," the nurse can indirectly intensify the patient's anxiety (as well as block any further discussion).

Fostering Optimism

As noted, patients with acute myocardial infarction frequently deny their emotional feelings as a means of coping with stress. In many cases it may be beneficial to allow the patient to continue to use this defense mechanism, at least up to a certain point. Certainly this is not to say that the CCU team should ever let the patient believe that he has not in fact suffered a heart attack, or lie to him about the seriousness of his condition, but it does imply that allowing the patient to maintain an optimistic outlook by means of denial may be advantageous. In fact some studies have shown that patients who can effectively deny anxiety or depression during the acute phase of the illness have a better chance for survival than nondeniers. From a practical standpoint this suggests that it may be helpful to foster the patient's optimism by treating him with the conviction that recovery is fully anticipated. In other words, the CCU team should emphasize survival and recovery rather than risks and dangers. (It is important to point out that this concept applies to the management of acute myocardial infarction, but not necessarily to all other illnesses.)

Reassurance

The nurse can provide reassurance in two ways: by her own demeanor and by talking to the patient in the most encouraging fashion possible. Patients become more confident when the nurse acts in a calm, positive, efficient manner. If the nurse appears tense and anxious (a normal reaction in many instances) the patient's anxiety level is bound to increase. It is very reassuring for the patient to learn of any evidence of progress toward his recovery. For example, if it is apparent that the patient is able to tolerate increased activity without difficulty, the nurse should deliberately comment on this fact, and indicate that it represents a good sign. Broad promises such as, "Don't worry, everything will be all right," serve little purpose and should be avoided. It is also important for the nurse to offer the patient a hopeful outlook for the future, and make him aware that most patients can lead a useful, productive life despite a myocardial infarction. It is helpful to emphasize that normal activities after recovery from a heart attack are beneficial rather than dangerous.

Listening

By listening attentively and demonstrating genuine interest the nurse can assist the patient to ventilate his feelings. Expression of emotions is often an effective form of therapy since in describing his fears the patient may recognize the sources of the problem, and be able to deal with them. However, the nurse should not prod the patient to discuss his emotions since many times, particularly during the first few days, the patient is not able to sort out his feelings.

Manipulating the Environment

Maintaining a peaceful atmosphere in the CCU helps the patient to relax and regain his emotional equilibrium. The nurse should establish deliberate rest periods for the patient during which time he is not disturbed by visitors or the staff. Radio, television, and newspapers can prevent a feeling of isolation. Allowing the patient to sit in a bedside chair (if his condition permits) is usually a source of encouragement.

Anticipating Emotional Reactions

It is very helpful for patients to understand that many of the emotions they experience are normal, anticipated responses. The nurse can assist the patient by letting him know that being depressed, for example, is a common reaction during the coronary care period. The intensity of emotional reactions can often be reduced if they are anticipated.

Drug Therapy

As a general rule it is useful to administer tranquilizers during the first few days of hospitalization. However, the dosage should be adjusted so that the patient is not constantly drowsy or sleepy. Antidepressant drugs should not be used in patients with acute myocardial infarction because they may produce adverse cardiac effects.

7

The Major Complications of Acute Myocardial Infarction and the Related Nursing Role

There are five death-producing complications of acute myocardial infarction: heart failure, cardiogenic shock, thromboembolism, ventricular rupture, and cardiac arrhythmias.

As explained in previous chapters, the concept of intensive coronary care is based on the prevention or successful treatment of these complications; it is only in this way that lives can be saved. To accomplish this objective it is essential to understand the etiology, clinical manifestations, and principles of treatment of each complication.

HEART FAILURE

Acute myocardial infarction affects the pumping action of the heart in nearly all instances; however, the degree of impairment varies greatly. When the injured myocardium is unable to pump an adequate amount of blood to meet the metabolic needs of the body the condition is called *heart failure*. Approximately 60% of patients with acute myocardial infarction develop clinical signs of heart failure during the acute phase of the illness. The mortality rate in these patients is substantially higher than in those without heart failure. Indeed with the present ability to prevent arrhythmic deaths, advanced heart failure and cardiogenic shock (collectively called pump failure) have become the major cause of death among patients treated in coronary care units (CCUs).

Left Heart Failure

The heart consists of two separate but related pumping systems: the right heart, the pump for the pulmonary circulation, and the left heart, the pump for the systemic circulation. The relation of these two systems is shown in Figure 7.1.

Heart failure may involve the left heart, the right heart, or both sides of the heart. Because myocardial infarction affects the left ventricle almost exclusively, *left heart failure* is by far the more common form of failure in this situation. Right heart failure is nearly always secondary to left ventricular failure in patients with myocardial infarction; it rarely develops independently.

CIRCULATION THROUGH LEFT AND RIGHT HEART
Schematic Diagram

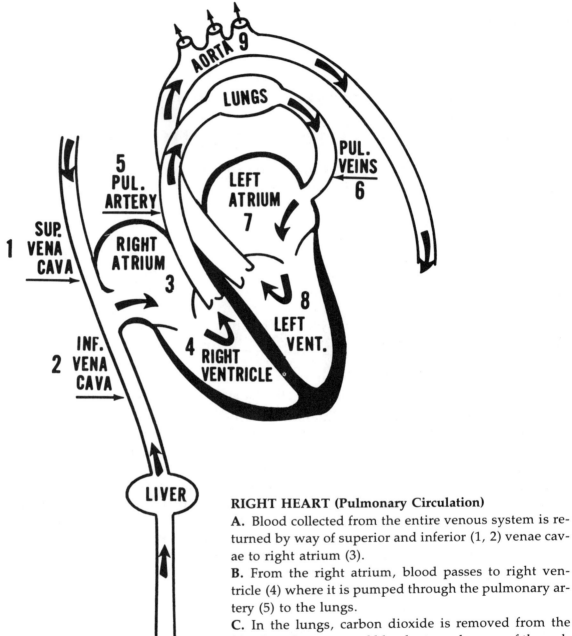

RIGHT HEART (Pulmonary Circulation)
A. Blood collected from the entire venous system is returned by way of superior and inferior (1, 2) venae cavae to right atrium (3).
B. From the right atrium, blood passes to right ventricle (4) where it is pumped through the pulmonary artery (5) to the lungs.
C. In the lungs, carbon dioxide is removed from the blood, and oxygenated blood returns by way of the pulmonary veins (6) to the left heart.
LEFT HEART (Systemic Circulation)
A. Oxygenated blood from the pulmonary veins enters the left atrium (7) and passes to the left ventricle (8).
B. Contraction of the left ventricle propels the blood through the aorta (9) and to the systemic circulation.

Figure 7.1.

The primary cause of left heart failure after acute myocardial infarction is damage to the muscles of the left ventricle. The infarcted area and the surrounding zones of injury and ischemia do not contract normally, and as a result the pumping ability of the left ventricle is reduced.

This reduction in pumping performance is manifested by a decrease in the stroke volume and the cardiac output. *Stroke volume* is the amount of blood ejected from the ventricle with each contraction. *Cardiac output* represents the total amount of blood pumped from the ventricle per minute. The relation between stroke volume and cardiac output is expressed as follows:

$$\text{Cardiac output} = \text{stroke volume} \times \text{heart rate*}$$

The decrease in cardiac output may be modest or profound (depending for the most part on the size of the infarction); the degree of this hemodynamic deficit is an important factor in determining the severity of left ventricular failure.

Because of the reduction in pumping performance the left ventricle is no longer able to eject (empty) the full volume of blood it receives from the pulmonary circulation (right heart). Consequently an excess amount of blood remains in the left ventricle after each contraction (systole). This residual volume increases since the uninjured right ventricle continues to pump its normal quota of blood into the pulmonary circulation, but the incompletely emptied left ventricle cannot readily accept the volume delivered to it. Therefore the pressure rises in the left ventricle during diastole (the interval between contractions in which the ventricles fill with blood). This elevation in *ventricular diastolic pressure* impedes the subsequent flow of blood from the pulmonary circulation into the left heart, causing the pressure to increase in the left atrium and, in turn, the pulmonary veins and pulmonary capillaries. In effect, a backward pressure develops throughout the pulmonary venous system. The engorged (congested) veins and capillaries impose on the available air space within the lungs and also reduce the lungs' distensibility. More significantly, the increased pulmonary venous pressure forces fluid through the walls of the pulmonary capillaries into the lung tissues. This exudation of fluid into the lungs produces the clinical state known as *left ventricular failure*.

At first, the fluid collects in the interstitial tissues which surround the air cells (alveoli) of the lungs; this is called *interstitial edema*. This early manifestation of left ventricular failure does not produce symptoms nor can it be detected by physical examination of the chest. Therefore the condition is designated incipient or *subclinical left ventricular failure*. However, the presence of interstitial edema can be identified by a chest x ray, as shown in Figure 7.2. (This is one of the reasons that x-ray examination of the chest is a standard procedure in CCUs.) As left ventricular failure progresses, edema fluid is forced into the alveoli themselves; this collection of fluid within the air spaces is called *alveolar edema*. It produces distinct signs and symptoms which characterize the serious complication known as *overt left ventricular failure*. The chain of events leading to overt left ventricular failure are summarized in Figure 7.3.

Before describing the clinical manifestations of left ventricular failure, it is important to point out that the cardiovascular system utilizes several compensatory mechanisms in an attempt to maintain an effective circulation and to avert heart failure. These compensatory mechanisms produce many of the clinical findings of left ventricular failure. For example, as soon as the cardiac output begins to fall, the sympathetic nervous system is stimulated (by reflex means). This stimulation results in an increase in the heart rate and in the strength of myocardial contraction, which help to preserve an

---

*If, for example, the stroke volume is 60 cc and the heart rate is 70/minute, the cardiac output is 4200 cc. Normally, the cardiac output at rest is about 4000–6000 cc. The normal stroke volume is 70–80 cc.

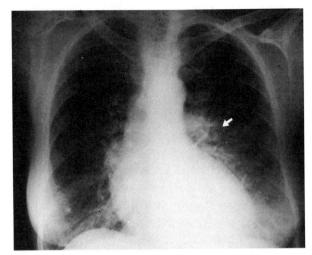

Figure 7.2. X-Ray film of chest demonstrating inter-stitial edema (arrow).

adequate cardiac output, at least temporarily. (For instance, if the stroke volume falls to 40 cc but the heart rate increases to 120 per minute, the cardiac output is still maintained at 4800 cc despite the reduction in pumping performance.) Thus a rapid heart rate (tachycardia) is a characteristic feature of early heart failure. In addition to these sympathetic nervous system effects, the heart itself attempts to compensate for its decreased pumping ability. This is accomplished as follows: When the residual volume and pressure in the left ventricle increase during diastole, the ventricle dilates and its muscle fibers stretch (lengthen). This stretching has a beneficial effect because the strength of ventricular contraction depends on the length of the myocardial fibers just before they contract (in much the same way as a rubber band contracts more forcefully when it is stretched fully). These (and other) compensatory mechanisms are effective up to a certain limit, but finally they cannot counteract the failing heart and, in fact, become self-defeating. At this stage (called decompensation) signs and symptoms of overt failure develop.

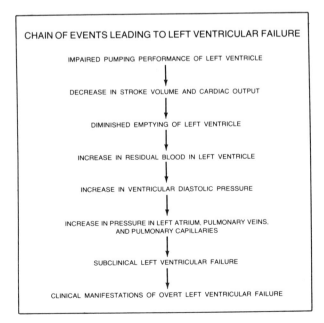

Figure 7.3.

Clinical Manifestations of Left Ventricular Failure

Symptoms

Dyspnea.   Shortness of breath (dyspnea) is the earliest and most common symptom of left ventricular failure. It results primarily from congestion of the pulmonary venous network which, as explained, reduces the elasticity (distensibility) of the lungs and diminishes the available air space. The problem is intensified when alveolar edema develops because the edema fluid interferes with the exchange of oxygen and carbon dioxide in the alveoli, causing a reduction in the oxygen saturation of the blood. At first, dyspnea occurs only on exertion and therefore may not be apparent except during physical activity (e.g., when the patient gets out of bed or washes himself). As heart failure worsens, dyspnea occurs even at complete rest. Mild dyspnea may be difficult for the observer to detect (since it is a subjective symptom), and for this reason the nurse should ask the patient specifically if he feels short of breath, particularly during activity.

Orthopnea.   If dyspnea occurs when the patient is in the recumbent position and is relieved by sitting up, the condition is called *orthopnea*. This more advanced form of dyspnea can be suspected when the patient requests extra pillows or asks that the head of his bed be raised. With severe orthopnea the patient may prefer to be propped straight up in bed or to sit in a chair. These positions relieve orthopnea by diminishing pulmonary congestion and improving the ventilatory capacity of the lungs.

Paroxysmal Nocturnal Dyspnea.   For reasons that are not wholly clear, marked shortness of breath sometimes develops abruptly while the patient is asleep; hence the condition is called *paroxysmal nocturnal dyspnea*. These episodes of sudden dyspnea represent decompensation of the left ventricle following an acute increase in pulmonary venous congestion. The usual clinical story of paroxysmal nocturnal dyspnea is that about an hour or two after falling asleep the patient awakens *suddenly* with marked dyspnea and respiratory distress. He complains of suffocation, and great anxiety is usually evident. Paroxysms of coughing associated with loud wheezing accompany the dyspnea. (Because of the wheezing character of respiration, which resembles an asthmatic attack, the term *cardiac asthma* is sometimes used to describe the episode.) Breathing is improved in the sitting position, and most patients assume this posture immediately or leave the bed and attempt to reach a nearby window, believing that fresh air will help their breathing. The attack may subside after a few minutes in a sitting position or the episode may worsen progressively, with dyspnea, coughing, and wheezing becoming more intense. Although paroxysmal dyspnea develops in most instances with dramatic suddenness, it is quite likely that subclinical left ventricular failure existed previously and progressed insidiously.

Acute Pulmonary Edema.   The most advanced stage of acute left heart failure is *pulmonary edema*. This condition develops because of a massive accumulation of fluid in the alveolar and interstitial tissues of the lungs. The fluid interferes with oxygenation of the blood and results in *hypoxia* (a decrease in the oxygen content of the blood). Unless hypoxia is corrected the vital organs become deprived of oxygen, and finally irreversible arrhythmias develop and death occurs.

The clinical picture of acute pulmonary edema is distinctive and seldom poses a problem in diagnosis. The characteristic features are severe dyspnea, orthopnea, incessant cough (producing frothy, blood-tinged sputum), and extreme anxiety. Cyanosis may be present, and gurgling sounds are audible from the respiratory tree. In conjunction with these obvious signs of respiratory difficulty, a rapid pulse rate and profuse sweating are noted. (The latter findings are due to a marked increase in sympathetic nervous system activity.) The total picture leaves no doubt that the patient is in acute distress and that emergency treatment is essential.

Physical Signs

Rales.   The cardinal physical sign of overt left ventricular failure is the presence of rales. These abnormal breath sounds are produced by fluid in the alveoli and can be detected by auscultation of the chest. At first, rales are confined to the bases of the lungs (basilar rales), but as left ventricular failure progresses the rales extend higher and higher in the lung fields. Thus the height of the rales in the lungs is an index of the extent of heart failure. Coarse, bubbling rales may be heard throughout the entire chest with acute pulmonary edema.

Gallop Rhythm.   The second classic sign of left ventricular failure is a gallop rhythm which is identified by stethoscopic examination of the heart. Normally the heart has two distinct sounds described simply as the first and second heart sounds (or as S_1 and S_2). When the left heart fails and the ventricle dilates (in order to accommodate the increased diastolic volume) a third heart sound usually appears. Because the cadence of the three sounds resembles the sound of a galloping horse, the rhythm is descriptively termed a *gallop rhythm*. This extra heart sound (called S_3) occurs just after the second heart sound, as illustrated in Figure 7.4. It is heard best with the bell of the stethoscope placed over the apex of the heart. The presence of this type of gallop rhythm (known as a ventricular gallop) indicates dilation of the left ventricle and is a distinct sign of left ventricular failure even if rales cannot be heard.

There is a second type of gallop rhythm known as an atrial gallop. It differs from a ventricular gallop in that the extra heart sound is heard just before the first heart sound instead of after the second sound. In this circumstance the extra sound is called a fourth heart sound to distinguish it from the S_3 of a ventricular gallop. An atrial gallop (also described as an S_4 gallop) is a less serious finding than a ventricular gallop (an S_3 gallop) and may sometimes occur even in the absence of left ventricular failure. It is believed that an atrial gallop is caused by resistance to ventricular filling during diastole.

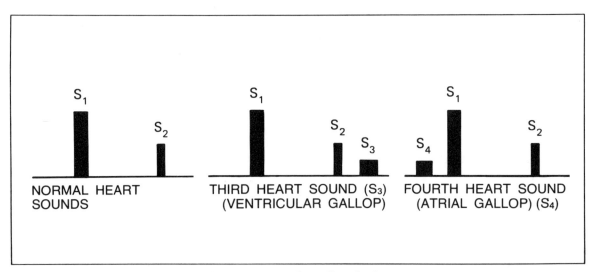

Figure 7.4. Normal heart sounds and components of a gallop rhythm.

Nonspecific Signs.   Although rales and a ventricular gallop rhythm are the only two definite diagnostic signs of left ventricular failure, other physical findings usually develop when the heart fails. For example, tachycardia, sweating, a reduction in blood pressure, and restlessness are often observed during acute left ventricular failure. The latter signs are not specific indications of left ventricular failure, but they do contribute to the overall clinical picture. Moreover, these nonspecific findings may be the earliest manifestation of left ventricular failure and therefore are important diagnostic cues.

Treatment of Left Ventricular Failure

There are three fundamental objectives in the overall treatment program for left ventricular failure:

1. To improve the pumping performance of the left ventricle. This is accomplished primarily by the use of digitalis.
2. To reduce the volume of blood returning to the left ventricle in order to lower pulmonary venous pressure. Diuretic therapy is used for this purpose. With acute pulmonary edema morphine and other measures are also required.
3. To improve oxygen saturation so that adequate tissue oxygenation can be maintained. This is achieved by means of oxygen inhalation therapy.

The actual sequence of treatment and the methods used depend on the severity of left ventricular failure and the urgency of the clinical situation. The treatment of acute pulmonary edema is of greatest concern and is described below.

Treatment of Acute Pulmonary Edema

Morphine.   This narcotic is one of the most important drugs in the treatment program for acute pulmonary edema and should be administered immediately, preceding all other forms of therapy. Morphine has several beneficial effects in this circumstance: not only does it relieve the intense anxiety associated with acute pulmonary edema but, more significantly, it depresses the respiratory centers in the brain and reduces the number of respirations. As respiration slows, the volume of blood returning from the pulmonary circulation to the left ventricle is decreased. In addition, morphine reduces venous tone, which causes pooling of blood in the peripheral veins and thereby diminishes venous return to the heart. Morphine is usually administered intramuscularly in doses of 10–15 mg. In urgent situations the drug can be given intravenously.

Oxygen Therapy.   During the period of respiratory embarrassment the concentration (saturation) of oxygen in arterial blood is usually markedly reduced. Therefore it is essential to administer oxygen in order to preserve tissue function. The highest oxygen concentration is provided by the use of an intermittent positive-pressure apparatus which delivers 100% oxygen through a well-fitted face mask (with a nonrebreathing bag). Nasal catheters or cannulas deliver only 30–40% oxygen concentrations and therefore are the least desirable means of supplying oxygen in this critical situation. Oxygen should always be humidified prior to inhalation to prevent drying of the airway. Humidification can be accomplished by bubbling oxygen through water. A 30% solution of ethyl alcohol may be used instead of water; it has the added advantage of also reducing pulmonary secretions by its antifoaming action.

Diuretics.   Rapid-acting diuretics, such as furosemide (Lasix) or ethacrynic acid (Edecrin), administered intravenously usually produce dramatic clinical improvement; dyspnea abates within minutes, after which there is a copious diuresis. Theoretically these agents are effective because they promote excretion of fluid, thereby reducing the volume of blood returning to the heart. However, the extraordinary rapidity with which these drugs act in controlling pulmonary edema (even before diuresis occurs) suggests that other pharmacologic actions are also involved. It is believed that these agents have a direct effect on the venous system, causing the veins to dilate and hold a greater volume of blood. Furosemide (Lasix) is administered intravenously in doses of 40–80 mg. The usual intravenous dose of ethacrynic acid (Edecrin) is 50 mg. (Diuretic therapy is described in greater detail in the discussion of right heart failure.)

Digitalis.   Digitalis is extremely valuable in the treatment of acute left ventricular failure. Unlike morphine and diuretics, which exert their effect by reducing venous return, digitalis acts directly on the heart and increases the strength of myocardial contractility. The importance of improved myocardial contractility is readily apparent: the stroke volume and cardiac output increase while the residual volume of blood in the ventricle decreases. Thus digitalis helps to counteract the basic hemodynamic problems that produced left ventricular failure. Because of the urgency of the situation, rapid-acting digitalis preparations are administered intravenously in treating acute pulmonary edema. (With less severe forms of left ventricular failure digitalis usually is given orally.) The three most rapidly acting digitalis preparations are ouabain, lanatoside C, and digoxin; of these, digoxin is the most commonly used. The dosage schedule of the three drugs is shown in Figure 7.5. These preparations are administered intravenously at regular intervals (e.g., every 2–4 hours) until clinical improvement occurs or the maximum dose is reached. After this point daily maintenance doses are given orally. (The side effects and other important features of digitalis therapy are described in Chapter 18.)

RAPID-ACTING DIGITALIS PREPARATIONS

	INITIAL DOSE	AVERAGE ONSET OF ACTION	SUBSEQUENT DOSES
DIGOXIN	0.5 MG (IV)	15 MINUTES	0.25 MG EVERY 2–4 HOURS UNTIL A TOTAL DOSE NO GREATER THAN 1.5 MG IS REACHED
LANATOSIDE C (CEDILANID)	0.8 MG (IV)	10 MINUTES	0.4 MG EVERY 2–4 HOURS UNTIL A TOTAL DOSE NO GREATER THAN 2.0 MG IS REACHED
OUABAIN	0.20 MG (IV)	5 MINUTES	0.1 MG EVERY HOUR UNTIL A TOTAL DOSE NO GREATER THAN 1.0 MG IS REACHED

Figure 7.5.

Bronchodilators.   Acute pulmonary edema is accompanied by spasm of the bronchial tree. This bronchospasm (which creates the loud wheezing sounds heard during the acute attack) interferes with ventilation. In an effort to relieve bronchospasm, bronchodilator drugs are frequently used (in conjunction with oxygen therapy). The most popular drug for this purpose is aminophylline, which is administered intravenously in a dosage of 250–500 mg. The drug is diluted to 50 cc and injected *slowly*, over a 15-minute period. The dose may be repeated every 3–4 hours if needed. In addition to dilating the bronchioles, aminophylline also increases cardiac output and lowers venous pressure. The main disadvantage of the drug is that it may cause hypotension and arrhythmias, particularly if it is injected too rapidly. To avoid these undesirable effects, aminophylline is often administered by rectal suppository (500 mg.)

Rotating Tourniquets.   In the event that the measures just described are not successful promptly in controlling acute pulmonary edema, rotating tourniquets may be employed. The application of tourniquets traps venous blood in the extremities and thereby reduces venous return to the heart. The tourniquets are applied to the extremities with a pressure sufficient to impede venous return but not great enough to interfere with arterial blood flow to the limbs (i.e., the distal pulses must always remain palpable). The pressure is released in one extremity every 15 minutes in a rotating fashion (to prevent tissue damage). When the acute episode has subsided the tourniquets are removed, one at a time, at intervals of 15 minutes. Releasing all the tourniquets simultaneously may cause a sudden increase in venous return and again overload the pulmonary circulation.

Phlebotomy.   The circulating blood volume can also be reduced by means of phlebotomy, during which 500 cc of blood is withdrawn into a vacuum-type bottle. This method is used only when all other means of treatment have failed, and is seldom required.

Right Heart Failure

In acute myocardial infarction the right heart fails as a sequel to left heart failure; isolated right heart failure, as mentioned previously, is extremely rare. The sequence of events leading to right heart failure is outlined in Figure 7.6. When the left heart fails, significant backward pressure develops in the pulmonary veins and capillaries, as already noted. Therefore blood being pumped from the *right* ventricle through the pulmonary arteries meets resistance in the pulmonary capillaries, causing the pressure to rise in the main pulmonary artery. As the pulmonary artery pressure mounts, emptying of the right ventricle is impaired. The residual volume of blood within the right ventricle impedes the flow of blood from the right atrium. As a consequence, blood returning to the right atrium from the superior and inferior vena cavae meets resistance. This creates a backward pressure throughout the entire peripheral venous system, leading to congestion of the venous network. The clinical picture that results from this overloading of the venous system is called *congestive heart failure*.

Although this etiologic concept, described as *backward* heart failure, is logical and explains many of the clinical findings of right heart failure, it is certain that the problem of the failing heart is infinitely more complicated. For instance, it is well known that congestive heart failure is accompanied by the retention of sodium and water, and that kidney function is also disturbed. The latter changes cannot be explained fully on the basis of increased backward pressure, and it is apparent that renal and hormonal factors also contribute to the total picture of right heart failure. It is believed that the reduction in cardiac output that accompanies left heart failure results in a decrease in renal blood flow; this insufficiency of renal blood flow stimulates the production of salt- and water-retaining hormones (e.g., aldosterone). This theory, called *forward* heart failure, implies that part of the problem of congestive failure develops independently of backward pressure. It is very likely that backward and forward heart failure coexist, and that the various clinical findings of right heart failure are a combination of both causes.

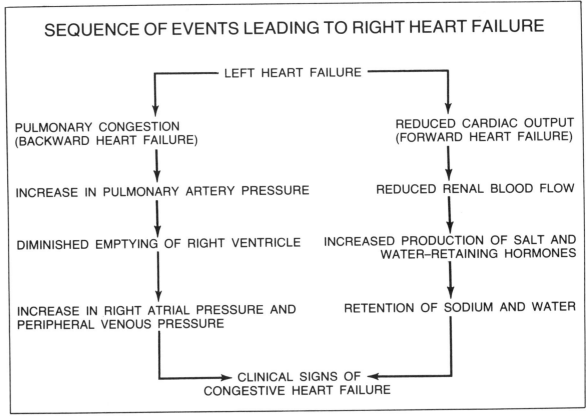

Figure 7.6.

Clinical Manifestations of Right Heart Failure

The signs and symptoms of right heart failure are related fundamentally to the retention of water and sodium within the body. The end result of this fluid entrapment is an overloading of the venous system which produces the following clinical findings.

Distended Neck Veins. Increased venous pressure in the superior vena cava causes distention of the veins in the neck. If the veins remain distended when the patient is placed in a semiupright (45-degree angle) position, it is very likely that right heart failure is present. (Neck veins may distend in the absence of heart failure, but in this circumstance the veins empty immediately when the patient's head is raised; therefore observation of the neck veins should always be made with the patient in a semiupright position.) Neck vein distention is one of the earliest signs of right heart failure and certainly the easiest to detect.

Peripheral Edema.   As the result of increased pressure in the venous system, fluid is forced from the capillaries into the subcutaneous tissues of the body. This fluid collection, called peripheral or subcutaneous edema, occurs primarily in the dependent areas of the body. In patients with acute myocardial infarction who are bedfast, the back (especially the sacral area) is dependent, and therefore edema is usually noted first in this area. (In patients who are ambulatory, the feet and legs are the usual sites of edema formation.) Rarely, peripheral edema is generalized and found throughout the entire body; this condition is called *anasarca*. The severity of peripheral edema is graded from 1+ to 4+. Mild edema (1+) is sometimes difficult to detect on physical examination; however, all forms of edema are accompanied by a gain in body weight. Therefore weighing the patient each day is a useful method of estimating the extent of edema fluid accumulation.

Pleural Effusion.   Edema fluid may also accumulate in the pleural cavity. This collection is described as a pleural effusion. It usually develops along with peripheral edema but can occur independently. Large pleural effusions compress the lungs and therefore may produce (or intensify) dyspnea. The presence of a pleural effusion can be suspected if diminished or absent breath sounds are noted while listening to the patient's lungs. The diagnosis is confirmed by x-ray examination of the chest (Fig. 7.7).

Enlarged and Tender Liver.   Backward pressure in the inferior vena cava and hepatic veins causes venous engorgement of the liver. As a result the liver enlarges, becomes tender, and can be palpated on physical examination. Hepatic enlargement may produce discomfort in the right upper quadrant of the abdomen and is often accompanied by loss of appetite and nausea. When the liver is engorged, pressure applied over the right upper quadrant of the abdomen causes the neck veins to distend. This phenomenon, known as the *hepatojugular reflux*, is a diagnostic sign of right heart failure. Abdominal compression increases the amount of blood returning to the heart, thus raising venous pressure and intensifying neck vein distention because the right heart is unable to handle the increased blood flow.

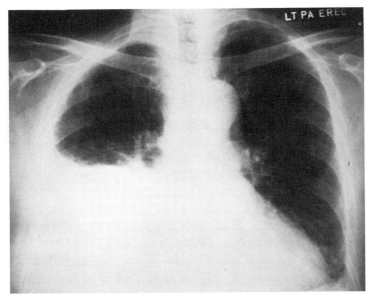

Figure 7.7. There is a very large pleural effusion noted on this chest x-ray film. In most instances pleural effusions are much less extensive than shown in this example.

Treatment of Right Heart Failure

Because right heart failure coexists with left heart failure (in patients with acute myocardial infarction) there is overlapping of the treatment programs. However, the two major objectives in the treatment of right (congestive) heart failure are to improve cardiac efficiency and to control sodium-water retention. The following measures are used to accomplish these aims.

1. Improvement in Cardiac Efficiency

a) **Reduction of Metabolic Needs of the Body.**   As noted previously, heart failure indicates that the cardiac output is insufficient to meet the needs of the body. Therefore it is highly desirable to reduce the body's needs, if possible, in order to assist the failing heart. Rest is one of the most effective ways to diminish the cardiac workload. Consequently, limitation of physical activity by bed rest or chair rest is a basic element in the treatment program. Total bed rest, however, is unnecessary, and patients can obtain adequate rest while sitting in a bedside chair. Also, patients should be permitted to use a bedside commode rather than a bedpan since the energy expenditure is less with a commode. Moreover, complete bed rest is undesirable because it tends to increase the risk of thromboembolism, as explained later in this chapter.

b) **Digitalis.**   Digitalis is the cornerstone of the treatment program for congestive heart failure. Because right heart failure is seldom an emergency problem digitalis preparations are usually administered orally rather than intravenously. In most instances digitalization is accomplished over a period of 24–48 hours; maintenance doses are continued thereafter. The most commonly used drugs are digoxin, digitoxin, and digitalis leaf. All digitalis preparations must be used cautiously because there is only a narrow zone between effective drug action and toxicity. Overdosage of digitalis (*digitalis toxicity*) may produce serious arrhythmias (as well as systemic symptoms, including anorexia, nausea, and vomiting).

2. Control of Sodium–Water Retention

a) **Restriction of Sodium Intake.**   Right heart failure is characterized by the retention of sodium and water. Although this disorder originates in the kidneys, restriction of sodium (salt) in the diet helps to alleviate the problem. When clinical signs of right heart failure develop, sodium intake is usually limited to 1000–2000 mg per day. (The normal daily diet contains 10,000 mg or more of sodium chloride.) Even when heart failure is not evident, many physicians prescribe low-sodium diets on a prophylactic basis for all patients with acute myocardial infarction.

b) **Diuretic Therapy.**   Diuretic agents are highly effective in promoting the urinary excretion of salt and water. In fact, edema and other signs of heart failure are so readily controlled in most instances with diuretics that these drugs are second in importance only to digitalis in the management of congestive heart failure. Despite their usefulness, diuretics are not meant to replace rest, diet, and digitalis in the treatment program; they should be used in conjunction with these other measures. There are several classes of diuretic agents with varying degrees of potency:

Thiazide diuretics. These drugs, which are moderately potent, act by blocking the reabsorption of sodium in the tubules of the kidneys.* By inhibiting the customary return of sodium to the body, thiazide diuretics allow large amounts of sodium and water to be excreted in the urine. These agents are administered orally and usually promote diuresis within 2 hours. The effectiveness of their action can be assessed by carefully measuring the urinary output and fluid input, along with recording the patient's body weight daily. The main problem encountered with the use of thiazide diuretics is *potassium depletion*. This occurs because thiazides also block the tubular reabsorption of potassium, and therefore excessive amounts of potassium are excreted in the urine. The loss of potassium resulting from this drug-induced mechanism is of particular concern in patients with acute myocardial infarction because low potassium levels (hypokalemia) can increase myocardial excitability and cause serious ventricular arrhythmias. Also, hypokalemia is dangerous in patients receiving digitalis since potassium depletion sensitizes the myocardium to digitalis and therefore predisposes to digitalis toxicity. Indeed, in the presence of hypokalemia even small doses of digitalis may produce digitalis toxicity. In addition to these adverse effects on the heart, hypokalemia also produces systemic signs and symptoms. With marked potassium depletion many patients develop lethargy, anorexia, mental confusion, and a decrease in urinary output. Hypokalemia can be determined by measuring serum potassium levels and, less dependably, by electrocardiographic (ECG) findings. If hypokalemia develops, replacement of potassium (either by intravenous infusion or orally, depending on clinical circumstances) is essential. (The use of potassium is considered in Chapter 18.)

Furosemide (Lasix) and ethacrynic acid (Edecrin). These agents are the most potent diuretics available. They exert their effect in the same way as the thiazides, by blocking tubular reabsorption of sodium. They can be administered intravenously or orally and produce a rapid and profound loss of sodium and water, far greater than that achieved by the use of thiazide diuretics. Because of their extreme potency, which may produce marked hypokalemia and excessive fluid loss, these drugs should be reserved for urgent clinical situations (e.g., acute pulmonary edema) or heart failure that is refractory to the thiazide diuretics. Potassium replacement therapy is nearly always required in patients treated with furosemide or ethacrynic acid.

Aldosterone antagonists. As mentioned, congestive heart failure is accompanied by an excessive production of *aldosterone*, a hormone that causes the body to retain salt. Spironolactone (Aldactone) is an aldosterone antagonist and therefore promotes the excretion of sodium. This drug is far less potent than the thiazide diuretics, and its onset of action is very slow (usually 2–5 days). Consequently this diuretic is used in nonurgent situations, particularly if other forms of therapy have failed. The main advantage of aldosterone antagonists is that they do not cause significant potassium loss, thus minimizing the risk of hypokalemia.

Triamterene (Dyrenium). This drug, also a weak diuretic, increases the excretion of sodium by acting on the renal tubular exchange mechanism. However, the urinary excretion of potassium is not affected by this agent, and therefore there is no danger of inducing hypokalemia. This potassium-sparing effect eliminates the need for supplemental potassium therapy.

---

*Fluid filtered through the glomeruli of the kidneys normally contains a large quantity of sodium; however, most of this sodium is reabsorbed by the tubules of the kidney and returned to the bloodstream (in order to maintain an adequate sodium level in the body). Only the amount of sodium not reabsorbed by the tubules is excreted in the urine.

Fluid Restriction. Usually it is not necessary to restrict fluid intake in patients with mild or moderate heart failure. However, with more advanced failure it is beneficial to limit water intake to 1000 cc daily. The reason for this restriction is that excessive water intake tends to dilute the amount of sodium in the body fluids and may produce a *low-salt syndrome* (hyponatremia). The latter condition is characterized by lethargy and weakness. It results most often from the combination of a restricted sodium diet, increased sodium loss during diuresis, and excessive water intake. The diagnosis of hyponatremia is established by measuring serum sodium levels.

Nursing Role in Heart Failure

There are two basic aspects of the nursing role in the management of patients with heart failure: 1) detection of the early signs of heart failure, and 2) participation in the treatment program.

Detection of Early Heart Failure

There is good reason to believe that the earlier acute heart failure is treated the better will be the result. Therefore recognition of the first signs and symptoms of heart failure assumes great importance in the total care of patients with acute myocardial infarction. Because the nurse is in constant attendance (unlike the physician) and has the opportunity of observing the patient's clinical course uninterruptedly, it is understandable that the detection of early heart failure has become an integral part of coronary care nursing. To this end the nurse is expected to assess the patient's status repeatedly and to advise the physician of significant findings. The evaluation should be based on planned observation, careful physical examination, and thoughtful interpretation of the clinical evidence. The nursing assessment includes the following observations, all of which may indicate early heart failure.

1. Respiration.   Observe the rate and character of respirations. A gradual increase in the number of respirations per minute is an important sign of heart failure. Is the patient short of breath? Is he more comfortable propped up in bed? It is important to ask the patient these questions since mild dyspnea and orthopnea cannot always be recognized by observation alone. Has the patient developed a cough? If so, the frequency of coughing and the type of sputum should be noted.

2. Pulse Rate.   Record the pulse rate regularly and compare with previous recordings. A pulse rate of greater than 100 per minute is cause for suspicion of left ventricular failure. (This possibility becomes more likely when other causes of tachycardia, e.g., temperature elevation or anxiety, are not present.) Because arrhythmias develop frequently during heart failure, careful observation of the rhythm of the heart on the cardiac monitor is necessary.

3. Sweating.   Observe the patient's skin for evidence of sweating. Very often sweating is a manifestation of increased sympathetic nervous system activity that accompanies acute heart failure.

4. Restlessness and Insomnia.   Determine the probable cause for restlessness, anxiety, or disturbed sleep patterns. In many instances these symptoms are the result of emotional distress; however, they may also represent subtle warnings of early left ventricular failure. The indiscriminate use of tranquilizers and sedatives without consideration of the underlying mechanism of the problem is unwise and may mask an important clue to the early diagnosis of heart failure.

5. Weakness and Fatigue.   Inquire if the patient feels unusually weak and fatigued. These symptoms are very common with heart failure, probably as a result of decreased tissue perfusion secondary to the reduction in cardiac output.

6. Physical Examination by the Nurse.   Examine the patient in a systematic way to detect signs of left and right heart failure. (As noted previously, signs of left heart failure precede signs of right heart failure in patients with acute myocardial infarction.) This examination, which should be conducted every 4 hours (at the time vital signs are ordinarily recorded) includes the following observations:

a. Rales at the bases of the lungs
b. Gallop rhythm
c. Distention of neck veins (in the semiupright position)
d. Peripheral edema (especially in sacral area and back)
e. Right upper quadrant abdominal tenderness (due to hepatic engorgement)
f. Hepatojugular reflux (neck vein distention while pressure is exerted over liver area)

Participation in the Treatment Program

The nurse has several important responsibilities in the overall treatment program for heart failure. These include initiating emergency treatment for acute pulmonary edema, assessing the effects of therapy, and helping the patient to understand the treatment measures that are taken.

Initiating Emergency Treatment for Acute Pulmonary Edema*.

1. Recognize the complication and notify the physician immediately. The clinical picture of acute pulmonary edema is so distinctive that diagnosis is seldom a problem.
2. Administer humidified oxygen by means of a tight-fitting face mask. The flow rate should be adjusted to 8–10 liters per minute. Face masks are usually frightening to patients in respiratory distress, and the nurse should make it clear that the mask will not interfere with breathing. Intermittent positive-pressure ventilation may be ordered by the physician.
3. Raise the head of the bed so that the patient is in a sitting (Fowler's) position. This position facilitates breathing by lowering the diaphragm and allowing the lung capacity to expand.
4. Prepare and administer drug therapy as ordered by the physician (or in accordance with the standard protocol of the CCU). The customary treatment program involves the immediate administration of morphine and a rapid-acting diuretic.
5. Apply rotating tourniquets to the extremities if the previous measures have not produced improvement.
6. Observe the cardiac monitor for the development of arrhythmias. Reduced tissue oxygenation and electrolyte disturbances resulting from heart failure commonly precipitate serious arrhythmias during this period.
7. Arrange for the collection of arterial blood samples (for blood gas determinations), if ordered.

---

*The scope of nursing intervention in emergency situations varies considerably among hospitals. In hospitals that do not have house officers or other physicians in full-time attendance it is a common practice for the medical staff to adopt a standard program for emergency treatment which the nurse may initiate if a physician is not immediately available.

Assessing the Effects of Therapy.   After the treatment program for heart failure is started it is essential to evaluate the patient's clinical condition at regular intervals in order to plan a subsequent course of action. Should diuretic therapy be continued? Are additional doses of digitalis required? Is oxygen therapy still required? Should other measures be instituted? The physician's decision about these and other questions regarding treatment depend on the patient's clinical response to therapy. The nurse participates in this assessment process in the following ways:

1. Recording vital signs with particular emphasis on changes in the heart rate and respiration
2. Examining the patient to detect reduction or progression of the signs of heart failure (As part of the examination, the patient should be weighed at the same time each day. Changes in body weight provide an accurate means of assessing fluid retention.)
3. Monitoring the heart to identify the development of arrhythmias
4. Questioning the patient about side effects of drug therapy
5. Recognizing signs and symptoms of digitalis toxicity, hypokalemia, or low-salt syndrome
6. Organizing laboratory data (e.g., electrolytes and arterial blood gases) in an orderly manner so that changes can be readily noted

Helping the Patient to Understand the Treatment Program.   Acute pulmonary edema is an extremely frightening experience; most patients feel that death is near. The nurse should reassure the patient that prompt improvement can be anticipated after treatment is started. A calm, confident attitude is often the best form of reassurance. Each step in the treatment program should be explained briefly to the patient, particularly when the use of equipment (e.g., positive-pressure breathing devices) is involved.

Even with less-severe forms of heart failure, it is important for the nurse to explain to the patient why certain measures are necessary. Not only does explanation help to relieve anxiety, it also serves to enlist the patient's cooperation. For example, salt-restricted diets are often unpalatable, and patients may refuse their meals. If the need for dietary control is understood by the patient, he is better able to accept the inconvenience.

CARDIOGENIC SHOCK

Cardiogenic shock is the most severe manifestation of decreased left ventricular pumping function; it occurs in approximately 15% of patients hospitalized with acute myocardial infarction. Until recently more than 80% of patients who developed the clinical syndrome of cardiogenic shock (also called power failure syndrome) could be expected to die during the period of hospitalization. Now there is hope that this awesome mortality can be reduced by the application of new methods of treatment.

The precise cause of cardiogenic shock is still uncertain, but it is known that this complication is associated with extensive destruction of the left ventricle. Autopsy studies have shown that in most patients who die of cardiogenic shock more than 50% of the myocardium is destroyed. This does not necessarily mean that all of the damage is produced by the initial infarction; it may be that the infarcted area continues to enlarge during the course of cardiogenic shock. Research studies now are being conducted to determine if the extent of myocardial damage can be controlled by drug therapy administered within the first few hours after the attack. [Among the drugs being tested are propranolol (Inderal), hyaluronidase (Alidase), and digoxin.] If it is possible to limit the ultimate size of an evolving myocardial infarction, the incidence of cardiogenic shock (and left ventricular failure) may decline.

The effects of this severe damage to the myocardium are depicted in Figure 7.8. As a result of extensive injury to the myocardium the stroke volume and cardiac output are reduced greatly. (This is accompanied by an increase in pressure in the left atrium, pulmonary capillaries, and pulmonary arteries, as noted in the discussion of left ventricular failure.) The marked decrease in cardiac output causes the systemic arterial blood pressure to fall (*hypotension*). In an effort to preserve effective circulation the small arterioles throughout the body constrict, in effect confining the circulating blood volume to the vital organs at the expense of peripheral tissues. This generalized *vasoconstriction*, mediated through the sympathetic nervous system, is beneficial at first; ultimately, however, it cannot compensate for the very low cardiac output, and sustained hypotension develops. When the systolic arterial blood pressure falls below a critical level the vital organs fail to receive adequate amounts of blood and oxygen to sustain normal cellular metabolism; this is called *inadequate perfusion*. This generalized perfusion deficit affects all of the organs of the body and produces the clinical findings of cardiogenic shock. Of particular importance is the effect of underperfusion on the heart itself. When the blood flow through the coronary arteries decreases during shock, the myocardium is further deprived of oxygen. This impairs myocardial contractility of the uninjured segment of the ventricle and at the same time promotes additional tissue destruction (thus increasing the size of the infarction). Consequently the cardiac output falls even more, and a vicious cycle is created. In summary, cardiogenic shock develops because the damaged left ventricle is unable to maintain the cardiac output at a level necessary for adequate tissue perfusion.

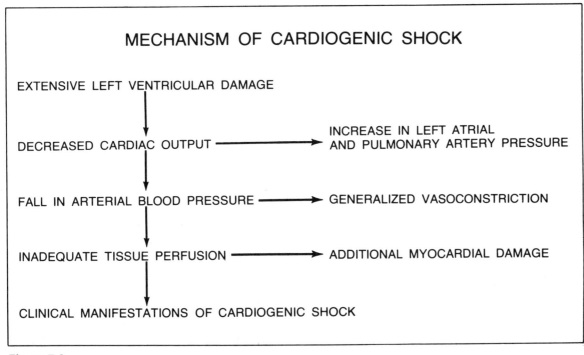

Figure 7.8.

Unless adequate perfusion can be restored promptly, the body cells deteriorate and die. Once the vital organs are destroyed in this way, treatment is to no avail and death must be anticipated; this latter state is called *irreversible shock*. The exact dividing line between irreversible and reversible shock is unknown, but it appears that reversibility is related primarily to the duration of the perfusion deficit. It is believed that certain enzyme systems concerned with utilization of oxygen by the tissues are irreparably damaged during cardiogenic shock and that death occurs from this cause. The end stage of cardiogenic shock is associated with profound vasodilation (circulatory collapse) and finally the development of ventricular fibrillation or ventricular standstill, which are unresponsive to treatment.

Clinical Manifestations of Cardiogenic Shock

Inadequate tissue perfusion results in a combination of clinical findings which *collectively* define cardiogenic shock. In other words, underperfusion affects all of the major organs of the body, and therefore the clinical picture of cardiogenic shock is characterized by involvement of multiple systems. The most important manifestations of cardiogenic shock are as follows.

Hypotension

A marked decrease in arterial blood pressure is an outstanding feature of acute circulatory insufficiency. In nearly all instances the systolic blood pressure falls below 90 mm Hg. However, it must be clearly understood that hypotension by itself is not synonymous with cardiogenic shock. Unless hypotension is accompanied by other clinical findings of inadequate perfusion (e.g., diminished urinary output or mental confusion, as described below) the diagnosis of cardiogenic shock is not justified. For example, if a patient has a blood pressure of 84/50 but the pulse rate is not rapid, urinary output is normal, and there is no evidence of mental confusion, it should not be assumed that cardiogenic shock is present. A more reasonable diagnosis of this condition is hypotension, a common occurrence in the early stages of acute myocardial infarction and of much less importance than cardiogenic shock.

As cardiogenic shock develops, the systolic pressure declines before the diastolic pressure; consequently it is not unusual to record a blood pressure, for example, of 70/60 in this circumstance. The numerical difference between the systolic and diastolic pressures is called the *pulse pressure* (e.g., 120/80 = pulse pressure of 40 mm Hg). Since narrowing of the pulse pressure is frequently an early sign of cardiogenic shock, it is essential to measure the systolic and diastolic pressures precisely in order to detect insidious changes. When cardiogenic shock worsens, the diastolic pressure falls along with the systolic pressure; and often the blood pressure becomes unobtainable. (In assessing blood pressure levels it is necessary to realize that the customary cuff-stethoscope method of measurement may produce spuriously low readings, particularly in the presence of cardiogenic shock. Therefore when blood pressure readings are very low or cannot be obtained, *direct* blood pressure measurement may be required; this is accomplished by inserting an indwelling catheter into the arterial system and recording the intraarterial pressures directly.)

Mental Changes

One of the earliest features of cardiogenic shock is mental apathy and lassitude: the patient seems disinterested in his surroundings and often just stares into space. Other common findings that occur at the same time or later are disorientation, confusion, agitation, and restlessness. All of these mental changes reflect ineffective perfusion of the brain. As the shock state progresses, seizures may occur and finally coma develops.

Oliguria

As a result of diminished renal blood flow, the kidneys fail to function effectively and the urinary volume decreases markedly. With adequate perfusion the kidneys normally excrete at least 1 cc of urine per minute (or 60 cc per hour). During cardiogenic shock the urinary output falls below 20 cc per hour (*oliguria*), or it may cease entirely. This latter condition (*anuria*) is an ominous sign and generally signals irreversible shock.

Cold, Moist Skin

Because of peripheral vasoconstriction which usually accompanies cardiogenic shock, there is a marked reduction in blood flow to the skin. Consequently the skin becomes cold and pale. Along with this vasoconstrictive response there is an increase in sympathetic nervous system activity, which causes profuse sweating. The combination of vasoconstriction and sympathetic stimulation produces the cold, pale, clammy skin that characterizes cardiogenic shock.

Metabolic Acidosis

Adequate oxygenation is essential for normal cellular metabolism and function. In cardiogenic shock the supply of oxygen available to the tissues is drastically reduced. In an attempt to preserve cellular function and life the body employs a temporary, alternate metabolic pathway which does not demand oxygen; this is called *anaerobic* metabolism, in contrast to the normal *aerobic* pathway, which uses oxygen. The end product of aerobic metabolism is carbonic acid, which is excreted as carbon dioxide by the lungs; the end product of anaerobic metabolism is *lactic acid*. Unlike carbon dioxide, which is readily removed from the body, lactic acid cannot be excreted by the lungs or kidneys and therefore accumulates in the blood. This retention of lactic acid results in *lactic acidosis*. Lethal arrhythmias, which are refractory to treatment, develop in the presence of lactic acidosis and cause death.

Treatment of Cardiogenic Shock

Over the years a variety of methods have been used to treat cardiogenic shock. That the present mortality rate remains greater than 80% clearly indicates that no mode of therapy has been consistently successful in combating this complication. However, ongoing research has provided several important leads regarding an improved plan of treatment. The plan is based on the following concepts: 1) the earlier cardiogenic shock is recognized and treated, the greater is the chance for survival; 2) therapeutic decisions must be based on repeated assessment of the patient's physiological status; 3) a standardized treatment program for all patients is defeating because the clinical course has many variations; 4) drug therapy should be selected and altered according to the hemodynamic and clinical response; 5) in many patients the only hope for survival rests with mechanical assistance of the failing circulation; 6) surgical treatment may be feasible if other measures have failed. According to these current concepts a logical approach to the treatment of cardiogenic shock should involve the following steps.

1. Early Recognition of Cardiogenic Shock

Because there is very little hope for survival once cardiogenic shock reaches an advanced stage (e.g., complete cessation of urinary output), the primary focus of the treatment program must be directed toward early detection and treatment of the complication. Occasionally cardiogenic shock develops soon after acute myocardial infarction has occurred, but far more often the shock state evolves gradually, usually several hours after the attack. Consequently in most instances there is an opportunity to recognize the first clinical manifestations of shock. Early detection can be achieved only by planned, repeated observation of the patient's clinical condition. Any evidence suggesting impending shock such as diminished mental alertness, a modest reduction in blood pressure, narrowing of the pulse pressure, a gradual decrease in urinary output, or coolness and paleness of the skin is cause for prompt investigation of the patient's physiological status and the initiation of supportive treatment.

2. Basic Physiological Measurements

In order to evaluate the extent of the problem and to plan a logical treatment program it is necessary to monitor the following physiological parameters at the onset of cardiogenic shock.

Arterial Blood Pressure. As noted, blood pressure measurements made with a standard sphygmomanometer are frequently inaccurate in the presence of cardiogenic shock. Therefore, if the systolic pressure is low (e.g., less than 80 mm Hg) or if the pressure is difficult to determine, it is advantageous to insert an intraarterial catheter (usually through the radial artery) to permit direct blood presssure measurements. In this way the blood pressure can be measured precisely and recorded continuously.

Urinary Output. Accurate measurement of urinary output is of such great importance in assessing the patient's physiological status that an indwelling (Foley) catheter should be placed into the bladder in the early stages of cardiogenic shock. The urinary volume is measured at 30-minute intervals.

Arterial Blood Gases. Cardiogenic shock, as noted, is accompanied by inadequate oxygenation and metabolic acidosis. The extent of these two disturbances is determined by arterial blood gas studies (pO_2 and pH). If an intraarterial catheter is used to monitor blood pressure, arterial blood samples can be collected through the tube; otherwise arterial puncture must be performed each time.

Central Venous Pressure. It has been a standard procedure for many years to measure the central venous pressure (CVP) in patients with cardiogenic shock (or advanced left ventricular failure) as a means of estimating the extent of circulatory insufficiency. As explained previously, when left ventricular pumping performance decreases, a backward pressure develops throughout the pulmonary circulation; this pressure impedes right ventricular emptying and in turn causes a rise in the right atrium and vena cavae. The latter pressure (called the central venous pressure) can be measured readily by inserting a long polyethylene tube (catheter) into the superior vena cava by way of an arm, neck, or subclavian vein. The free end of the catheter is attached to a water manometer; the height of the water column in the manometer indicates the CVP. That the catheter is in proper position can be ascertained by having the patient cough. Coughing causes an increase in intrathoracic pressure and results in a sudden rise (and then fall) in CVP. The normal CVP ranges between 5–10 cm H_2O. It is important to realize that CVP reflects the ability of the *right* ventricle to handle venous return but offers much less information about left ventricular performance, which is of course the critical factor in cardiogenic shock. Unfortunately, the relationship between the right heart and left heart pressures is not always consistent, and therefore the CVP is not a truly accurate index of left ventricular function. In fact, in some instances the CVP may be normal or slightly elevated despite the presence of cardiogenic shock. Nevertheless measurement of CVP is still a useful and valuable procedure, particularly in CCUs unprepared for more sophisticated methods. In the vast majority of patients with cardiogenic shock the CVP is markedly elevated, usually to levels of 15–20 cm H_2O or more.

Pulmonary Artery Pressure.   An effective and very useful method for evaluating left ventricular pumping performance is to measure the pressure in the pulmonary artery. The basis of this measurement is as follows: As noted earlier, when myocardial contractility is impaired the ventricle cannot empty adequately; therefore the volume (and pressure) of blood in the left ventricle at the end of the filling period (diastole) increases significantly. This increase in *left ventricular end-diastolic pressure* (LVEDP) is one of the earliest and most important expressions of diminished left ventricular function. Therefore it is highly desirable to measure LVEDP as a means of evaluating the severity of cardiogenic shock, as well as the effects of treatment. However, *direct* measurement of LVEDP is a formidable procedure. The catheter must be inserted into a surgically exposed artery and threaded backward through the aorta and the aortic valve, and into the left ventricle. The procedure is performed in a cardiac catheterization laboratory with the use of fluoroscopy. Furthermore, placing a catheter in the left ventricle is hazardous in patients with acute myocardial infarction because of the risk of inducing myocardial irritability and ventricular fibrillation. In 1970 it was shown that LVEDP could be measured *indirectly* by means of a balloon-tipped catheter (Swan-Ganz catheter) inserted into the pulmonary artery by way of a peripheral vein. Unlike direct left ventricular catheterization, this method is safe and simple, and can be performed at the patient's bedside. Pulmonary artery pressure (PAP) is more accurate than CVP in assessing left ventricular function because the measurements are made nearer to the left heart. Moreover, alterations in left ventricular hemodynamics can be detected much sooner in the pulmonary artery than in the superior vena cava.

The procedure for monitoring PAP involves the use of a double-lumen catheter. The larger lumen measures the pressure in the pulmonary artery. The smaller lumen leads to a small balloon just proximal to the tip of the catheter. When inflated, the balloon serves to guide the catheter through the right atrium, right ventricle, and into proper position in the pulmonary artery. The catheter is inserted through an arm (antecubital) vein and advanced to the superior vena cava. After the catheter enters the vena cava the balloon is fully inflated with air and allowed to float through the right atrium and right ventricle into the pulmonary artery. The balloon finally wedges in a small branch of the pulmonary artery; this is called the *pulmonary wedge position*. The course the catheter traverses in reaching the wedge position is illustrated in Figure 7.9. Continuous pressure recordings are made during passage of the catheter to verify its location. As shown in Figure 7.10 the pressure waves are distinctly different in the right ventricle, pulmonary artery, and pulmonary wedge position. The pressure recorded in the pulmonary wedge position is termed the *pulmonary capillary wedge pressure* (PCWP). It represents the pressure in the pulmonary capillary bed, which reflects the left ventricular end-diastolic pressure. PCWP cannot be measured continuously because the inflated balloon obstructs the flow of blood through a segment of the lung and can cause pulmonary embolism. Consequently, as soon as the PCWP is determined the balloon is deflated. Deflation of the balloon (with the catheter still in the wedge position) permits the pulmonary artery pressure (PAP) to be measured. In most instances there is a close correlation between pulmonary artery (diastolic) pressure and PCWP. Therefore by monitoring PAP (which can be performed continuously because the balloon is deflated), left ventricular performance may be evaluated constantly. These hemodynamic measurements are extremely important in determining a logical plan of treatment and should be utilized whenever possible.

POSITION OF THE SWAN-GANZ CATHETER

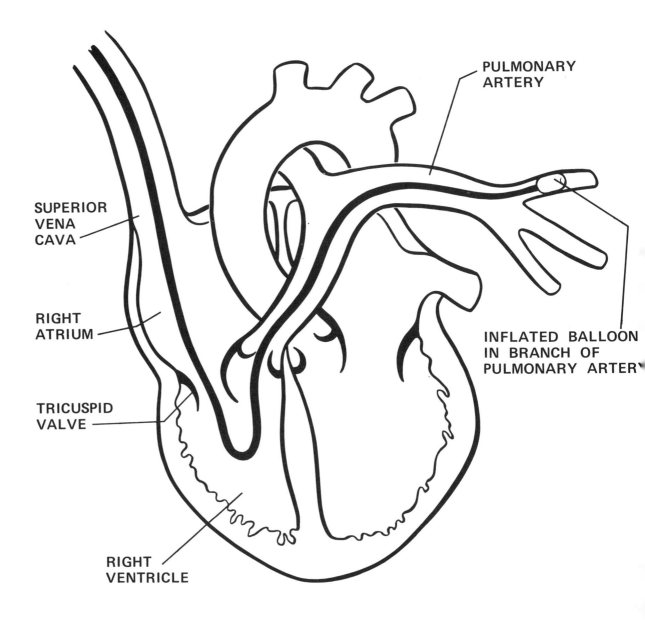

Figure 7.9. The course of catheter traverses in reaching the pulmonary wedge position for recording pulmonary artery pressure.

PRESSURE RECORDINGS DURING PASSAGE OF SWAN-GANZ CATHETER

Right Ventricle

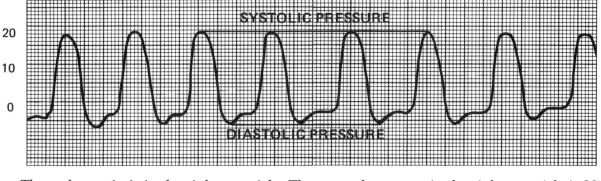

The catheter tip is in the right ventricle. The normal pressure in the right ventricle is 20 mm Hg systolic and 5 mm diastolic (20/5). In this example the pressure is 20/0 mm Hg.

Pulmonary Artery

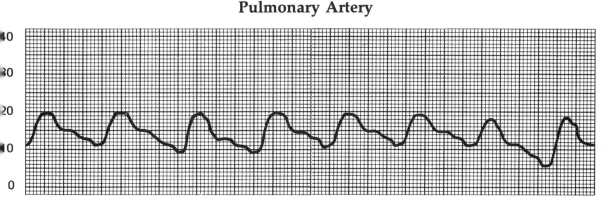

The catheter tip is in the pulmonary artery. The normal PAP is 25/10 mm Hg. In this case the systolic pressure is 20 mm Hg and the diastolic pressure between 10–12 mm Hg. The *diastolic* pulmonary artery pressure is used to assess left ventricular function; the pressure increases above 12 mm when the left ventricle begins to fail.

Pulmonary Capillary Wedge Pressure

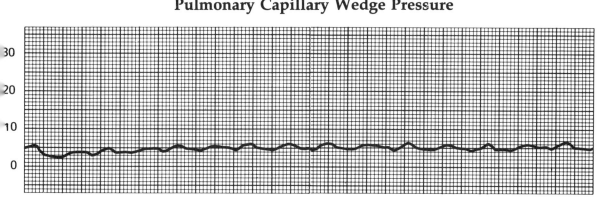

The catheter tip (with the balloon inflated) is in a small branch of the pulmonary artery. A PCWP of 5–12 mm Hg is considered normal. Levels above 12 mm Hg indicate reduced left ventricular emptying. The PCWP in this instance is about 5 mm Hg.

Figure 7.10

3. Supportive Therapy

With the appearance of the first signs of cardiogenic shock, several general measures are undertaken in an effort to preserve vital organ function until specific treatment can be instituted to improve cardiac performance (based on the results of hemodynamic studies). These initial steps, categorized as supportive therapy, include the following.

Administration of Oxygen. Oxygen is administered initially by means of a tight-fitting face mask. Arterial blood gas studies should be performed while the patient is receiving oxygen. If the results indicate inadequate arterial oxygenation (pO_2 levels of less than 75), assisted respiration may be necessary.

Relief of Pain. Patients with cardiogenic shock frequently develop ischemic chest pain because of reduced coronary blood flow and inadequate myocardial perfusion. Small doses of morphine (5–10 mg) should be administered intravenously to relieve this pain. (Intramuscular or subcutaneous injections are not advisable in this circumstance since drug absorption may be very slow in the presence of diminished circulation.)

Correction of Acidosis. As explained previously, inadequate tissue perfusion leads to lactic acidosis, a condition that even when of moderate severity adversely affects cardiac performance and contributes to the development of lethal arrhythmias. Consequently it is essential to detect and correct acidosis promptly. The presence of acidosis is determined by measurement of arterial blood pH. (The normal arterial blood pH is 7.35–7.45; levels lower than 7.35 indicate acidosis.) Lactic acidosis is treated with intravenous sodium bicarbonate (an alkali).

4. Specific Treatment

Infusion of Fluids. Hypotension, oliguria, and other signs of cardiogenic shock sometimes develop in patients with acute myocardial infarction as the result of a reduction in the circulating blood (plasma) volume. The volume depletion (*hypovolemia*) is usually caused by a combination of factors including inadequate fluid intake, anorexia, vomiting, profuse sweating, and excessive fluid loss from vigorous diuretic therapy. This form of shock is characterized by *normal (or low)* pulmonary artery and central venous pressures (in contrast to the high levels that are expected with typical cardiogenic shock). The condition can be corrected by the administration of adequate amounts of intravenous fluids to expand the plasma volume. Consequently, if the PAP or CVP is not elevated, plasma volume expansion should be undertaken as the first step in treatment. Usually 200 cc of 5% dextrose solution is administered intravenously over a 10-minute period (20 cc/minute). If hypovolemia is a contributory factor in shock, this trial of fluid loading usually causes the blood pressure and urinary volume to increase promptly. Additional fluids are then infused according to clinical and hemodynamic responses. With marked volume depletion, albumin, whole blood, or low-molecular-weight dextran may be required to expand the intravascular volume sufficiently. As a general rule patients who respond to volume expansion have a good chance for recovery.

Inotropic Drugs. Unless cardiogenic shock responds to plasma volume expansion (which happens in approximately 10% of cases), drug therapy is initiated in an attempt to increase the strength of myocardial contraction (and to raise the blood pressure). A variety of drugs are available for this purpose, but none is ideal. The main problem with these agents (categorized as intropic drugs) is that in achieving their effect they increase myocardial oxygen consumption. An increase in myocardial oxygen consumption is especially dangerous in the presence of cardiogenic shock since additional oxygen deprivation may cause the area of infarction to enlarge, thus reducing pumping function even more. Despite this (and other) adverse physiologic effects, inotropic drugs must be used when the blood pressure is very low and perfusion of vital organs cannot be maintained. One or more of the following drugs may be administered in this circumstance: levarterenol (Levophed), dopamine (Inotropin), isoproterenol (Isuprel), glucagon, digitalis. Although it is beyond the scope of this discussion to describe the precise pharmacologic actions and methods of administration of each of these agents, several general conclusions regarding inotropic therapy should be noted. First, the results of treatment vary from patient to patient, and therefore trials with different drugs (or different dosages) may be necessary. Second, no attempt should be made to restore blood pressure to normal, preshock levels. As a general rule the systolic pressure should be maintained in the range of 90–100 mm Hg; higher levels create an excessive myocardial oxygen demand. Third, inotropic drugs frequently induce serious arrhythmias; consequently careful ECG monitoring is mandatory during the period of treatment. Fourth, inotropic drugs usually act very promptly, and if definite improvement does not occur within an hour or two mechanical assistance of the circulation may be required.

Vasodilator Drugs. As noted previously, when cardiogenic shock develops the peripheral arterioles constrict (as a compensatory mechanism) to preserve adequate circulation to the vital organs. Although vasoconstriction is highly desirable at first, it may ultimately lead to a reduction in cardiac output because the left ventricle must pump against strong resistance in the arterial system (peripheral vascular resistance). In other words, increased peripheral vascular resistance can impede ventricular emptying and thereby diminish cardiac output. On this basis it has been proposed that *vasodilator* drugs be used to improve cardiac output if there is evidence of increased peripheral vascular resistance (as calculated from hemodynamic measurements). Unfortunately this concept has limited application in the treatment of cardiogenic shock because vasodilator drugs tend to lower the blood pressure. Occasionally, however, patients with cardiogenic shock exhibit systolic blood pressure above 100 mm Hg, in which case vasodilating agents may be administered cautiously. The two agents that appear most effective in increasing cardiac output in the presence of marked vasoconstriction are sodium nitroprusside and phentolamine. It must be emphasized that these vasodilating agents should *not* be used if the systolic blood pressure is less than 100 mm Hg.

Regulation of Heart Rate. An important measure in the treatment of cardiogenic shock is to maintain the heart rate above 60/minute but less than 120/minute, if possible. Heart rates beyond this range are ineffective and reduce the cardiac output. Therefore, in patients with abnormally slow or fast heart rates every effort must be made to control the rate as a means of improving cardiac output. This is achieved by the use of drugs or by electrical means (cardiac pacing or cardioversion), as described in subsequent chapters.

5. Mechanical Assistance of the Circulation

As apparent from the foregoing discussion drug therapy is designed primarily to increase cardiac output. However, for drugs to succeed in their purpose, the heart must receive an adequate amount of oxygen in order to preserve myocardial function; otherwise the infarcted area increases and treatment is to no avail. Thus the outcome of cardiogenic shock depends finally on the amount of oxygen available to the myocardium. Attempting to increase myocardial perfusion with inotropic drugs is often a lost cause because these agents also increase myocardial oxygen consumption. For this reason many cardiologists now believe that if patients in cardiogenic shock do not respond promptly to drug therapy mechanical assistance of the circulation should be undertaken without delay. The object of mechanical assistance is to increase coronary blood flow and at the same time to decrease the workload of the heart. In this way myocardial function can be maintained, at least temporarily.

The best known and probably the most effective method of mechanical cardiac assistance involves the use of an *intraaortic balloon pump*. The principle of intraaortic balloon pumping (IABP) is as follows: When blood is ejected from the left ventricle into the aorta during systole, only a small amount of aortic blood flows through the coronary arteries. By far the greatest flow through the coronary circulation occurs during diastole (when the myocardium is in a resting state). The underlying purpose of IABP is to raise the diastolic pressure in the aorta momentarily after each contraction so that a larger volume of blood will flow through the coronary arteries. This is achieved by inserting a long, narrow balloon through a femoral artery into the thoracic aorta (Fig. 7.11) and inflating it rapidly (with helium) at the onset of diastole. At the end of diastole (just before systole) the balloon is instantly deflated by a vacuum pump. The sudden decrease in aortic pressure lowers resistance to left ventricular pumping, thereby reducing the workload of the ventricle. The inflation–deflation system is automatically synchronized with the heartbeat, and IABP can be continued for many hours, if necessary. Drug therapy is used concomitantly with IABP, and if the patient's condition stabilizes mechanical assistance is gradually decreased and finally withdrawn. There have been several reports indicating impressive improvement with IABP, and the method appears promising in reducing mortality from cardiogenic shock.

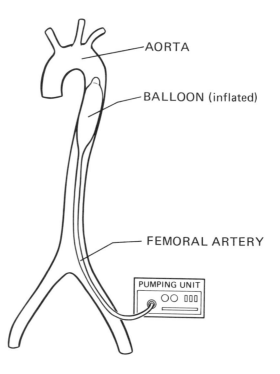

Figure 7.11. Position of an intraaortic balloon pump.

Nursing Role in Cardiogenic Shock

Early Recognition of Cardiogenic Shock

The importance of early detection and treatment of cardiogenic shock cannot be overemphasized. Indeed the main hope for survival depends on improving tissue perfusion as soon as possible. To this end the nurse must be alert for any changes in the patient's clinical condition which suggest that cardiogenic shock is developing. *Early signs of cardiogenic shock can be recognized only by repeated, planned observation at the bedside.* In examining the patient it is essential to remember that inadequate cardiac output (and organ perfusion) produces multiple signs—all of which must be considered in evaluating the problem. Particular attention should be given to the following clinical findings:

1. A decrease in systolic blood pressure, especially if associated with narrowing of the pulse pressure
2. Mental confusion, apathy, anxiety, or lethargy
3. A reduction in urinary volume
4. Cool, moist skin

Initial Treatment Program

When signs of cardiogenic shock appear (or if they are present on admission) the nurse should proceed promptly to initiate supportive therapy. The following measures are taken:

1. Notify the physician at once of the clinical findings.
2. Administer oxygen by means of a well-fitted face mask; the flow rate should be 8–10 liters/minute.
3. Inquire if the patient is experiencing chest pain. If so, intravenous morphine (5 mg) is usually ordered.
4. Adjust the flow rate of the intravenous infusion (5% dextrose in water) in accordance with the physician's instructions.
5. Insert an indwelling catheter into the urinary bladder. Measure and record the urinary volume every 20 minutes.
6. Measure the blood pressure every 15 minutes. By comparing serial readings, a continual fall in pressure can be distinguished from a stabilized level.
7. Observe the cardiac monitor carefully to identify changes in the heart rate and the development of arrhythmias. Because ventricular fibrillation is common in the presence of cardiogenic shock, a defibrillator should be at the bedside.
8. Place the patient in a supine position with a pillow under the head. The Trendelenburg position (used in hemorrhagic shock) is disadvantageous in cardiogenic shock.
9. Arrange for arterial blood gas studies.
10. Record all clinical and laboratory findings sequentially (on a flow sheet) so that changes in the patient's condition can be readily observed.

Subsequent Treatment Program

The specific treatment program for cardiogenic shock is conducted jointly by physician and nurse members of the CCU team. The most important nursing duties include the following:

1. Mobilizing all necessary equipment, drugs, and materials at the onset so that efficient care can be provided uninterruptedly

2. Assisting the physician in performing hemodynamic studies (e.g., insertion of central venous, pulmonary artery, and intraarterial catheters)

3. Measuring and recording blood pressure, urinary output, PAP (or CVP) at regular intervals in order to assess the effectiveness of treatment

4. Monitoring the heart rate and rhythm (cardiac monitoring)

5. Preparing and administering drug therapy in accordance with physicians' orders

6. Checking the patency of all intravenous and intraarterial lines, and adjusting the flow rate of intravenous fluids

7. Arranging for repeated laboratory studies (particularly arterial blood gases)

8. Preparing for assisted ventilation and endotracheal intubation if hypoxia cannot be controlled with nasal oxygen administration

9. Assembling and recording physiological and laboratory data in an organized way

10. Changing the patient's position at least every hour by tilting (slipping a pillow under one side) or elevating the head of the bed slightly

11. Staying with the patient to support him during this critical period

THROMBOEMBOLISM

Patients with acute myocardial infarction are especially prone to develop intravascular clots (thrombi); the reason for this is uncertain, but several factors are thought to contribute to the problem. Venous stasis which accompanies prolonged bed rest and muscular inactivity probably plays an important role in promoting clot formation. However, recent studies (using radioactive isotopes to detect clots in the leg veins) indicate that thrombi often develop within the first 3 days after acute myocardial infarction, suggesting that immobilization itself is not the primary cause of intravascular clotting. There is suspicion that the increased clotting tendency may be inherent in patients with coronary disease and is related to certain blood factors which induce abnormal coagulation (hypercoagulability). Another cause for thrombus formation after acute myocardial infarction is injury to the endocardial lining of the heart by the infarction process. In this circumstance, circulating blood cells adhere to the damaged area and form clots within the chambers of the heart. These intracardiac clots are called mural thrombi. The majority of thrombi, however, arise in the deep veins of the lower extremities (peripheral thrombi). It is estimated that approximately 40% of all patients with acute myocardial infarction develop clots in the calf veins during the period of hospitalization. However, in only a small percentage of cases do these thrombi produce symptoms or affect the clinical course of myocardial infarction. The incidence of peripheral thrombosis is highest in elderly patients and in those with heart failure.

When a peripheral or mural thrombus breaks loose from its site of origin it migrates through the circulatory system as an *embolus*. Depending on where they ultimately lodge, emboli are classified as pulmonary, cerebral, or peripheral. These three types of embolization are discussed separately.

Pulmonary Embolism

Pulmonary emboli nearly always originate in the *deep veins of the legs*. When the thrombus is dislodged from the vein it travels through the inferior vena cava, right atrium, and right ventricle, and finally occludes a branch of the pulmonary artery. There is little chance of mural thrombi causing pulmonary embolism since these latter clots are confined almost exclusively to the *left* heart and consequently remain in the systemic rather than the pulmonary circulation. (In this sense pulmonary embolism is not a direct result of acute myocardial infarction; the problem develops because of secondary factors.)

Of the three types of thromboembolic complications, pulmonary embolism is by far the most common. Autopsy studies indicate that pulmonary embolism occurs in about 25% of patients with acute myocardial infarction. However, these embolic episodes are seldom death-producing; the total mortality from pulmonary embolism (in patients with acute myocardial infarction) is 1–2% at most.

Clinical Manifestations of Pulmonary Embolism

The clinical response to pulmonary embolism depends on the size of the embolus and the degree of obstruction it produces in the pulmonary circulation. Most pulmonary emboli are small and do not produce distinct signs or symptoms; indeed the majority of embolic episodes go unnoticed. With a large pulmonary embolus (which occludes a major branch of the pulmonary artery) patients usually develop clinically recognizable findings. The typical features consist of sudden chest pain, dyspnea, cough (sometimes with hemoptysis), tachycardia, and marked anxiety. The chest pain, often described as crushing or oppressive in quality, may be located substernally or in the right or left side of the chest. The pain pattern frequently resembles that of acute myocardial infarction but differs in that ordinarily it does not radiate to the arms or jaws and is usually increased by inspiration. Rapid respiration and tachycardia are observed in nearly all cases soon after the onset of the episode. Physical examination of the chest may reveal wheezing or rales, but these findings are inconstant. With a massive pulmonary embolus (obstructing more than 50% of the main pulmonary artery), hypotension and circulatory collapse develop; in this circumstance death usually occurs rapidly.

Several diagnostic tests are used to identify pulmonary embolism. X-ray examination of the chest, probably the most common method, is of minimal diagnostic help immediately after an embolic episode because the characteristic findings rarely appear at once. A normal chest x ray offers no assurance that embolization has not occurred. A more reliable diagnostic procedure is the lung scan. By injecting a radioactive isotope intravenously and scanning the lung fields, the segment of the lung deprived of oxygen can be identified at an early stage. A comparison of a normal lung scan with one demonstrating a large pulmonary embolism is shown in Figure 7.12. The diagnosis of pulmonary embolism can sometimes be suspected from acute ECG changes that indicate an acute strain pattern of the right heart (which develops from resistance in the pulmonary circulation created by the embolus). Arterial blood gas determinations may also be useful in establishing the diagnosis. Nearly all patients with large pulmonary emboli exhibit arterial oxygen undersaturation (while breathing room air).

The onset of pulmonary embolism is by no means constant or predictable; however, its sudden occurrence after straining during defecation or when the patient first gets out of bed after prolonged inactivity is common enough to merit special precautions.

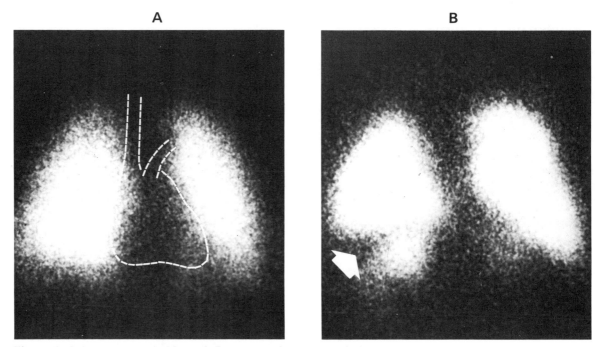

A　　　**B**

Figure 7.12. Lung scans. **A:** Normal. **B:** Large pulmonary embolism.

Cerebral Embolism

Cerebral emboli, unlike pulmonary emboli, originate as *mural* thrombi. Clots from the injured wall of the left ventricle travel through the aorta and occlude arteries in the brain, producing cerebral infarction. In some instances the embolic episode occurs very soon after acute myocardial infarction so that it is not uncommon for patients to be admitted to a hospital with typical findings of a stroke when the underlying problem is in fact an acute myocardial infarction. In this situation the effects of the stroke usually dominate the clinical picture and obscure cardiac symptoms. For this reason it is a wise practice to record an ECG routinely in all patients with sudden cerebrovascular events.

Clinical Manifestations of Cerebral Embolism

The most characteristic feature of cerebral embolism is the *sudden* onset of the stroke. In contrast to customary (nonembolic) strokes, there are no premonitory warnings, and the neurologic findings appear abruptly. Therefore if a patient with acute myocardial infarction suddenly develops signs of a stroke, it can be assumed that cerebral embolism has developed as a complication of myocardial infarction. The clinical course after the attack depends on the location of the cerebral infarction and the extent of the neurologic deficit it produces. Motor weakness, paralysis, and speech disturbances are the most common findings; many patients develop loss of consciousness. Diagnostic studies are seldom necessary. Death does not occur suddenly, but the prognosis is extremely poor. The combination of an acute myocardial infarction and a stroke is usually overwhelming, particularly in elderly patients.

Peripheral Embolism

Like cerebral emboli, peripheral emboli arise from clots formed within the left heart. Although these mural thrombi may lodge anywhere in the systemic arterial system, the most frequent site of peripheral embolism is in the femoral or iliac arteries supplying the lower extremities. The outcome of peripheral embolism depends on the artery involved and whether the embolus can be removed surgically (embolectomy).

Clinical Manifestations of Peripheral Embolism

Embolic occlusion of the major arteries to the lower extremities produces a distinctive clinical picture. There is a sudden onset of pallor, coldness, and numbness of the involved extremity. Within minutes, the patient develops pain in the leg along with decreased sensation. Physical examination reveals an absence of arterial pulsations in conjunction with a cold, pale extremity. In some instances both extremities are involved simultaneously, indicating that the embolus is at the bifurcation of the aorta. Unless embolectomy can be performed promptly, gangrene develops.

Treatment of Thromboembolism

Because emboli originate as thrombi the ideal method of treatment for all forms of embolism is to *prevent* thrombus formation. Prevention can often be accomplished by means of prophylactic anticoagulant therapy; however, the value of this approach is a subject of controversy. Before the era of CCUs it was customary to administer anticoagulant drugs prophylactically to most patients with acute myocardial infarction. When it was demonstrated that thromboembolic complications accounted for only a small percentage of the total mortality, the routine use of anticoagulant therapy was all but abandoned by most physicians. At present, prophylactic anticoagulant treatment is reserved primarily for patients with the highest risk of developing thromboembolism (i.e., the elderly and those with circulatory failure). Even this practice is not fully endorsed since many clinicians believe that the danger of anticoagulant therapy—particularly uncontrolled bleeding—outweighs the benefit of attempting to prevent clot formation. A second method of reducing the incidence of thrombus formation is to avoid venous stasis whenever possible. This can often be achieved by exercising the extremities, changing the body position frequently, and minimizing the duration of complete bed rest.

If embolism does occur, anticoagulant therapy is usually started immediately. In this situation the purpose of anticoagulants is not to treat the embolus but to prevent further clot formation at the site of origin and in turn to prevent additional emboli. Also, anticoagulant therapy may inhibit extension of the embolus. Heparin, which becomes active immediately after intravenous injection, is administered as soon as a thromboembolic complication is detected. This anticoagulant is continued for 5–7 days, after which oral agents are used.

Peripheral emboli involving the lower or upper extremities may be treated surgically. Although the operative risk is high in patients with acute myocardial infarction, embolectomy has been performed successfully in many instances.

Nursing Role in Thromboembolism

Prevention

The incidence of thrombus formation in the deep veins of the lower extremities can be reduced by thoughtful nursing care. The basic objective is to prevent venous stasis. Several measures are used for this purpose. During the period of bed rest after myocardial infarction the nurse should assist the patient in performing passive exercises at regular intervals. In addition, the patient should be encouraged to flex and extend his feet against a footboard. Elastic stockings may be applied to prevent venous pooling. If support stockings are used it is important to verify that they remain in proper position and do not produce a tourniquet effect. Placing pillows (or elevating the gatch of the bed) under the knees must be avoided, since they can obstruct venous flow in the extremities. The nurse should caution the patient about straining at defecation, and provide stool softeners or laxatives if needed.

Recognition of the Problem

Because pulmonary embolism often resembles acute myocardial infarction the nurse must consider the possibility that recurrent chest pain may be due to an embolic complication. Whenever pulmonary embolism is suspected, the nurse should record a 12-lead ECG and prepare for arterial blood gas studies. Careful inspection of the legs for signs of thrombophlebitis (warmth, tenderness, or swelling) is important, particularly in high-risk patients.

Cerebral infarction can be recognized without difficulty. If the patient suddenly develops motor weakness, paralysis, or a speech disturbance, the physician should be notified at once.

Survival after peripheral embolism depends for the most part on the rapidity with which arterial blood flow can be surgically reestablished after occlusion has occurred; therefore the nursing role in detecting this complication at its onset is of crucial importance. Any delay in recognizing the problem increases the likelihood of irreversible tissue damage.

Treatment Program

With few exceptions, anticoagulant therapy is used in treating thromboembolic complications. The most rapid and effective method of anticoagulation involves the use of intravenous heparin. A continuous intravenous drip containing 200–300 mg heparin in a solution of 500 cc dextrose in water is administered at a rate that will achieve and maintain a venous clotting time of two to three times the normal control value. Intravenous heparin may also be administered intermittently by way of a heparin lock inserted into a peripheral vein. The usual dosage with this method is 50–100 mg every 4 hours, depending on the patient's clotting time.

During the course of anticoagulant therapy the nurse must observe the patient carefully for signs of bleeding. Excessive doses of anticoagulant drugs can cause hemorrhage anywhere in the body, but the most common bleeding sites are the skin, kidneys, and gastrointestinal tract. Careful examination of the body surface should be made during routine nursing care to detect evidence of ecchymosis. The urine and stools must be observed on each occasion. Any evidence of bleeding should be reported to the physician promptly. Anticoagulant therapy may have to be discontinued or anticoagulant antagonists (protamine sulfate or vitamin K_1 administered.)

VENTRICULAR RUPTURE

Rupture of the ventricle is the least common of the major complications of acute myocardial infarction; however, it is the most lethal and probably accounts for 5% of all hospital deaths from myocardial infarction.

Ventricular rupture is nearly always associated with extensive transmural infarction involving through-and-through myocardial necrosis. The perforation, which develops suddenly, occurs in the center of the necrotic area and is apparently due to softening and weakening of the muscle fibers. The rupture may involve either the outer wall of the left ventricle or the interventricular septal wall; the former site is far more common.

When the outer ventricular wall ruptures, blood rushes through the ventricle and instantly fills the surrounding pericardial sac. This extravasation of blood into the closed pericardium produces compression of the heart *(cardiac tamponade)* and prevents ventricular filling. Death usually occurs within minutes. When the rupture involves the interventricular septum (rather than the outer ventricular wall) the outcome is not necessarily fatal immediately, but the prognosis is very poor. In this situation blood from the left ventricle is forced into the right ventricle (because of the difference in pressures of the respective ventricles) and produces abrupt right ventricular overloading, and in turn severe right heart failure.

For many years it was believed that physical activity during the early period after infarction was a major factor in causing ventricular rupture. It now appears that this concept is incorrect since many ruptures occur despite complete bed rest. Moreover, about one-third of cardiac ruptures develop within the first 2 days after hospitalization. Sustained hypertension and the use of anticoagulant therapy have also been incriminated as possible causes of ventricular rupture, but there is little evidence to substantiate these relationships. Perhaps the most significant factor in the development of ventricular rupture is the size and extent of the infarction and the degree of collateral circulation to the involved area. Curiously, ventricular rupture occurs more frequently in women than in men and is the only complication of acute myocardial infarction with a female preponderance; the reason for this is uncertain.

Clinical Manifestations of Ventricular Rupture

Rupture of the outer ventricular wall is nearly always manifested by *sudden* death. Occasionally the patient may complain of recurrent chest pain just before the event, and a sudden fall in blood pressure and abrupt slowing of the heart rate is noted. Clinically, the picture is that of an arrhythmic death. Although the mechanical (pumping) action of the heart ceases immediately after cardiac rupture, the heart's electrical activity may persist for many minutes or longer (because electrical impulses continue to be generated although the ventricles cannot contract). Thus during resuscitation attempts electrical activity may be noted on the cardiac monitor even though the patient is dead.

When the interventricular septum perforates, the diagnosis can often be suspected by the sudden appearance of a loud systolic murmur which was not present previously. This finding coupled with the abrupt development of *right* heart failure (due to the opening between the left and right ventricles) strongly suggests septal rupture. The diagnosis can be confirmed with the use of the Swan-Ganz catheter. A marked increase in oxygen saturation is found in the right heart (reflecting the passage of oxygenated blood from the left ventricle into the right ventricle).

Treatment of Ventricular Rupture

Rupture of the outer ventricular wall almost invariably produces death before any corrective measures can be attempted. Indeed the only hope for survival is immediate repair of the rupture site with excision of the infarcted area (infarctectomy). This procedure has been attempted very rarely, but with the growing availability of heart surgery teams it is conceivable that this form of emergency surgery may be used more often.

Unlike rupture of the ventricular wall, rupture of the septum does not necessarily result in immediate death, and there is an opportunity for surgical intervention in many cases.

Nursing Role in Ventricular Rupture

If sudden death occurs from ventricular rupture the nurse must make certain that the catastrophe is not in fact due to a treatable and reversible cause, specifically ventricular fibrillation or standstill. Cardiopulmonary resuscitation should be attempted immediately and continued until it is definitely ascertained that an arrhythmia is not responsible for the death-producing event.

Because of the potential ability to repair an interventricular septal repture, the nurse should notify the physician immediately in the event a patient suddenly develops right heart failure associated with the appearance of a loud systolic precordial murmur. Preparation should be made promptly for the insertion of a Swan-Ganz catheter since the physician will confirm the diagnosis by measuring the pressure and arterial oxygen saturation in the right ventricle by means of this device.

CARDIAC ARRHYTHMIAS

Arrhythmias are by far the most frequent complication of acute myocardial infarction. At least 90% of all patients with acute infarction develop some disturbance in the rate, rhythm, or conduction of the heartbeat. Prior to the introduction of the system of intensive coronary care, nearly half of all myocardial infarction deaths were due to this single cause. Because of the extreme importance of arrhythmic complications, the remaining chapters of this book are dedicated to the identification and treatment of each of the common arrhythmias.

8

Cardiac Monitoring

Curious as it now seems, as late as 1960 arrhythmias were not considered to be a particularly common complication of acute myocardial infarction. However, the reason for this erroneous impression is understandable: there was no practical method available until that time for detecting arrhythmias on a continuous basis; instead, arrhythmia detection depended for the most part on routine electrocardiograms (recorded perhaps once or twice a day) and on physical examination. Because of the intermittent nature of these observations a high percentage (the majority) of arrhythmias went unnoticed, and more than 40% of deaths from acute infarction were due to arrhythmic complications. Then electronic equipment was developed (as a byproduct of space age engineering) which permitted a *continuous* display of the patient's electrocardiogram. With these instruments, appropriately called cardiac monitors, it became possible to observe the heart's electrical activity at all times and in this way to identify any arrhythmic disturbance the instant it occurred. Cardiac monitoring became the cornerstone of intensive coronary care.

This chapter describes the principles and methods of cardiac monitoring as a prelude to the subjects of electrocardiography and the interpretation of arrhythmias.

THE BASIS OF CARDIAC MONITORING

Each heartbeat is the result of an electrical stimulus. This impulse, which originates normally in a specialized area of the right atrium, is conducted through a network of fibers within the heart (the conduction system) and finally stimulates the myocardium to contract. This same electrical force spreads outward from the heart and reaches the surface of the body where it can be detected with electrodes attached to the skin. The purpose of the cardiac monitor is to pick up the electrical signals generated by the heart and to display them on a screen (oscilloscope) in the form of a continuous electrocardiogram. By analyzing the electrocardiographic wave forms, any disturbance in cardiac rate, rhythm, or conduction can be identified (as explained in the following chapters).

MONITORING EQUIPMENT

There are dozens of different types of cardiac monitors currently available. While these machines vary in size, design, dependability, elegance, and cost, their fundamental components are the same. A basic monitoring system works in the following way:

1.   Electrodes attached to the patient's chest wall pick up the electrical impulses initiated by the heart.

2.   These original waves are too small to be seen on the monitor screen, and for this reason they are directed through an amplifier where their height is increased about 1000 times.

3.   The amplified impulses pass through a magnetic field (galvanometer), where a series of wave forms are established. These deflections, reflecting each phase of the heart's electrical activity, comprise an electrocardiogram.

4.   The electrocardiogram is then displayed continuously on an oscilloscopic screen (similar to a small television screen). The size, position, and brightness of the electrocardiogram can be adjusted as necessary to obtain the clearest "picture."

5.   In addition, the monitor counts each heartbeat and displays the average heart rate per minute on a rate meter. (Actually, the machine counts the electrical waves associated with ventricular activation, called R waves, and not the ventricular contractions themselves.) With each heartbeat a light (pulse light) flashes and a sound ("beep") is heard. (The "beeper" may be turned off if the sound is annoying.)

6.   Integrated with the rate meter is an alarm system, which sounds a loud audio signal and causes a light to flash if the patient's heart rate falls below or exceeds preset levels. For example, if the lower-limit alarm is set at 50 per minute and the upper limit at 120 per minute, any decrease or increase in the heart rate beyond this particular range will cause the alarm to be triggered. Thus the onset of slow-rate or fast-rate arrhythmias can be recognized even though the nurse may not be observing the monitor at the time. A diagrammatic representation of a basic cardiac monitor is shown in Figure 8.1.

In addition to these fundamental components cardiac monitors may also include a variety of accessory devices.* Perhaps the most useful of these additional modules are those designed to enhance the detection of early warning signs of lethal arrhythmias. (As noted previously, the underlying theme of intensive coronary care is to *prevent* lethal arrhythmias by recognizing and treating warning arrhythmias.) That it may be difficult to identify specifically a transient warning arrhythmia from the electrocardiographic pattern seen on an oscilloscopic screen can be readily appreciated: the electrocardiogram moves across the screen rapidly, and the observer has only one fleeting glance of the pattern and no chance to analyze it in detail. The most popular mechanisms used to facilitate arrhythmia detection are direct write-out devices, memory systems, and components to hold or "freeze" the oscilloscopic pattern for closer inspection.

* In recent years there has been an attempt to make monitoring equipment more and more sophisticated by adding various accessories to the basic system. Some of these additions are valuable and improve monitoring capabilities, but others are no more than unnecessary luxuries. It is unwise to assume that a monitor will necessarily be more effective or do a better job just because the machine has a large number of dials, knobs, switches, or lights; indeed our own experience indicates exactly the opposite.

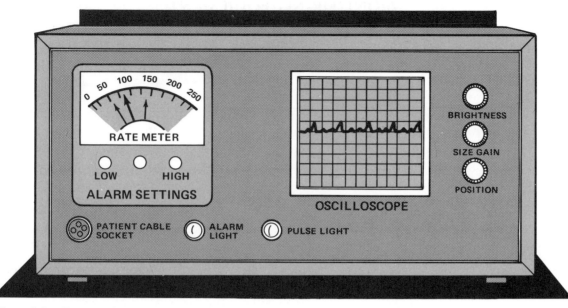

Figure 8.1. Basic cardiac monitor.

A direct write-out mechanism provides a printed record of the electrocardiogram seen on the oscilloscope. This documentation (in the form of a rhythm strip) permits precise identification of an arrhythmia and is also valuable for comparing electro-cardiographic changes over a period of time. The recording can be obtained on demand as well as automatically (whenever the alarm system is triggered).

Memory systems are designed to store and play back the electrocardiogram of the preceding 15–60 seconds (or more). This "instant replay" technique is useful in two circumstances. First, if a transient arrhythmia is noted on the oscilloscope but there is insufficient time to activate the direct write-out device, the episode can be recaptured and recorded by using the memory system. Second, if an observer is not near the monitor when an alarm is triggered, the memory mechanism will replay the events that *preceded* the occurrence.

Hold or "freeze" devices stop the movement of the electrocardiogram across the oscilloscopic screen, keeping a particular pattern in place until it can be interpreted. These modules do not print out an electrocardiogram (from which precise measurements can be made), and for this reason they may be less useful than direct write-out or memory mechanisms.

THE OPERATION OF CARDIAC MONITORS

Four steps are involved in cardiac monitoring: 1) attaching electrodes to the patient's chest wall; 2) connecting the wires from the electrodes to the monitor (by way of a "patient" cable); 3) adjusting the monitor to obtain an effective electrocardiogram; 4) setting the high-rate and low-rate alarm system at desired levels. Each of these aspects will be discussed separately.

Electrodes and Their Attachment

Electrodes serve to pick up the heart's electrical signals at the skin surface. It is apparent that unless the signals are detected properly the remaining phases of cardiac monitoring will have little meaning. Therefore the electrodes themselves and the manner in which they are attached to the skin is of critical importance.

Three types of electrodes have been used for cardiac monitoring. Although two of these electrode systems are no longer popular, it is worthwhile to discuss these earlier models in order to understand some of the problems that may be encountered with electrodes.

The first electrodes, called direct-contact electrodes, were round, metal plates about 1.5 inches in diameter, which were anchored to the skin by layers of adhesive tape. Because of electrical resistance between the skin and electrode surface, it was necessary to apply a layer of conductive jelly (gel) at the interface. These direct-contact metal electrodes presented several problems: first, they could not usually remain in place for more than 8–12 hours because the conductive jelly would dry (under the adhesive tape blanket) and skin irritation was common; second, the electrodes were cumbersome and often annoying to the patient; third, because of their large surface area the electrodes picked up extraneous electrical currents present within the skin itself, thus distorting the actual electrocardiogram. Lastly, preparing the electrodes and taping them in place was time-consuming, a serious handicap in emergency situations.

In an effort to get rid of most of these difficulties many coronary care units began to use hypodermic needles as electrodes. Small, 0.5-inch 25-gauge, metal hubbed needles were inserted directly under the skin surface for this purpose. In principle, needle electrodes were splendid: electrode jelly was not required, contact with the skin was perfect, electrical interference was minimal, and the needles could be placed very rapidly in emergencies. Unfortunately, however, these electrodes were difficult to keep in place, and many patients found them uncomfortable.

The third form of electrode was the disc type or "floating" electrode. These electrodes differ from direct-contact electrodes in that they are deliberately separated from the skin by a built-in "spacer" (Fig. 8.2). Conductive jelly is placed in the spacer, and the electrode is then attached to the skin by means of a surrounding ring of adhesive material. The main purpose of separating the electrode from the skin is to reduce local electrical interference at the skin surface, thus improving the quality of the electrocardiogram. In addition, disc electrodes do not have to be changed more than once a day since the electrode jelly remains moist in the spacer. Furthermore, these electrodes are lightweight, simple to apply, and seldom annoy the patient.

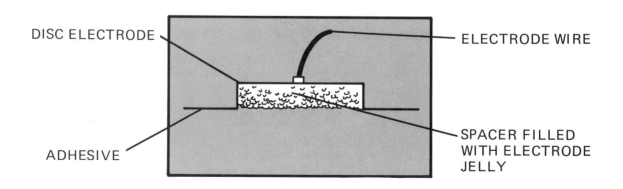

Figure 8.2.   Disc-type or "floating" electrode.

Most CCUs now use a modified version of the basic disc electrode. These are pre-packaged, pregelled, and disposable. The main advantage of the new electrodes is that they greatly shorten the time required for electrode preparation and application, and therefore allow cardiac monitoring to be instituted without delay. By simply peeling off a paper backing from a foam adhesive pad the electrode is ready for use. Because the gel does not dehydrate after application or produce significant skin irritation, the electrodes can remain in place and function reliably for several days.

Location of Electrodes

Three electrodes are required for cardiac monitoring. Two of these serve to detect the heart's electrical activity; the third is a ground electrode, which carries off ("grounds") extraneous electrical currents from sources other than the heart. (With some monitoring equipment four or even five electrodes may be used; the purpose of these additional electrodes is to obtain multiple electrocardiographic views of the heart.)

In positioning the electrodes on the chest wall the object is to select locations that will provide the clearest electrocardiographic wave forms, permitting arrhythmias to be identified readily. The two most common positions are the so-called conventional position and the modified chest lead position.

With the conventional position (Fig. 8.3), the right (R) electrode is placed on the right side of the sternum below the clavicle and medial to the pectoral muscles. The left (L) electrode is situated at the level of the lowest palpable rib on the left side of the chest in the anterior axillary line. The ground (G) electrode is placed at the lower right rib cage area, opposite the left (L) electrode. With the electrodes in these positions the monitor records the electrical activity between the R and L electrodes. This particular path (or lead) normally produces the tallest ventricular complexes (R waves) and is chosen primarily for this reason.

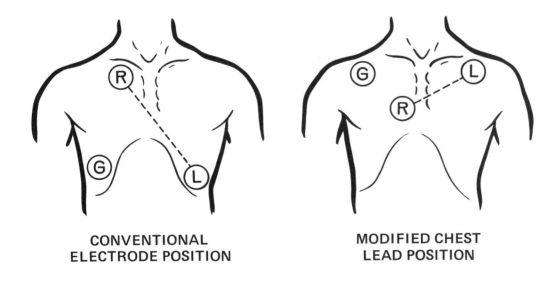

CONVENTIONAL ELECTRODE POSITION

MODIFIED CHEST LEAD POSITION

Figure 8.3. The two most common electrode positions.

With the modified chest lead (MCL) position the right (R) electrode is placed in the fourth interspace at the right border of the sternum (or over the sternum itself). The left (L) electrode is located near the left shoulder, just under the outer portion of the clavicle. The ground (G) electrode is situated in the right shoulder area. Because the path between the R and L electrodes in this position is different than that of the conventional lead, the resultant electrocardiographic pattern is also different (as will be explained in the next chapter).

The choice of electrode positions is a matter of individual preference. Some clinicians believe that the MCL position may be more useful in identifying certain arrhythmias; others favor the conventional position. However, strict reliance on one method for all patients is ill-advised. The nurse should be allowed to select the position that provides the clearest and most informative electrocardiogram for each individual patient.

Attachment of Electrode to Skin

Proper attachment of the electrodes to the skin is undoubtedly the one most important step in effective cardiac monitoring. Unless there is excellent contact between the skin and the electrodes, the electrocardiographic wave form will be distorted and artifacts will appear. In addition, the electrodes must be anchored firmly to prevent movement or displacement. The procedure for attaching electrodes is as follows:

1. Prepare the skin areas designated for electrode placement.

    a. If necessary, chest hair should be shaved in 4-inch areas around the intended electrode sites.

    b. The area is cleansed with alcohol to remove skin oils and tissue debris, and then rubbed dry with a towel or gauze sponge. (In some instances it may be necessary to abrade the skin to obtain a clear electrocardiographic signal. If so, the area should be rubbed with abrasive electrode paste.)

    c. If the chest wall is damp or wet with sweat, the electrode site should be dried thoroughly so the adhesive pad will adhere to the skin. (If sweating continues and the area cannot be kept dry, an antiperspirant spray can be used and a thin coat of tincture of benzoin applied to the peripheral area.)

2. Prepare the electrodes for use and attach to skin.

    a. When pregelled, disposable electrodes are used, the sealed package is opened just before the electrode is applied. (If the foil package remains open too long, the conductive gel may dry.)

    b. The protective paper covering is peeled from the electrode, exposing the adhesive backing and the gel-covered disc.

    c. The electrode is attached by simply pressing the adhesive foam pad firmly to the skin surface.

    d. If the electrodes are not pregelled, conductive jelly is placed in the spacer before application. Excessive amounts of jelly should be avoided because the conductive medium may spread and interfere with the adhesion of the electrode.

3. Change electrodes as necessary.
    a. Pregelled disposable electrodes may remain in place for several days. However, if the electrocardiographic pattern becomes less distinct (often due to drying of the electrode gel), if the patient is diaphoretic, or if skin irritation develops, the electrode must be changed and reapplied.
    b. Nondisposable electrodes are generally changed at least once a day. In many instances it is necessary to change electrodes every 8 hours because of drying of the electrode gel and skin irritation. When these electrodes are changed, freshly cleaned electrodes should be used rather than adding more gel to the used electrode.

Connecting the Wires from the Electrodes to the Monitor

The signals detected by the electrodes are transmitted to the monitor through an electrical cable known as the patient cable (in contrast to the monitor cable, which goes to a wall socket for electrical power). The electrodes are connected to the patient cable by means of thin wires, 12–18 inches in length. These connecting wires snap on or clamp on to the electrodes; the other end of the wire plugs into a receptacle on the patient cable. The receptacle has designated openings for the respective electrode wires. Depending on the monitoring equipment being used, one opening is marked either R (right) or RA (right arm). The second opening is designated L (left) or LA (left arm). The third opening is identified as G (ground) or RL (right leg). Figure 8.4 illustrates these openings.

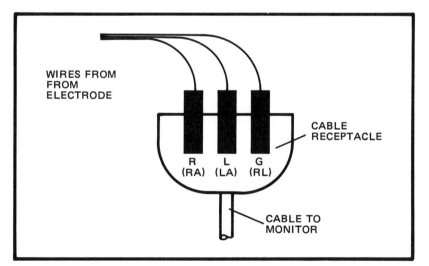

Figure 8.4.   Connections for electrode wires.

The following steps are involved in connecting the electrodes to the patient cable and finally to the monitor:

1. After the electrodes are firmly attached to the skin, the connecting wires are snapped or clamped into place on the electrode.
2. When the conventional electrode position is used for monitoring, the wires from the right (R), left (L), and ground (G) electrodes are inserted into the corresponding R, L, and G terminals of the cable receptacle.
3. In contrast, when the modified chest lead position is used, the electrode wire from the right (R) electrode is inserted into the L opening and the wire from the left (L) electrode into the R opening. In other words, the R and L electrode wires are placed in a reversed position in the receptacle. The ground (G) electrode is placed in the G terminal.
4. After verifying that the connection sites are all secure and that there is no tension on the electrode wires, the patient cable receptacle is pinned to the patient's gown.
5. The monitor end of the patient is then inserted into the cable socket of the monitor.

Adjusting the Monitor

If the electrodes have been applied properly and all wires connected securely, the electrocardiographic pattern appearing on the oscilloscopic screen should be clear and distinct. Failure to obtain clear signals is due, in most instances, to faulty technique during the first two steps of the monitoring procedure or to external electrical interference (as described in the following pages).

Even with flawless technique, three monitor adjustments may be necessary: brightening (or darkening) the display, centering the pattern on the screen, and adjusting the height of the wave forms, particularly the waves of ventricular activation (R waves).†
The amplitude of the ventricular complexes is of great importance because if these waves are too small the rate meter will not recognize and count them and therefore the heart rate will appear falsely low. In this circumstance the height (gain) control dial is adjusted to increase the amplitude of the wave forms. If the height of the waves cannot be increased sufficiently by adjusting the dial, the electrode positions must be changed to obtain a greater electrical potential. An alternative method of augmenting wave height is to switch the electrode wires in the cable receptacle. For example, by placing the wire from the R electrode in the G terminal and vice versa, a different electrical lead will be recorded, which may produce taller waves.

Setting the Alarm System

As noted previously, the high- and low-rate alarms are integrated with the rate meter and are triggered when the heart rate displayed on the meter falls below or exceeds predetermined levels. The alarm limits should be set according to the patient's prevailing heart rate. If the heart rate is between 60 and 100, it is customary to set the low alarm at 50 per minute and the high alarm at 140 per minute. However, if the patient's heart rate is either very slow or very fast, the range for the alarm settings should be

---

† The exact methods for making these adjustments may vary with different monitors; therefore it would be impractical to attempt to describe a uniform set of instructions. The manufacturer's manual, provided with the equipment, explains these procedures in detail and should be studied carefully.

narrowed. For instance, if the patient's rate is 50 per minute, the low-rate alarm should be set at 40 and the high-rate alarm at about 80. In this way the observer would be alerted to even slight rate changes, which may be very significant in this situation.

Because of false alarms (described in the following paragraphs), there may be a temptation to set the alarm limits widely apart (e.g., 40–180) or, worse, to turn off the alarm mechanism entirely. This practice defeats the purpose of the alarm system and should *never* be adopted.

PROBLEMS WITH CARDIAC MONITORING

Many different problems may be encountered during cardiac monitoring; some of these are due to limitations of the monitoring system itself, but the great majority are the result of improper technique. The most common difficulties are discussed here.

False High-Rate Alarms

The alarm system is dependent on the accuracy of the rate meter. In principle, the meter is meant to count the average number of heartbeats (ventricular complexes) per minute; but most meters are not this specific and actually count *all* high deflections on the electrocardiogram assuming that these are ventricular waves. Unfortunately, contraction of skeletal muscles also produces tall waves (called muscle potentials), which the rate meter is unable to distinguish from ventricular complexes. Consequently if a patient turns in bed, moves his extremities suddenly, or has a muscle tremor—all of which may produce rapid, tall muscle potentials—the rate meter will misinterpret these spikes as heartbeats and cause a *false* high-rate alarm (Fig. 8.5).

Attempts have been made to control this problem by adding electronic filters to "absorb" muscle potentials and by programming rate meters to count only waves of a particular configuration rather than all tall spikes. Despite these measures, false high-rate alarms are still common occurrences in actual practice.

One simple method for reducing interference from muscle potentials is to place the electrodes in positions that are not directly over large muscle masses (e.g., not over the pectoral or shoulder muscles).

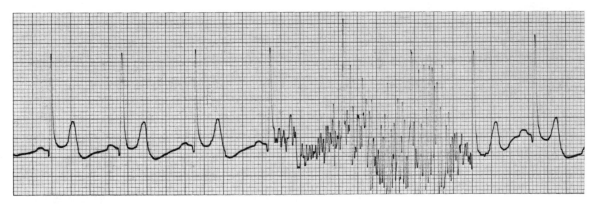

Figure 8.5.   False high-rate alarm caused by muscle potentials.

False Low-Rate Alarms

Any disturbance in the transmission of electrical signals between the skin surface and the monitor can produce a false low-rate alarm. This problem is caused most often by ineffective skin-electrode contact resulting from separation of an electrode, profuse

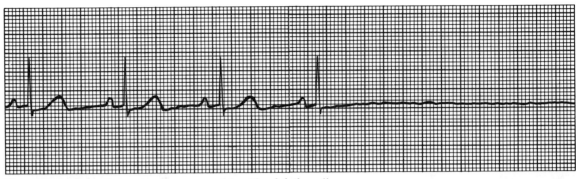

Figure 8.6. False low-rate alarm caused by "lead failure."

sweating, or drying of the conductive jelly. Disconnection of an electrode wire (or the patient cable) is another common source of false low-rate alarms. In all of these situations no electrical activity will be transmitted to the rate meter and oscilloscope, and it might appear at first glance that the heartbeat has stopped (Fig. 8.6). The danger of mistaking this technical error for ventricular standstill is obvious and of serious consequence. To prevent this particular problem specific alarms have been incorporated in some monitoring systems to distinguish "lead failure" from lethal arrhythmias.

False low-rate alarms can also occur if the ventricular waves are not tall enough to activate the rate meter. For example, if an arrhythmia develops in which every other ventricular complex is oriented in an opposite direction to the normal beats (R waves) and is of reduced amplitude (Fig. 8.7), the rate meter may not be able to detect the smaller complexes. In the electrocardiogram in Figure 8.7, the actual heart rate is 64 per minute; however, if the rate meter detected only the taller upright waves, just 32 beats per minute would be counted. This would create a *false* low-rate alarm. This problem can be corrected by either increasing the amplitude of the complexes or by changing the lead position.

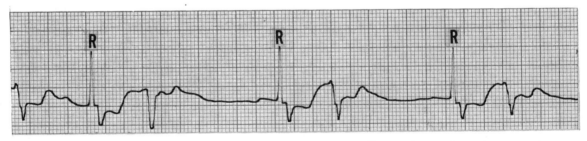

Figure 8.7. False low-rate alarm caused by ventricular waves not tall enough to activate the rate meter.

Electrical Interference

Electrical current from external sources, such as power lines or other electronic equipment, may create interference with the monitor signal. This form of interference appears on the oscilloscopic screen as a series of fine, rapid spikes (60 per second because alternating current has 60 cycles per second) which distort the base line of the electrocardiogram. The effect of electrical interference is shown in Figure 8.8A. Note the difference in clarity of the pattern once the interference from external voltage had been eliminated (Fig. 8.8B). Electrical interference may arise from improper grounding of equipment or from loose connections.

When electrical interference occurs, the first step is to determine if electrode contact is secure and if all connecting wires are firmly in place. Failure to eliminate interference with these measures suggests improper grounding of other electrical equipment being used. Frequent or persistent electrical interference may indicate a defect in the wiring system in the CCU. (An electrical engineer should be consulted in this circumstance, particularly since the problem may represent an electrical hazard to the patient.)

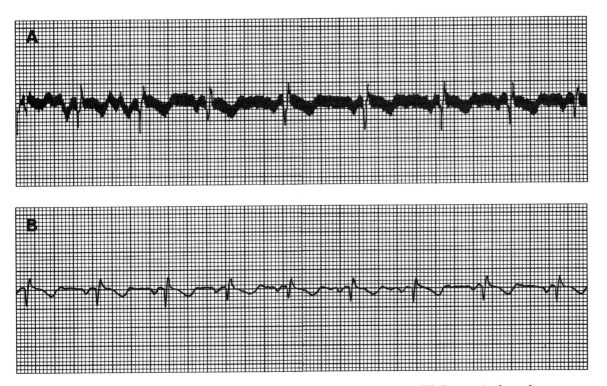

Figure 8.8(A). Interference from an external source such as a power line. **(B).** Pattern is clear after interference is eliminated.

Wandering Base Line

At times the electrocardiographic pattern displayed on the oscilloscope may wander up and down on the screen (Fig. 8.9). This movement, called a wandering base line, makes it difficult to identify arrhythmias, particularly when part of the pattern moves completely off the screen. These excursions are generally produced by motion of the patient (e.g., turning in bed) or simply by respiration. When the problem is caused by body movement, the fluctuation is transient and can be corrected by adjusting the "po-

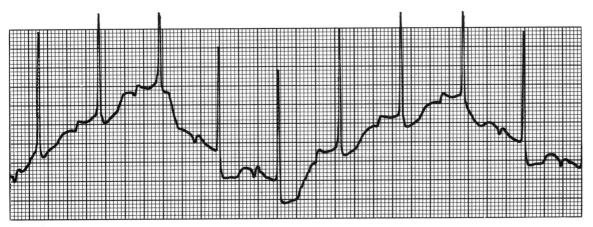

Figure 8.9. Wandering base line.

sition" dial to center the electrocardiogram. A wandering base line caused by respiratory motion usually has a cyclic pattern related to inspiration and expiration. In such cases the electrodes should be repositioned away from the lowest ribs to minimize the effect of chest wall movement.

Skin Irritation

Because electrodes must remain attached to the skin for several days, inflammatory reactions at these sites are not uncommon. This skin irritation may develop from the adhesive that secures the electrodes or from the conductive jelly. Disposable electrodes are less likely to produce skin reactions because the adhesive material is usually hypoallergenic and the jelly less irritating. If inflammation does develop about the electrode site, the area should be treated with an emollient or anesthetic cream, and the electrode repositioned a few inches away. Regardless of the electrode used it is important to examine the electrode sites at regular intervals to determine if skin irritation is present.

Electrical Hazards

Until recently there were no uniform safety standards for electronic equipment, and therefore with some monitors (particularly older models) patients may be exposed to electrical hazards. The main threat is that leakage current may pass from the monitor to the patient, particularly when more than one piece of equipment is being used. For example, if a temporary transvenous pacemaker has been positioned in the heart, leakage current from the monitor may travel down the pacing catheter to the heart and induce ventricular fibrillation! It is mandatory that *all* electrical equipment be designed in a way to avoid electrical hazards of this kind. Moreover, the grounding system within the coronary unit must be wholly effective in its purpose. As a safety precaution, electrically powered beds should not be used for patients who are being monitored.

TELEMETRIC MONITORING

It is possible to record the heart's electrical activity without direct wires from the electrodes to the monitor. This method is called telemetric monitoring. It works as follows: the wires from the skin electrodes are connected to a small battery-operated radio (FM) transmitter, about the size of a cigarette package, which is attached to the patient's gown or worn around the neck. The transmitter sends the electrical signals to a receiver by means of a radio beam. The receiver then feeds the signal into a standard monitor. The major value of this technique is that the patient can be monitored even though he is not in the CCU; in fact, he can be on a different floor of the hospital far removed from the recording equipment. Many institutions use telemetric monitoring to detect unexpected arrhythmias that may develop after the patient has been transferred from the CCU.

Electrocardiograms can also be transmitted by telephone so that monitoring can be accomplished from hundreds of miles away if necessary. The telephone number of the receiving station in the CCU is dialed and a special transmitter sends the signals through the telephone line to the monitor. Rescue squads sometimes use telephonic monitoring when assistance or advice is needed from hospital personnel.

9

The Electrocardiographic Basis of Arrhythmias

Because arrhythmias can be positively identified only by means of an electro-cardiogram (ECG) it is essential that CCU nurses acquire a fundamental, usable knowledge of electrocardiography. The object of this and the following chapters is to provide a basic understanding of the electrocardiographic detection and interpretation of arrhythmias.*

FUNDAMENTALS OF ELECTROCARDIOGRAPHY

Impulse Formation

Each normal heartbeat is the result of an electrical impulse that originates in a specialized area in the wall of the right atrium called the *sinoatrial (SA) node*. This island of tissue serves as a "battery" for the heart and normally discharges an electrical force 60 to 100 times a minute in rhythmic fashion. Because the SA node controls the heart rate it is designated the *pacemaker*. However, most other areas of the heart have the potential ability to initiate impulses (an inherent property of cardiac muscle), but they assume this role only under abnormal circumstances. Whenever the SA node is replaced in its normal pacemaking function the new site of impulse formation is called an *ectopic* pacemaker.

Conduction of Impulse

The original impulse is transmitted through the heart to the ventricles along an orderly path called the *conduction system*. When the impulse reaches the ventricular muscles, contraction occurs.

The electrical conduction from the SA node to the contractile cells of the ventricle is seen in Figure 9.1.

---

* When we conceived the nurse-centered system of intensive coronary care it was our impression that nurses required a comprehensive course in electrocardiography not unlike that offered to house officers. Experience has shown, however, that an overly detailed training program is unnecessary and that nurses can fulfill their roles successfully with considerably less instruction than we anticipated. The following discussion therefore focuses only on those aspects of electrocardiography that permit the nurse to assume clinical responsibilities in the CCU.

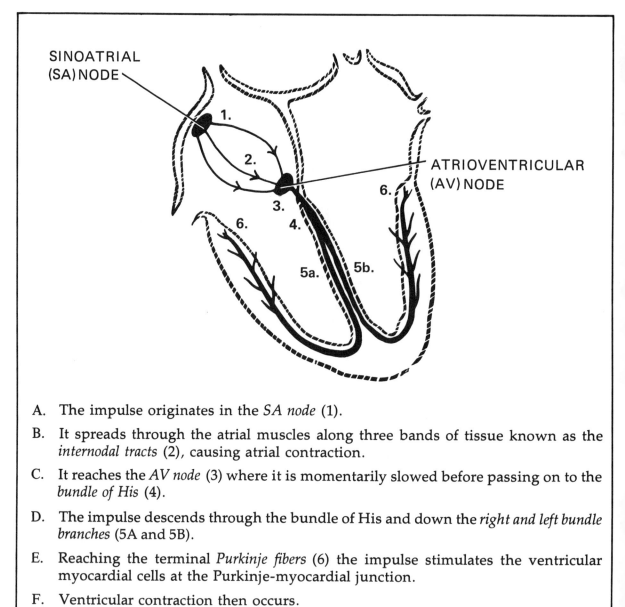

A. The impulse originates in the *SA node* (1).

B. It spreads through the atrial muscles along three bands of tissue known as the *internodal tracts* (2), causing atrial contraction.

C. It reaches the *AV node* (3) where it is momentarily slowed before passing on to the *bundle of His* (4).

D. The impulse descends through the bundle of His and down the *right and left bundle branches* (5A and 5B).

E. Reaching the terminal *Purkinje fibers* (6) the impulse stimulates the ventricular myocardial cells at the Purkinje-myocardial junction.

F. Ventricular contraction then occurs.

Figure 9.1.

The Cardiac Cycle

When the Purkinje-myocardial cells are stimulated there is a discharge of electrical forces stored within the myocardial cells. This electrical process is called *depolarization*; it results in ventricular contraction. After depolarization the muscle cells recover and re-store electrical energy. This recovery process is called *repolarization*. Under normal circumstances the next impulse from the SA node arrives when repolarization is complete; activation then occurs again. The combined periods of stimulation (depolarization) and recovery (repolarization) constitute the *cardiac cycle*.†

---

† The discharge and the storage of electrical forces within the myocardial cells during depolarization and repolarization is associated with a chemical process involving the exchange of sodium and potassium ions across the myocardial cell membrane. This subject is discussed in Chapter 18.

THE ELECTROCARDIOGRAM

Each portion of the cardiac cycle is characterized by changes in the electrical activity of the heart. The original impulse from the SA node, the conduction through the heart, the stimulation of muscles, and the recovery period can be correlated with the flow of electrical forces at the particular instant. That the heart's electrical activity could be detected and measured has been known since the early 1900s when Willem Einthoven used a sensitive string galvanometer—called an electrocardiograph—for this purpose.

The basis of electrocardiography is straightforward: The electrical forces within the heart are transmitted outward to the surface of the body where they can be detected with electrodes attached to the extremities. The ebb and flow of these forces cause upward and downward deflections in a galvanometer. The resultant waves are then amplified (for greater visibility) before being recorded on a moving piece of graph paper. In this way a continuous "picture" of the electrical activity during the cardiac cycle is achieved; this recording is called an electrocardiogram.‡

Electrocardiographic Leads

Because the electrical forces generated by the heart travel in multiple directions simultaneously it is necessary to record the flow of current in several planes if a comprehensive view of the heart's electrical activity is to be obtained. There are three major planes for detecting electrical activity, called lead I, lead II, and lead III, which are recorded by placing electrodes on the right arm, left arm, and left leg, respectively. (In practice, a fourth electrode is placed on the right leg; it serves as a ground electrode and is not part of an electrical lead.) Each of the three leads records the difference in electrical forces between two electrode sites. As shown in Figure 9.2, lead I is derived

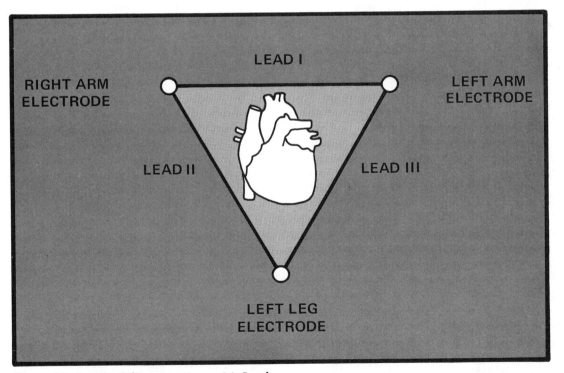

Figure 9.2. Standard Electrocardiographic Leads.

---

‡ The instrument which detects and amplifies the electrical waves from the heart is called an electrocardiograph. The printed record from the electrocardiograph is an electrocardiogram.

from electrodes on the right arm and left arm; lead II from electrodes on the right arm and left leg; and lead III from electrodes on the left arm and left leg. From an electrical standpoint, a hypothetical triangle (called the Einthoven triangle) is formed by these three leads with the heart in the center. In other words, each lead is electrically equidistant from the heart.

Since the leads record electrical forces in three different planes, it is understandable that an ECG obtained from each lead will have a different appearance. An example of the variation of electrocardiographic patterns in leads I, II, and III (recorded simultaneously) is depicted in Figure 9.3.

To understand why the electrocardiographic deflections (waves) differ in the three leads it is necessary to consider briefly a fundamental principle of electricity: Electrical current flows between two poles (or electrodes), one of which is positive (+) and the other negative (−).

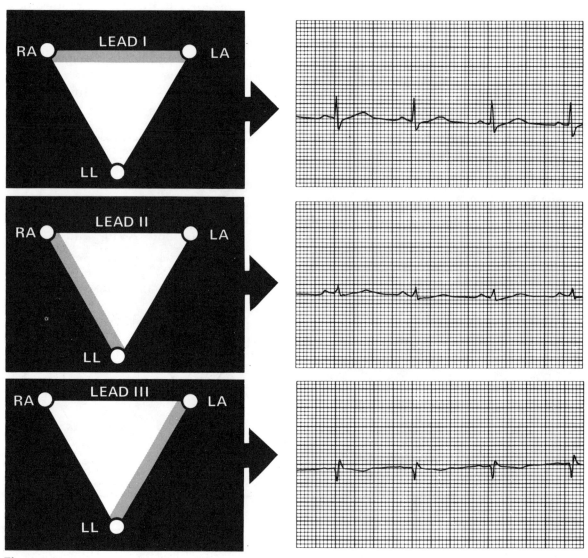

Figure 9.3.

When the current flows *toward* the positive pole, the electrocardiograph will record an upward (positive) deflection:

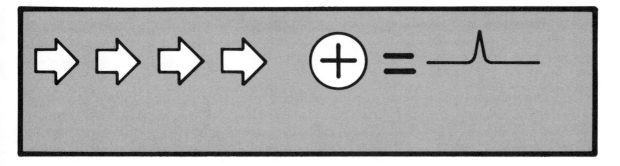

Conversely, when the current flows *away* from the positive electrode, the electrocardiograph will record a downward (negative) deflection:

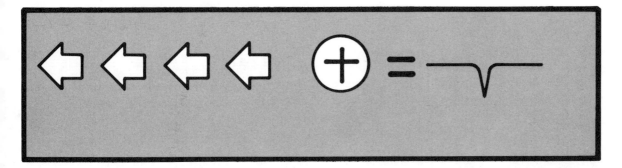

The respective positions of the positive (+) and negative (−) electrodes in leads I, II, and III are shown in Figure 9.4. Thus the deflections (waves) observed on an ECG depend on which lead is being recorded.

A complete electrocardiograph consists of 12 separate leads: the 3 standard leads (I, II, and III), 3 modified (augmented) leads (AVR, AVL, and AVF), and 6 leads positioned across the chest wall (V_1, V_2, V_3, V_4, V_5, and V_6). A full 12-lead electrocardiogram is reproduced in Figure 9.5. Note that each lead produces a different electrocardiographic pattern because of the variation of the electrode positions.

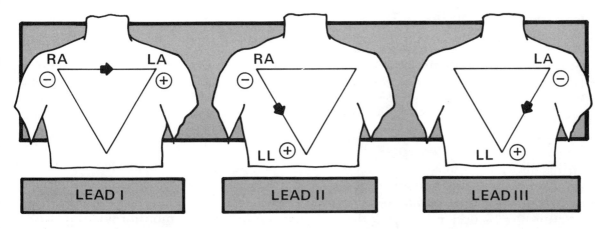

Figure 9.4. Positions of positive (+) and negative (−) electrodes for lead I, lead II, and lead III. *RA*, right arm. *LA*, left arm. *LL*, left leg.

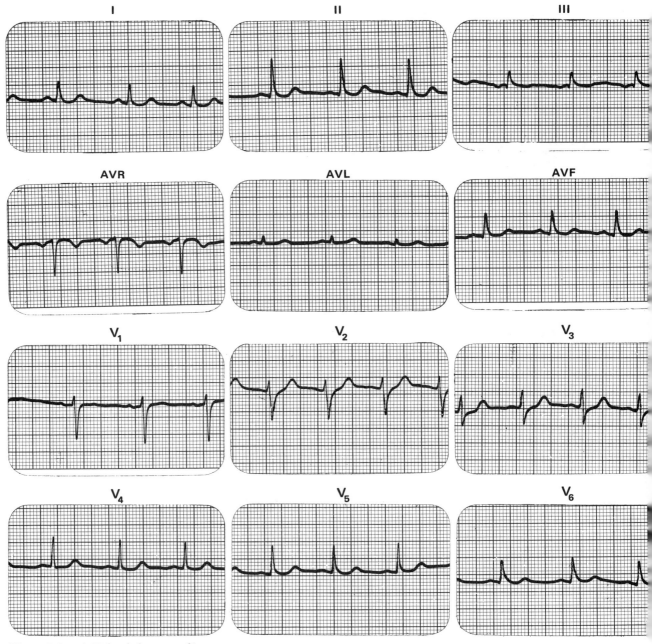

Figure 9.5. A 12-lead electrocardiogram.

Monitoring Leads

Cardiac monitors depict only a single lead, which is determined by the position of the positive and negative electrodes attached to the chest wall. Using the conventional electrode position the resultant lead is similar to standard lead II. With a modified chest electrode position the lead is equivalent to lead V_1. While these two chest leads are the most useful for detecting the majority of arrhythmias, by no means can they identify all rhythm disturbances. It is important to recognize this limitation of cardiac monitoring and when the interpretation of an arrhythmia is in doubt the chest leads may have to be repositioned (to obtain a more distinctive lead) or a 12-lead electrocardiogram should be obtained.

It must also be understood that the ECG seen on the cardiac monitor will depend on which particular lead is being used; therefore attempting simply to memorize certain patterns as a means of identifying arrhythmias is of no avail. For example, the ECGs shown in Figure 9.6 were recorded simultaneously from a conventional (lead II) monitoring lead and from a modified (V_1) lead. The difference in the appearance of the wave forms in the two leads makes it readily apparent that memorizing patterns is not a useful way to learn the interpretation of arrhythmias.

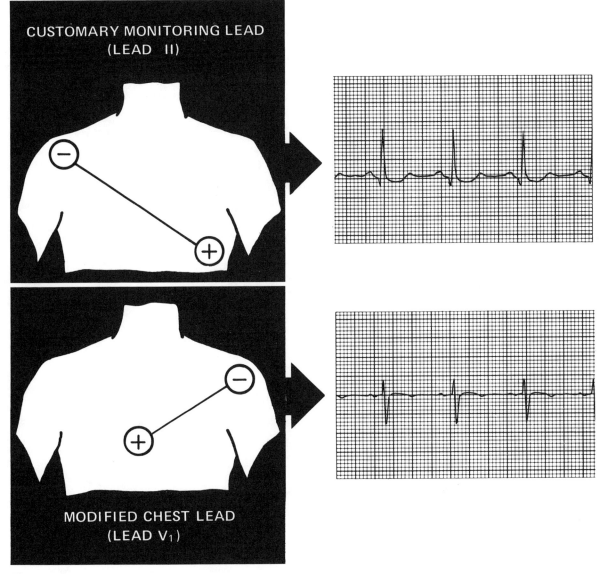

Figure 9.6.

ELECTROCARDIOGRAPHIC WAVE FORMS

The electrical activity during the cardiac cycle is characterized by five separate waves or deflections which are designated as P, Q, R, S, and T; these letters were arbitrarily selected and have no additional meaning. Before considering the meaning of each of these deflections it is necessary to discuss two key features of electrocardiographic waves: their amplitude (or voltage) and their duration.

Amplitude (voltage) is measured by a series of horizontal lines on the ECG. Each horizontal line is 1 millimeter apart and represents one-tenth of a millivolt (the basic

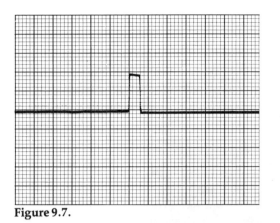

Figure 9.7.

unit of intensity of the heart's electrical activity). Thus in Figure 9.7 we see that the deflection extends nine lines (9 millimeters) above the baseline; this indicates that the voltage of the wave is 0.9 millivolt. The amplitude of the wave reflects only its electrical force and has no relation to the muscular strength of ventricular contraction.

Duration of a wave is measured by a series of vertical lines, also 1 millimeter apart. The time interval between each vertical line is 0.04 second. Accordingly, the width of the deflection shown in Figure 9.7 extends for 3 millimeters and represents 0.12 second (0.04 × 3).

The relationship between voltage and time is demonstrated in the ECG in Figure 9.8.

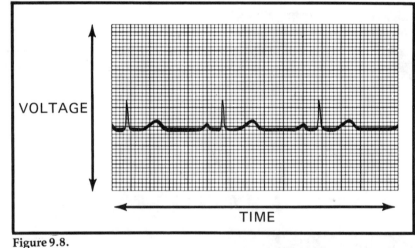

Figure 9.8.

To simplify the measurement of the wave forms, every *fifth* line, both horizontally and vertically, is inscribed boldly, producing a series of larger squares. These large squares then represent 0.5 millivolts vertically and 0.20 second horizontally, as shown in Figure 9.9.

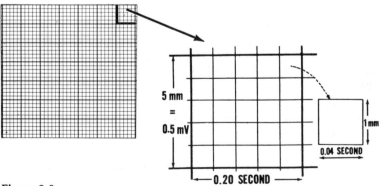

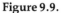

Figure 9.9.

Configuration of the Normal Electrocardiogram

The electrical pattern of the normal cardiac cycle is seen in Figure 9.10.

The meaning and significance of each of the waves and time intervals must be thoroughly understood in order to interpret an ECG.

P Wave

This wave represents electrical activity associated with the original impulse from the SA node and its passage through the atria.

If P waves are present and are of normal size and shape it can be assumed that the stimulus began in the SA node. If these waves are absent or abnormally positioned, it implies the impulse originated outside the SA node. Therefore the identification of P waves is of critical importance in differentiating normal sinus rhythm from *ectopic* rhythms.

PR Interval

The period from the start of the P wave to the beginning of the QRS complex is designated as the PR interval. It represents the time taken for the original impulse to pass from the SA node, through the atria and AV node, to the ventricles.

With normal conduction the duration of this interval is 0.20 second or less. If the duration of the PR interval exceeds 0.20 second it can be reasoned that a conduction delay (block) exists in the area of the AV node (or less likely, below the AV node). In some instances the PR interval is unusually short (less than 0.12 second), which indicates that the impulse reached the ventricle through a shorter-than-normal (accessory) pathway (Wolff-Parkinson-White syndrome).

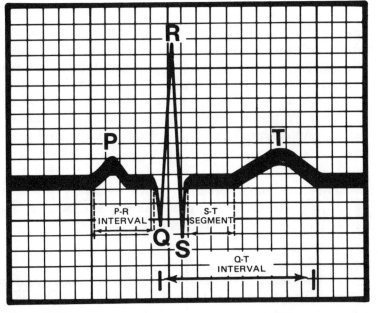

Figure 9.10.

QRS Complex

These waves represent depolarization of the ventricular muscle. The depolarization process starts at the endocardium of the ventricle and progresses outward to the epicardial surface. This results in a complex consisting of an initial downward deflection (Q wave), a tall upward deflection (R wave), and a second downward deflection (S wave). These three deflections comprising the QRS complex vary in size according to the lead being recorded. For example, there may be a tall R wave and a small S wave (Fig. 9.11A) or a small R wave and a deep S wave (Fig. 9.11B). In many instances, again depending on lead placement, one or more of the three components of the QRS complex may not be seen. For instance, in Figure 9.11C the complex does not include a Q wave.

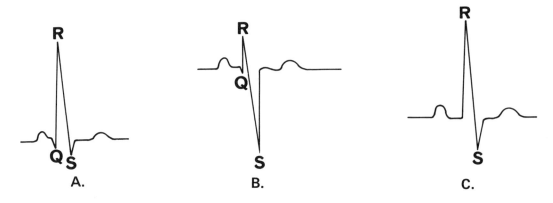

A. B. C.

Figure 9.11.

The QRS interval is measured from the beginning of the Q wave to the end of the S wave. (If a Q wave, R wave, or S wave is absent the QRS complex is measured from the beginning to the end of the remaining waves.) The normal duration of the QRS complex is always *less* than 0.12 second. When the duration of the complex is 0.12 second or more it indicates that the ventricles have been stimulated in a delayed or abnormal manner (e.g., a bundle branch block).

ST Segment

This interval describes the period between the completion of depolarization and the beginning of repolarization (recovery) of the ventricular muscles. Normally this segment is *isoelectric*, meaning it is neither elevated nor depressed because the positive and negative forces are equally balanced during this period. Elevation or depression of the ST segment indicates an abnormality in the onset of recovery of the ventricular muscle, usually because of injury (e.g., acute myocardial infarction). Examples of isoelectric, depressed, and elevated ST segments are shown in Figure 9.12.

T Wave

This wave represents the major portion of the recovery phase after ventricular contraction. Any condition which interferes with normal repolarization (e.g., myocardial ischemia) may cause the T waves to invert.

QT Interval

This interval defines the total duration of the combined phases of depolarization and repolarization of the ventricular muscle. In other words, it represents the total period of ventricular stimulation and recovery.

The QT interval is measured from the *beginning* of the QRS complex to the *end* of the T wave. The interval varies with heart rate, but with normal sinus rhythm the duration seldom exceeds 0.40 second.

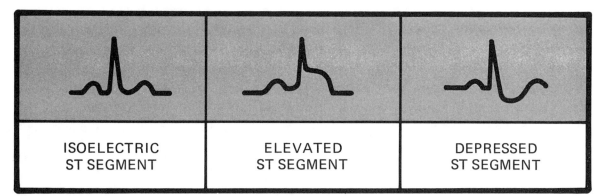

| ISOELECTRIC ST SEGMENT | ELEVATED ST SEGMENT | DEPRESSED ST SEGMENT |

Figure 9.12.

Significance of the Electrocardiogram

By analyzing the wave forms and intervals just described certain deductions can be made which offer indirect information about the heart. It is important to realize that the ECG does not depict the actual physical condition of the heart or its function; it simply reveals the electrical activity of the heart. Thus an ECG may be normal in the presence of heart disease unless the pathologic process actually disturbs the electrical forces. For example, a patient may have coronary atherosclerosis which has not produced myocardial ischemia or injury and, consequently, no abnormality will be seen on the ECG.

The ECG does, however, have a relationship with the systolic and diastolic phases of ventricular action as shown in Figure 9.13. Note that ventricular contraction (systole) begins at the peak of the QRS complex after electrical stimulation has occurred and ends near the completion of the T wave. Diastole commences at this time and continues until the next R wave.

Electrocardiography has many valuable uses in medical practice, but its major importance is in the diagnosis of acute myocardial infarction and the identification of abnormal cardiac rhythms.

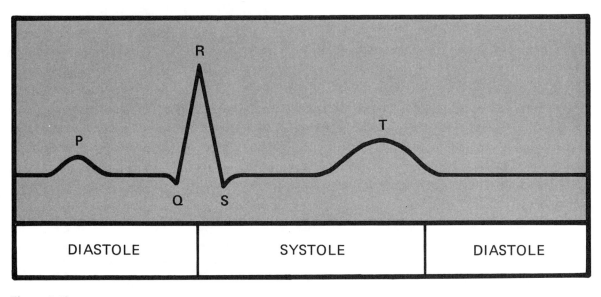

| DIASTOLE | SYSTOLE | DIASTOLE |

Figure 9.13.

ARRHYTHMIAS

The normal ECG consists of a repetitive series of P, Q, R, S, and T waves, all conforming to established standards for size and shape, and occurring at regular intervals at a rate of 60–100/minute. If these conditions exist it can be concluded that there are no abnormalities in the heart's electrical activity and that the heart is in normal sinus rhythm (Fig. 9.14). When either the rate, rhythm, or contour of the individual waves does not meet normal standards, the disorder is called an *arrhythmia.*§

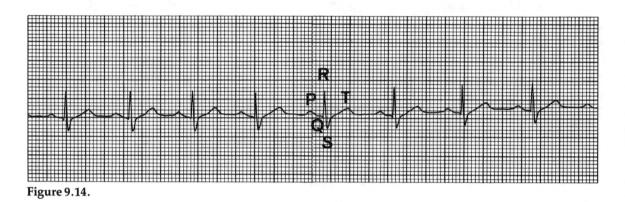

Figure 9.14.

Classification of Arrhythmias

There are several ways to categorize arrhythmias, but perhaps the most logical method is to separate the disorders into two main classes:

1. disturbances of impulse formation
2. disturbances of conduction

The basis of this classification is readily understandable. We know that under normal conditions the SA node generates impulses rhythmically at a rate of 60–100/minute and that each impulse is transmitted to the ventricles causing a ventricular contraction. Therefore if the heart rate is slower than 60/minute or faster than 100/minute, or if the heartbeat is irregular, the problem can be attributed to one of two primary causes: Either the impulses are not being *formed* properly (i.e., too fast, too slow, or irregularly) or else there is a disturbance in the *conduction* system which interferes with the passage of the impulse to the ventricle.

Disturbances of Impulse Formation

Arrhythmias due to disturbances of impulse formation are classified according to the site of origin and the mechanism of the disturbance.

The major sites of origin of impulse formation arrhythmias are:

SA node (sinus rhythms)
Atria (atrial rhythms)
AV nodal area (nodal or junctional rhythms)
Ventricles (ventricular rhythms)

---

§ In a strict sense the term arrhythmia indicates the absence of a normal rhythm and might be restricted to this one type of disturbance. In practice, however, the term is used collectively to describe all forms of abnormalities of the heartbeat, including disturbances in rate, rhythm, and conduction. Nevertheless, some linguists feel that the well-established term *arrhythmia* should be discarded and replaced with the broader word *dysrhythmia*. It seems to us that a change in terminology at this late date for the sake of linguistic purism serves no purpose and can only lead to confusion. Therefore throughout this book we have retained the term arrhythmia.

The major mechanisms are:

Tachycardia (rate greater than 100 beats/minute)
Bradycardia (rate less than 60/minute)
Premature beats
Flutter
Fibrillation

On this basis, the term *sinus tachycardia* indicates that the impulse originated normally in the SA node but that the heart rate is greater than 100 beats/minute (tachycardia). By comparison, *ventricular tachycardia* also describes a rapid-rate arrhythmia but one that originated in the ventricle rather than the SA node.

A full classification of arrhythmias due to disturbances in impulse formation and to disturbances of conduction appears in Table 9.1. Each of these arrhythmias is considered individually in Chapters 10 through 16.

Disturbances of Conduction

A conduction disturbance refers to an abnormal delay or block in the passage of the cardiac impulse from the SA node through the Purkinje fibers in the ventricle. Blocks may occur at any point along the course of the conduction system, but it is customary to classify these defects according to three main anatomic sites:

1. Blocks within the SA node or atria (SA blocks)
2. Blocks between the atria and ventricles (AV blocks)
3. Blocks within the ventricles (intraventricular blocks)

These major blocks are subgrouped as shown in Table 9.1.

Table 9.1. Classification of the Most Common Cardiac Arrhythmias

Arrhythmias Due to Disorders in Impulse Formation	Arrhythmias Due to Conduction Disturbances
Sinoatrial (SA) Node Arrhythmias	***Sinoatrial Block***
Sinus Tachycardia	
Sinus Bradycardia	***Atrioventricular (AV) Blocks***
Sinus Arrhythmia	First-Degree AV Block
Wandering Pacemaker	Second-Degree AV Block
Sinoatrial Arrest	Third-Degree (Complete) AV Block
Atrial Arrhythmias	***Intraventricular Blocks***
Premature Atrial Contractions	Left Bundle Branch Blocks
Paroxysmal Atrial Tachycardia	Right Bundle Branch Blocks
Atrial Flutter	Bilateral Bundle Branch Blocks
Atrial Fibrillation	*Ventricular Standstill*
Atrial Standstill	
AV Nodal Area (Junctional) Arrhythmias	
Premature Junctional Contractions	
Passive Junctional Rhythm	
Paroxysmal Junctional Tachycardia	
Nonparoxysmal Junctional Tachycardia	
Ventricular Arrhythmias	
Premature Ventricular Contractions	
Ventricular Tachycardia	
Ventricular Fibrillation	

Classification of Arrhythmias by Prognosis

In addition to the method just described, arrhythmias can also be classified in a general way (but not categorically) according to their seriousness or prognosis (Table 9.2). This division of arrhythmias is useful to nurses caring for patients with acute myocardial infarction since it describes the relative importance of various arrhythmias from a clinical standpoint. It is essential to realize, however, that this classification offers no more than a broad index of seriousness and is not truly dependable. Using this classification arrhythmias may be considered in three general groups.

Minor Arrhythmias

These disorders are not of *immediate* concern because they usually do not affect the circulation nor do they warn of the development of more serious arrhythmias.

Major Arrhythmias

These disturbances either reduce the pumping efficiency of the heart or herald the onset of lethal arrhythmias. They require prompt treatment.

Death-Producing Arrhythmias

These are lethal arrhythmias and require immediate resuscitation in order to prevent death.

Table 9.2. Classification of Arrhythmias According to Prognosis

Minor Arrhythmias
  Sinus Tachycardia
  Sinus Bradycardia
  Sinus Arrhythmia
  Wandering Pacemaker
  Premature Atrial Contractions
  Premature Junctional Contractions
  Premature Ventricular Contractions (when infrequent)

Major Arrhythmias
  Sinus Tachycardia (when persistent)
  Sinus Bradycardia (when rate is 50 or less per minute)
  Sinoatrial Arrest or Block
  Atrial Tachycardia
  Atrial Flutter
  Atrial Fibrillation
  Passive Junctional Rhythm
  Paroxysmal Junctional Tachycardia
  Nonparoxysmal Junctional Tachycardia
  Premature Ventricular Contractions (when frequent or in pairs)
  Ventricular Tachycardia
  First-Degree AV Heart Block
  Second-Degree AV Heart Block
  Third-Degree (Complete) Heart Block
  Bundle Branch Block

Death-Producing Arrhythmias
  Ventricular Fibrillation
  Ventricular Standstill

Interpretation of Arrhythmias from the Electrocardiogram

There are five basic steps which assist in the identification of arrhythmias. The ECG should be studied in an orderly fashion in the following manner:

Step 1. Calculate the heart rate. Three methods can be used to obtain the rate per minute:

a. Count the number of R waves in a 6-inch strip of the ECG tracing (which equals 6 seconds). Multiply this sum by 10 to get the rate per minute. Since the electro-cardiographic paper is marked into 3-inch (3-second) intervals (at the top margin), the approximate heart rate can be rapidly calculated.

b. Commercially available rate calculators, which measure the distance between R waves, may be placed on the ECG and the heart rate read directly from the scale.

c. Divide the number of large squares (0.20 second) between two R waves into 300 to obtain the approximate rate per minute.

On the basis of heart rate alone, arrhythmias can be classified as: a) slow rate *(bradyar-rhythmias)*, where there are less than 60 beats/minute; b) normal rate arrhythmias, where the rate is between 60–100 beats/minute; and c) fast rate *(tachyarrhythmias)*, where there are more than 100 beats/minute. Since several arrhythmias are character-ized only by rate changes, rate calculation is essential in interpreting any ECG.

Step 2. Measure the regularity (rhythm) of the R waves. This can be done by simple ob-servation or by actually measuring the intervals. If the R waves occur at regular intervals (with a variance of less than 0.12 second between beats) the ventricular rhythm is nor-mal. When the difference in R-R intervals is greater than 0.12 second, the ventricular rhythm is said to be irregular. This division of ventricular rhythm into regular and ir-regular categories assists in identifying the mechanism of many arrhythmias.

Step 3. Examine the P waves. If P waves are present, are of normal shape, and precede each QRS complex, the heartbeat originates in the sinus node and a sinus rhythm exists. The absence of P waves or an abnormality in their configuration or their position with respect to the QRS complex indicates that the impulse started outside the SA node and that an ectopic pacemaker is in command.

Step 4. Measure the PR interval. Normally this interval should be between 0.10–0.20 second. Prolongation or reduction of this interval beyond these limits indicates an ab-normality in the conduction system between the atria and the ventricles.

Step 5. Measure the duration of the QRS complex. If the width between the onset of the Q wave and the completion of the S wave is greater than 0.12 second (three fine lines on the ECG paper), an intraventricular conduction defect exists.

The Interpretation of Specific Arrhythmias

By following the five steps just outlined arrhythmias can be categorized as due to disturbances in impulse formation or disturbances in conduction and then identified specifically by name.

The application of the orderly analysis of an electrocardiogram is shown in the following example (Fig. 9.15):

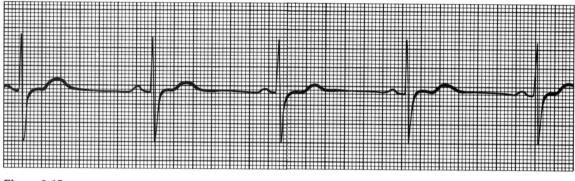

Figure 9.15.

1. *Rate.* Note that there are five R waves in the 6-inch ECG strip. This means that the heart rate is about 50/minute (5 × 10). Since this rate is less than the normal range of 60–100/minute, a slow-rate arrhythmia (bradyarrhythmia) is present.

2. *Rhythm.* The R-R intervals are equal. We know therefore that this arrhythmia is characterized by a regular rhythm.

3. *P waves.* A P wave appears before each QRS complex and is normal in shape. This means that the impulse originated in the SA node.

4. *PR interval.* This interval measures 0.18 second, which is within the normal limits (0.10–0.20 second). On this basis we can conclude that conduction from the SA node to the ventricle was not disturbed.

5. *QRS complex.* These complexes are 0.10 second in duration, indicating that there is no defect in conduction through the bundle branches or Purkinje network.

Analyzing these facts we can conclude that the only abnormality noted on the ECG is a rate of less than 60/minute. Since there are no disturbances in conduction (the PR interval and QRS complexes are normal), we know that the slow rate is the result of a *disturbance in impulse formation*. Because of the presence of normal P waves before each QRS complex the problem can be localized to the SA node, which is discharging at a rate that is too slow. Therefore the interpretation of the arrhythmia is sinus bradycardia.

Another demonstration of the five basic steps used in arrhythmia interpretation is presented below (Fig. 9.16):

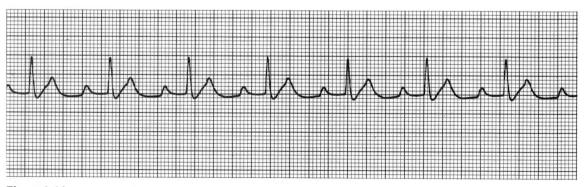

Figure 9.16.

1. *Rate.* The heart rate is about 70/minute (seven R waves in 6 seconds × 10) and is normal.

2. *Rhythm.* The R waves occur at regular intervals, and therefore the rhythm is regular.

3. *P waves.* These waves are readily apparent before each QRS complex, indicating a normal sinus rhythm.

4. *PR interval.* The time from the beginning of the P wave to the onset of the QRS complex measures 0.24 second. This time interval is prolonged, exceeding 0.20 second.

5. *QRS complex.* These complexes are 0.08 second in duration.

Based on this information it can be reasoned that impulse formation was normal since the impulses originated in the SA node in a regular rhythm at a rate of 80/minute. However, the PR interval is definitely prolonged (0.24 second), which indicates that there was a delay in conduction of the impulses somewhere between the SA node and the ventricles. That the duration of the QRS complex is normal tells us that once the impulse reached the intraventricular network ventricular activation proceeded normally thereafter. The problem in this case is a *disturbance in conduction* called a first-degree atrioventricular (AV) block, the details of which are described subsequently.

Specific Arrhythmias

Chapters 10 through 16 describe and give examples of arrhythmias due to impulse formation disorders and conduction disturbances in the following sequence:

Impulse Formation Disturbances
1. Arrhythmias originating in the SA node (Chapter 10).
2. Arrhythmias originating in the atria (Chapter 11).
3. Arrhythmias originating in the AV nodal area (Chapter 12).
4. Arrhythmias originating in the ventricles (Chapter 13).
5. Ventricular fibrillation (Chapter 14).

Conduction Disturbances
1. Blocks originating in the SA node or atria (Chapter 15).
2. Blocks originating in the AV node (Chapter 15).
3. Blocks originating below the AV node (Chapter 15).
4. Ventricular standstill (Chapter 16).

The ECGs depicted in these chapters were taken directly from cardiac monitors by a direct write-out mechanism; they represent the patterns the nurses actually observed when documenting the arrhythmias.

It is important to realize that all of the patients from whom these ECGs were recorded had acute myocardial infarction, and that many of them were receiving various drugs when the tracings were taken. As a result, most of the electrocardiographic examples show these effects in addition to the arrhythmia itself. While "pure" forms of the arrhythmias could have been used for these teaching purposes, we believe it is much wiser to present the arrhythmias as they are actually seen in a CCU.

The methods of treatment for the individual arrhythmias described in the following chapters are those we currently employ on our own service and should not be construed as universally accepted regimens. Although these forms of treatment have been widely adopted there is nevertheless a difference of opinion in some centers about the ideal treatment for several of the arrhythmias. A detailed description of the actions and methods of use of the most common antiarrhythmic drugs is found in Chapter 18.

10

Arrhythmias Originating in the Sinoatrial (SA) Node

Sinus Tachycardia
Sinus Bradycardia
Sinus Arrhythmia
Wandering Pacemaker
Sinoatrial Arrest (and SA Block)

This group of arrhythmias results from disturbances of impulse formation in the SA node.

The SA node retains its normal role as pacemaker, but instead of discharging impulses at regular intervals 60–100 times/minute the rate either exceeds 100/minute (sinus tachycardia) or is less than 60/minute (sinus bradycardia), or the node does not discharge rhythmically (sinus arrhythmia). In some instances the pacemaker site wanders from the SA node to nearby areas (wandering pacemaker). If the SA node fails to discharge an impulse, the arrhythmia is called sinus arrest.

Impulse formation in the SA node is under the control of the sympathetic and parasympathetic nervous systems. Overactivity of one of these normally balanced forces leads to disturbances in rate, rhythm, or site of impulse formation. When the sympathetic system is dominant the heart rate speeds, and when the parasympathetic system (vagal influence) is in control the rate slows. The node itself is seldom the source of these arrhythmic disturbances.

As a general rule sinus node disorders are not dangerous and can be considered as minor arrhythmias. However, if the heart rate is very slow (less than 50/minute) or very fast (greater than 130/minute) the risk is significantly increased, in which case the arrhythmia would be classified as a major arrhythmia.

SINUS TACHYCARDIA

Etiology

The SA node is the pacemaker and discharges impulses at a rate faster than 100/minute. This acceleration in heart rate often reflects overactivity of the sympathetic nervous system resulting from fever, anxiety, or physical activity. Of greater importance, sinus tachycardia may be a manifestation of heart failure. In this situation the heart rate increases through reflex mechanisms to compensate for reduced stroke volume.

Clinical Features

1. Occasionally the patient may describe palpitations and dyspnea; however, in most instances sinus tachycardia does not produce any symptoms.
2. The only pertinent finding is a rapid, regular heart rate, usually 100–150 beats/minute. An ECG is required to distinguish sinus tachycardia from other fast-rate arrhythmias.
3. When sinus tachycardia returns to normal rhythm it does so gradually, in contrast to other tachycardias (e.g., paroxysmal atrial tachycardia), which may cease abruptly.

Danger in Acute Myocardial Infarction

1. Tachycardia tends to increase the work of the heart and its oxygen consumption. This expenditure may lead to left ventricular failure or additional myocardial ischemia (angina).
2. *RISK:* The danger depends primarily on the etiology of the rapid heart rate. When sinus tachycardia is due to anxiety, fever, or physical activity, the risk is usually not great. On the other hand, if sinus tachycardia develops as a consequence of left ventricular failure, the danger is distinctly increased and the prognosis then varies with the cardiac reserve and the duration of the tachycardia.

Treatment

1. The first step in treatment is to identify the underlying cause of the arrhythmia rather than attempt to slow the rate. Always to be considered is the possibility that sinus tachycardia represents a sign of early left ventricular failure.
2. Once the cause of sinus tachycardia is recognized, treatment is directed at correction of the basic problem. For example, when the rapid rate is due to temperature elevation, aspirin may be effective; or if the tachycardia is secondary to anxiety, tranquilizers or sedatives may be helpful in reducing the rate.
3. If sinus tachycardia leads to ischemic pain (angina), opiates may be indicated.
4. When sinus tachycardia is due to left ventricular failure, administration of digitalis is usually effective in controlling the heart rate (as well as increasing the force of myocardial contraction).
5. Drug therapy aimed solely at reducing the heart rate, without consideration of the underlying cause of sinus tachycardia, is ill advised and of little use.

Nursing Role

1. Identify the rapid-rate arrhythmia as sinus tachycardia and document it with a rhythm strip.
2. Examine the patient at regular intervals, always seeking possible causes for the arrhythmia (e.g., elevated temperature, apprehension).
3. When the source of sinus tachycardia cannot be readily identified, be suspicious that left ventricular failure exists and attempt to elicit other evidence of early heart failure (e.g., orthopnea, cough, restlessness).
4. If the patient develops symptoms secondary to the arrhythmia or if the clinical signs vary, the physician should be notified.
5. Discuss the use of sedatives, tranquilizers, aspirin, and digitalis with the physician.
6. If anxiety seems to be the cause of sinus tachycardia, attempt to alleviate the emotional stress through nursing intervention.

Case History

A 42-year-old male had been in the CCU for 2 days with a stable pulse rate ranging from 75–90/minute. An ECG showed an acute anterior infarction with normal sinus rhythm. While his wife was visiting, the patient became obviously upset and the monitor showed sinus tachycardia at a rate of 130/minute. The nurse assessed the clinical condition of the patient and could find no change other than the rapid heart rate. She calmed the patient by talking with him and continued to assess the heart rate. In addition she administered an ordered sedative. One hour later the pulse rate was 90/minute.

SINUS TACHYCARDIA—IDENTIFYING ECG FEATURES

1. **Rate:** Usually 100–150 beats/minute.
2. **Rhythm:** Regular.
3. **P waves:** Normal. (If the rate is very rapid, the P waves may not be clearly identified because they may encroach on the preceding T waves.)
4. **PR interval:** Normal, indicating that conduction from the SA node through the ventricles is not disturbed.
5. **QRS:** Normal.

EXAMPLE: Sinus Tachycardia (Fig. 10.1)

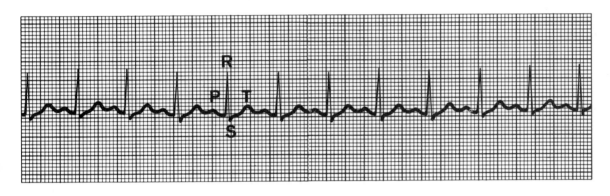

INTERPRETATION OF ECG

Rate:	About 120/minute.
Rhythm:	Regular.
P waves:	Normal.
PR interval:	Normal (0.16 second), and each P wave is followed by a normal QRS complex.
QRS:	Normal (width is 0.06 second).
Comments:	Other than the rapid rate there are no abnormalities.

EXAMPLE: Sinus Tachycardia (Fig. 10.2)

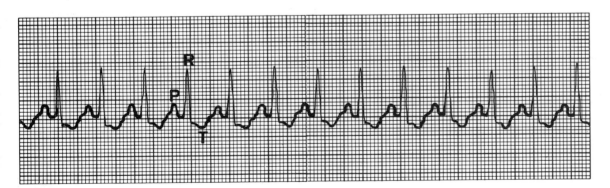

INTERPRETATION OF ECG

Rate:	About 130/minute.
Rhythm:	Regular.
P waves:	Normal.
PR interval:	Normal (0.16 second).
QRS:	Normal (0.06 second).
Comments:	The T waves are inverted, reflecting myocardial ischemia.

SINUS BRADYCARDIA

Etiology

The SA node is the pacemaker and discharges at a rate slower than 60 times/minute. Sinus bradycardia is particularly common during the first few hours after acute infarction. The slow rate is usually the result of parasympathetic (vagal) dominance of the SA node secondary to either myocardial ischemia, pain, drugs, or other factors.

Clinical Features

1. Sinus bradycardia seldom produces symptoms unless the rate is slow enough to reduce cardiac output.
2. The only physical sign is a slow, regular heart rate, usually 40–60 beats/minute.

Danger in Acute Myocardial Infarction

1. The greatest threat of sinus bradycardia is that it may allow a faster ectopic focus to take over as pacemaker. In this way serious ventricular arrhythmias may develop when a slow heart rate is present.
2. If the cardiac output falls because of the slow rate, cerebral and coronary blood flow may become insufficient and result in syncope and angina.
3. Sinus bradycardia, when extreme, may be a prelude to SA node arrest; however, this sequence is not common.
4. *RISK:* Sinus bradycardia is associated with several potential arrhythmic and hemodynamic complications (especially within the first few hours of the attack) and for this reason must be regarded as an important *warning* arrhythmia.

Treatment

1. Sinus bradycardia should be treated under the following circumstances:
   a. if there are any signs or symptoms indicating a reduction in cardiac output (syncope, hypotension, angina, or heart failure)
   b. if premature ventricular contractions develop during the period of bradycardia
   c. if the rate is less than 50/minute, particularly in elderly patients or those with previous myocardial damage
2. Atropine, which blocks the vagal effect on the SA node, is highly effective in accelerating the heart rate and should be the initial therapy. The drug is given intravenously in a dosage of 0.5–1.0 mg.
3. If atropine is unsuccessful, isoproterenol (Isuprel) will often increase the heart rate. This agent is administered by a slow intravenous infusion containing 1 mg isoproterenol in 500 cc glucose solution.
4. If drug therapy fails, or if its effect is short lived, temporary transvenous pacing may be required to maintain a normal heart rate.
5. Drugs with known bradycardic effects such as digitalis, reserpine, morphine, or propranolol (Inderal) should be avoided or discontinued in the presence of sinus bradycardia.

Nursing Role

1. Carefully review the ECG to ascertain that the slow rate is due to sinus bradycardia rather than another cause such as heart block or nodal (junctional) rhythm. Document the arrhythmia.
2. Record the heart rate at frequent intervals for comparative purposes; this is particularly important after drug therapy is initiated.
3. Assess the patient's clinical course in a planned manner to determine if there are signs or symptoms of decreased left ventricular performance.
4. Observe the ECG pattern repeatedly for evidence of premature ventricular contractions. If these occur, notify the physician immediately.
5. If the heart rate falls below 50/minute, advise the physician.

Case History

A 78-year-old man was brought to the CCU 1 hour after an episode of severe chest pain. On admission the blood pressure was 90/60 and the pulse rate 48/minute. On the monitor frequent premature ventricular beats were noted. The nurse notified the physician of these findings. Atropine (0.6 mg) was administered intravenously and within 5 minutes the blood pressure rose to 114/76, the heart rate increased to 76/minute, and the premature ventricular contractions lessened.

SINUS BRADYCARDIA—IDENTIFYING ECG FEATURES

1. **Rate:**   Usually 40–60/minute, but may be slower.
2. **Rhythm:**   Regular.
3. **P waves:**   Normal.
4. **PR interval:** Normal, and each P wave is followed by a normal QRS complex.
5. **QRS:**   Normal.

EXAMPLE: Sinus Bradycardia (Fig. 10.3)

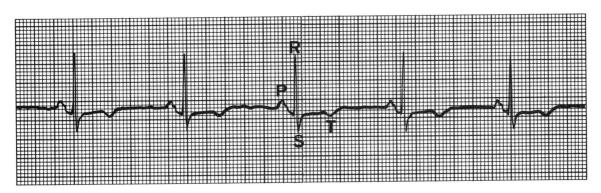

INTERPRETATION OF ECG

Rate: About 50/minute.
Rhythm: Regular.
P waves: Normal.
PR interval: Normal (0.16 second).
QRS: Normal (0.08 second).
Comments: The inverted T waves are not related to the arrhythmia; they result from myocardial ischemia.

EXAMPLE: Sinus Bradycardia (Fig. 10.4)

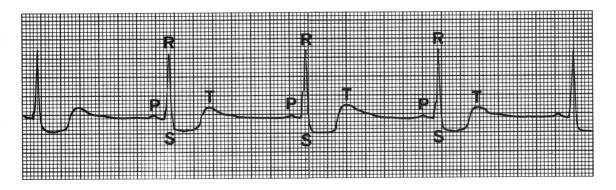

INTERPRETATION OF ECG

Rate: About 50/minute.
Rhythm: Regular.
P waves: Normal.
PR interval: Normal (0.14 second), and each P wave is followed by a QRS complex.
QRS: Normal (width is 0.08 second).
Comments: There is deep sagging of the ST segment, representing myocardial injury.

SINUS ARRHYTHMIA

Etiology

In sinus arrhythmia the impulses arise from the SA node but not in a completely regular rhythm. The irregularity of discharge is due to variation of vagal influence on the SA node, resulting in *alternating* periods of slow and fast rates. In most instances this effect is related to the phases of respiration with the rate increasing with inspiration and slowing with expiration.

Clinical Features

1. The pulse is irregular, but the patient is unaware of this minor disturbance in rhythm.
2. The diagnosis of sinus arrhythmia can only be verified with an ECG but it may be suspected clinically if a change in heart rate occurs with deliberate breath-holding.

Danger in Acute Myocardial Infarction

1. Sinus arrhythmia causes no hemodynamic effects, nor does it warn of more serious arrhythmias. Consequently it can be regarded as an unimportant and nondangerous arrhythmia.
2. *RISK:* None.

Treatment

No treatment is indicated.

Nursing Role

1. Ascertain that the irregular rhythm is due to sinus arrhythmia and document with an ECG strip.
2. Make certain that the irregularity is not a manifestation of a more serious arrhythmia (e.g., atrial fibrillation).

Case History

A 70-year-old woman was admitted to the unit with a typical history of acute myocardial infarction. While taking the patient's pulse the nurse noted an irregular rhythm. From the monitor she recognized that the problem was sinus arrhythmia and recorded this finding on the admission sheet. The arrhythmia persisted all during the patient's stay in the CCU. No treatment was given for this minor arrhythmia.

SINUS ARRHYTHMIA—IDENTIFYING ECG FEATURES

1. **Rate:** The heart rate per minute is normal (60–100); however, the rate increases during inspiration and then slows during expiration.
2. **Rhythm:** Irregular. There is a variation of at least 0.12 second between the longest and shortest R-R intervals.
3. **P waves:** Normal.
4. **PR interval:** Normal. Each P wave is followed by a normal QRS complex.
5. **QRS:** Normal width.

EXAMPLE: Sinus Arrhythmia (Fig. 10.5)

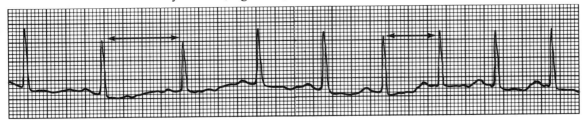

INTERPRETATION OF ECG

Rate: About 90/minute.
Rhythm: Irregular. The time varies more than 0.12 second between the longest and shortest R-R intervals. (Compare distance between arrows indicating R-R intervals.)
P waves: Normal.
PR interval: Normal (0.20 second), and each P wave is followed by a QRS complex.
QRS: Normal.
Comments: The flat or inverted T waves are due to myocardial ischemia and are unrelated to the arrhythmia.

EXAMPLE: Sinus Arrhythmia (Fig. 10.6)

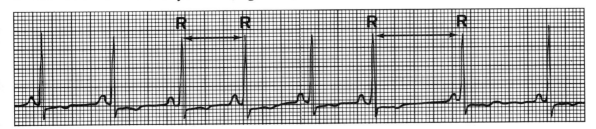

INTERPRETATION OF ECG

Rate: About 80/minute.
Rhythm: There is a variation in R-R intervals of more than 0.12 second.
P waves: Normal.
PR interval: Normal (0.12 second).
QRS: Normal (0.04 second).
Comments: The short R-R intervals occur during inspiration, and the long R-R intervals during expiration.

WANDERING PACEMAKER

Etiology

The SA node remains the basic pacemaker, but at times the impulse may originate in different portions of the node, or the pacemaker may actually wander from the SA node to the atria or the AV nodal area. This shifting of the impulse site within the SA node to the atria or the AV nodal tissue is usually related to vagal influences, and a wandering pacemaker is a variant of sinus arrhythmia in this respect.

Clinical Features

A wandering pacemaker produces no symptoms or signs and can be recognized only by ECG.

Danger in Acute Myocardial Infarction

1. There is no particular danger from a wandering pacemaker. The arrhythmia usually reflects fluctuating depression of the SA node by vagal influence.
2. *RISK:* None.

Treatment

1. No treatment is needed in most instances.
2. If depression of the SA node permits the AV node (junctional tissue) to dominate the pacemaker role, atropine can be used to block the vagal influence.
3. If a wandering pacemaker develops during digitalis therapy, the drug may be withheld temporarily to see if the arrhythmia is drug related and will disappear with cessation of digitalis.

Nursing Role

1. When a wandering pacemaker is noted on the monitor, document the arrhythmia with a rhythm strip.
2. Observe the ECG subsequently to verify that the SA node has not relinquished complete control to the atria or AV nodal area.

Case History

On the second day after admission to the CCU a 56-year-old man with an acute inferior wall infarction developed ECG evidence of a wandering pacemaker. The nurse noted that the configuration of the P waves varied at different times and realized that the pacemaker site was changing during these periods. Because these episodes were infrequent and since the SA node remained the dominant pacemaker, the nurse concluded that the problem was not serious and no treatment was given.

WANDERING PACEMAKER—IDENTIFYING ECG FEATURES

1. **Rate:** Usually normal but may be slow (because of vagal dominance).
2. **Rhythm:** Regular.
3. **P waves:** As the pacemaker wanders within the SA node or to the atria or AV node, the shape and position of the P waves vary, reflecting the different sites of origin of the impulse.
4. **PR interval:** The conduction time to the AV node depends on the site of impulse formation. Therefore the PR interval may vary slightly depending on the location of the pacemaker.
5. **QRS:** Normal. Conduction from the AV node to the ventricle is normal, so there is a normal QRS complex regardless of the size, shape, or position of the P waves.

EXAMPLE: Wandering Pacemaker (Fig. 10.7)

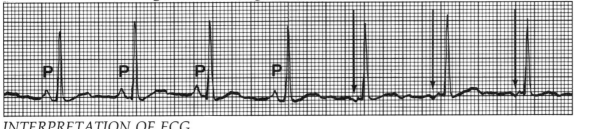

INTERPRETATION OF ECG

Rate: About 70/minute.
Rhythm: Regular.
P waves: The first four beats show normal P waves originating in the SA node. The last three complexes show abnormal P waves; the pacemaker has left the SA node.
PR interval: Normal (0.16 second).
QRS: Normal (0.06 second).
Comments: The pacemaker wanders between the SA and AV nodes as indicated by the change in P waves.

EXAMPLE: Wandering Pacemaker (Fig. 10.8)

INTERPRETATION OF ECG

Rate: About 70/minute.
Rhythm: Regular.
P waves: There is a change in shape and position of the P waves from the first to the last complexes.
PR interval: The PR interval varies in the last four beats. The interval cannot be measured in the first three beats because the pacemaker is in the AV nodal area and the P waves are obscured.
QRS: Normal (0.10 second).
Comments: The pacemaker was originally in the AV nodal area and moved progressively to the SA node.

SINOATRIAL ARREST (AND SA BLOCK)

Etiology

Under certain circumstances the SA node fails to initiate an impulse at the expected time in the cardiac cycle. In the absence of this impulse neither the atria nor ventricles are stimulated and the entire PQRST complex drops out for one beat. This is called *sinoatrial (SA) arrest*. In other instances the impulse is initiated normally but is blocked *within* the node and fails to reach the atria. Again, the complete PQRST complex is absent. This condition is designated as *SA block*. Although SA arrest is a disturbance of impulse formation and SA block a disturbance of conduction, they cannot be clinically distinguished from one another, and the two terms are used interchangeably. Sinoatrial arrest (or block) may result from excessive vagal dominance of the node or digitalis toxicity; however neither of these factors are probably as important as ischemic injury of the SA node.

Clinical Features

1. Patients may notice prolonged pauses in the heartbeat and describe this sensation; however, most are unaware of the arrhythmia.
2. The only physical finding is a prolonged pause detected while taking the pulse or listening to the heartbeat.
3. If the missed beats occcur frequently or consecutively, cerebral insufficiency manifested as syncope or vertigo may develop.

Danger in Acute Myocardial Infarction

1. When infrequent, SA arrest is not of great importance and usually reflects vagal overactivity.
2. Repeated episodes of SA arrest or very prolonged pauses between beats suggests ischemic damage to the SA node, a condition that is potentially dangerous.
3. When related to overdosages of digitalis (or quinidine), the arrhythmia assumes special significance since the drug may lead to further depression of SA node activity and result in atrial standstill.
4. *RISK:* SA arrest is usually not serious, but it is potentially dangerous when the episodes are repetitive or prolonged as the result of ischemic damage or drug overdoses.

Treatment

1. If SA arrest occurs only occasionally the condition is usually self-limiting and requires no treatment.
2. If the periods of SA arrest are frequent or prolonged, atropine (0.5–1.0 mg intravenously) will frequently restore normal SA impulse formation or conduction by inhibiting vagal effect on the SA node. Isoproterenol can also be used for this purpose.
3. If SA arrest does not subside spontaneously or fails to respond to drug therapy, a transvenous pacemaker should be inserted.
4. If SA arrest occurs in patients receiving digitalis or quinidine, these drugs should be discontinued promptly.

Nursing Role

1. When SA arrest is noted, document the arrhythmia with a rhythm strip.
2. If SA arrest becomes frequent or if more than two consecutive beats are missed, notify the physician promptly.
3. If SA arrest develops in patients receiving digitalis or quinidine, further dosages of these drugs should be withheld until reordered by the physician.

Case History

   A 61-year-old man was admitted to the CCU with an acute inferior infarction. On examining the patient the nurse noted that the pulse was 50/minute and occasionally irregular. The ECG revealed sinus bradycardia with episodes of SA arrest. In some instances there were as many as three missed beats in a row. The physician ordered atropine (1 mg intravenously), which promptly accelerated the heart rate and restored normal sinus function.

SINOATRIAL ARREST (AND SA BLOCK)—IDENTIFYING ECG FEATURES

1. **Rate:**   Usually slow (40–70/minute) but may be normal.
2. **Rhythm:**   The basic rhythm is normal except for the missing beats.
3. **P waves:**   No P wave with the missed beat since the SA node either did not discharge or the impulse failed to reach the atrium.
4. **PR interval:** The entire PQRST complex is missing for one or more beats during sinus arrest.
5. **QRS:**   No QRS complex is produced when the SA node impulse is absent or blocked.

EXAMPLE: Sinoatrial Arrest (or Block) (Fig. 10.9)

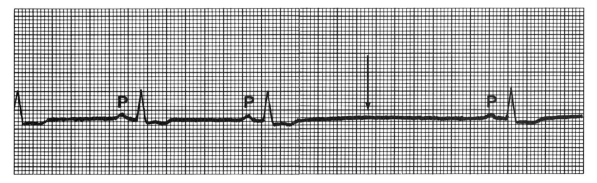

INTERPRETATION OF ECG

Rate: About 45/minute.
Rhythm: Sinus bradycardia with irregularity due to missed beat.
P waves: The P wave anticipated after the third complex is absent (see arrow).
PR interval: One PQRST complex is missing because of sinus node arrest or block.
QRS: There is no QRS complex in the absence of SA node impulses.
Comments: The SA node failed to discharge for one beat and then resumed its function.

EXAMPLE: Sinoatrial Arrest (or Block) (Fig. 10.10)

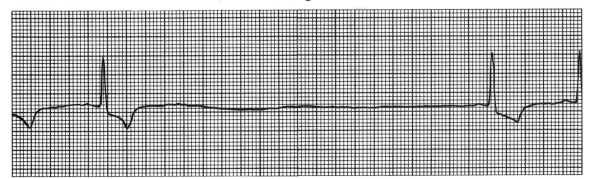

INTERPRETATION OF ECG

Rate: The underlying rate is about 60/minute.
Rhythm: The period of SA arrest creates an irregular rhythm.
P waves: Following the second QRS complex, P waves do not appear during a period equivalent to three anticipated beats.
PR interval: Three entire PQRST complexes are missing (missed beats).
QRS: Absent when the SA node failed to discharge.
Comments: The prolonged pause probably reflects serious ischemia of the SA node.

11

Arrhythmias Originating in the Atria

Premature Atrial Contractions
Paroxysmal Atrial Tachycardia
Atrial Flutter
Atrial Fibrillation
Atrial Standstill

As noted previously, the atria, the AV nodal area, and the ventricles all have the *potential* capacity to serve as pacemaker, but the SA node retains control because it normally discharges impulses at an inherently faster rate than the other sites. If for some reason a focus in the atrial walls initiates impulses more frequently than those arising from the SA node, the ectopic site in the atria replaces the SA node as pacemaker. This may occur for only one beat (premature atrial contraction) or continuously (atrial tachycardia, atrial flutter, or atrial fibrillation), depending on the degree and persistence of irritability of the abnormal focus.

When impulses originate in the atria, outside the SA node, at rates of *less than 200/minute*, the P waves are usually visible but are distorted in shape, indicating that the SA node is not in command. In this situation each impulse reaches the AV node and passes through to the ventricles without difficulty. Consequently a normal QRS complex follows each P wave (atrial tachycardia).

When the atria are stimulated *200–400 times/minute*, the AV node is unable to accept each impulse and blocks every second, third, or fourth atrial beat. The impulses that do pass the AV node are conducted normally thereafter to the ventricles. For example, in atrial flutter the atrial rate is two, three, or four times greater than the ventricular response and there are two, three, or four P waves between each normal QRS complex.

If the atria are stimulated at extremely fast rates (400–1000 times/minute), the atrial muscles are no longer capable of responding to these repetitive impulses and the individual fibers comprising the atrial muscle merely twitch, or *fibrillate*. The atria do not actually contract in this circumstance, and P waves are not seen. Because of this chaotic atrial activity, impulses reach the AV node at a rapid, irregular rate. The AV node blocks most of these rapid impulses, and those that pass to the ventricles do so at irregular intervals. Consequently the ventricular rhythm is irregular (atrial fibrillation).

Atrial arrhythmias result primarily from irritability of the atrial muscle usually caused by ischemic damage or by overdistention (stretching) of the atrial wall. Atrial rhythm disturbances associated with a rapid ventricular rate are categorized as major arrhythmias because they increase myocardial oxygen demand and also reduce pumping efficiency of the heart. These latter arrhythmias must not be allowed to persist; drug therapy or precordial shock should be used to terminate them promptly.

PREMATURE ATRIAL CONTRACTIONS

Etiology

When an ectopic focus in the atrium supersedes the SA pacemaker for one beat, a *premature atrial contraction* (PAC) results. These ectopic beats reflect irritability of the atrial muscle. Except for these isolated premature contractions the SA node remains as the basic pacemaker.

Clinical Features

1. Normally the patient is unaware of PACs; however, with a stethoscope a beat that occurs sooner than expected may be heard.
2. Positive identification can be made only by ECG.

Danger in Acute Myocardial Infarction

1. By themselves PACs have no particular significance, but they do indicate atrial irritability and may forewarn of impending serious atrial arrhythmias, e.g., paroxysmal atrial tachycardia or atrial fibrillation. When PACs increase beyond 6/minute, the arrhythmia assumes more importance in this regard.
2. *RISK:* PACs pose no immediate danger but may herald the onset of atrial fibrillation or other atrial arrhythmias.

Treatment

1. If PACs occur rarely and do not increase in frequency, treatment is usually unnecessary.
2. If the number of PACs increases during a period of observation, it is advisable to use antiarrhythmic drugs to control these ectopic beats. Quinidine, administered orally, is probably the most effective drug in this situation.

Nursing Role

1. Distinguish PACs from other causes of irregular heart rhythm and document their presence on an ECG.
2. Carefully observe the frequency of these premature beats for comparative purposes and advise the physician of any increase in the number of these beats.
3. Be aware that atrial fibrillation or other serious atrial arrhythmias may develop in the presence of frequent premature atrial beats.

Case History

A 62-year-old woman had occasional PACs during the first 24 hours after her admission. These occurred at a rate of 1–2/minute and were duly noted by the nurse and recorded as such on each hourly ECG strip. Early in the morning of the second day, the frequency of PACs increased to 4–5/minute and remained at that rate. The nurse advised the physician of this change during his visit, and quinidine therapy was started. Within 12 hours the arrhythmia was no longer evident.

┌─ PREMATURE ATRIAL CONTRACTIONS—IDENTIFYING ECG FEATURES ─┐

1. **Rate:**   Usually normal.
2. **Rhythm:**   After a PAC there is a slight delay (compensatory pause) before the next normal beat. This pause creates a mild irregularity in the cardiac rhythm.
3. **P waves:**   Either abnormally shaped or inverted, and differ from normal P waves originating in the SA node.
4. **PR interval:** Conduction from the atria to the ventricles (PR interval) is usually normal.
5. **QRS:**   Usually normal, indicating that there is no disturbance in intraventricular conduction.

EXAMPLE: Premature Atrial Contraction (Fig. 11.1)

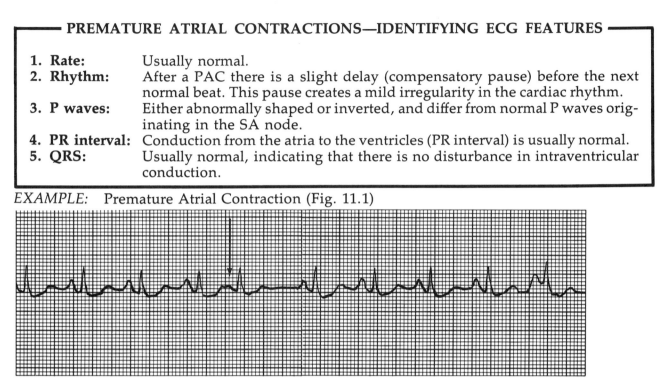

INTERPRETATION OF ECG

Rate: About 100/minute.
Rhythm: The premature complex and the pause that follows create a slight irregularity in the rhythm.
P waves: The P wave of the premature beat (arrow) is abnormally shaped and differs from the normal P waves originating in the SA node.
PR interval: Normal (0.12 second). The PAC originates in the atrium but is conducted normally through the His-Purkinje system.
QRS: Normal (0.08 second).
Comments: Isolated PACs are common and seldom pose a problem.

EXAMPLE: Premature Atrial Contraction (Fig. 11.2)

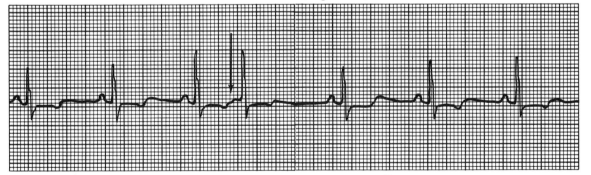

INTERPRETATION OF ECG

Rate: About 70/minute.
Rhythm: The normal rhythm is interrupted only by the premature beat.
P waves: Distorted with the premature beat (arrow); the remaining P waves are normal.
PR interval: Normal (0.16 second).
QRS: Normal (0.08 second).
Comments: A premature beat associated with a normal QRS complex indicates that the impulse originated in the atria (or AV nodal area). With a premature *ventricular* contraction the QRS complex is widened and distorted.

PAROXYSMAL ATRIAL TACHYCARDIA

Etiology

An irritable focus within the atrium but outside the SA node originates impulses at a rate of *150–250 times/ minute* and displaces the SA node as pacemaker. The ventricle is able to respond to each atrial impulse, and therefore the *atrial and ventricular rates are identical*.

Clinical Features

1. Characteristically paroxysmal atrial tachycardia (PAT) occurs *suddenly*, usually without warning, but may be preceded by premature atrial contractions.
2. Most patients are immediately aware of the rapid heart action and frequently describe a fluttering sensation in the chest or lightheadedness.
3. The arrhythmia is usually transient and ends *abruptly*, even without treatment.

Danger in Acute Myocardial Infarction

1. The rapid heart rate tends to reduce cardiac output because the volume of blood ejected with each contraction (stroke volume) is decreased as a result of the very short ventricular filling time between beats. The decrease in cardiac output may lead to left ventricular failure, particularly if the tachycardia is sustained.
2. The fast ventricular rate increases the demand for and consumption of oxygen by the myocardium. Consequently additional myocardial ischemia or angina may result. The longer that PAT persists, the greater the threat of further myocardial injury.
3. *RISK:* PAT is a dangerous arrhythmia with acute myocardial infarction but not an immediate cause of death. The risk is directly proportional to the duration of the arrhythmia.

Treatment

1. Initially an attempt should be made to terminate the arrhythmia by reflex vagal stimulation (e.g., carotid sinus massage). This technique is frequently effective.
2. If PAT cannot be terminated by vagal stimulation and the patient describes angina or symptoms of left ventricular failure, elective precordial shock (cardioversion) should be used promptly; this method seldom fails to restore sinus rhythm.
3. If the rapid rate does *not* produce obvious symptoms, drug therapy can be attempted. Morphine, given intravenously, or rapid-acting digitalis preparations (digoxin, Cedilanid-D) will often halt the arrhythmia.
4. If PAT occurs repetitively, prophylactic antiarrhythmia therapy is advisable. Quinidine, administered orally, is probably the most effective agent in this circumstance.

Nursing Role

1. The onset of PAT will trigger the high-rate alarm system of the monitor.
2. Examine the patient and verify the rapid pulse rate.
3. Document the arrhythmia with a rhythm strip.
4. Notify the physician immediately.
5. Assess the patient's clinical status, with particular reference to the presence of angina or signs of left ventricular failure. Record the blood pressure.
6. If the patient has signs or symptoms related to the arrhythmia, prepare for precordial shock (elective cardioversion).
7. Have appropriate drugs ready for use at the bedside.

Case History

A 55-year-old woman with an acute infarction had been in normal sinus rhythm for 48 hours after admission. At 4 PM the pulse rate was 82 and regular, and an hourly ECG strip taken by the nurse showed a normal sinus rhythm. At 4:10 PM the tachycardia alarm sounded and the monitor showed a heart rate of 160. At the bedside the nurse confirmed the rapid rate. The patient complained of chest pain and was obviously frightened. The nurse ran a rhythm strip and recognized PAT. She called the physician immediately and prepared for precordial shock. By the time the physician arrived several minutes later, the arrhythmia had stopped abruptly. In reviewing the rhythm strip it was apparent that the patient had a run of PAT which lasted for less than 3 minutes.

PAROXYSMAL ATRIAL TACHYCARDIA—IDENTIFYING ECG FEATURES

1. **Rate:**   150–250/minute.
2. **Rhythm:**   Regular.
3. **P waves:**   May not be visible (being buried in either the QRS complex or preceding T wave) or may be abnormally shaped.
4. **PR interval:** Typically a ventricular complex follows *each* P wave. The PR interval cannot be measured in many instances because the P waves are obscured.
5. **QRS:**   Usually normal but may be widened because of abnormal intraventricular conduction (aberrant conduction).

EXAMPLE: Paroxysmal Atrial Tachycardia (Fig. 11.3)

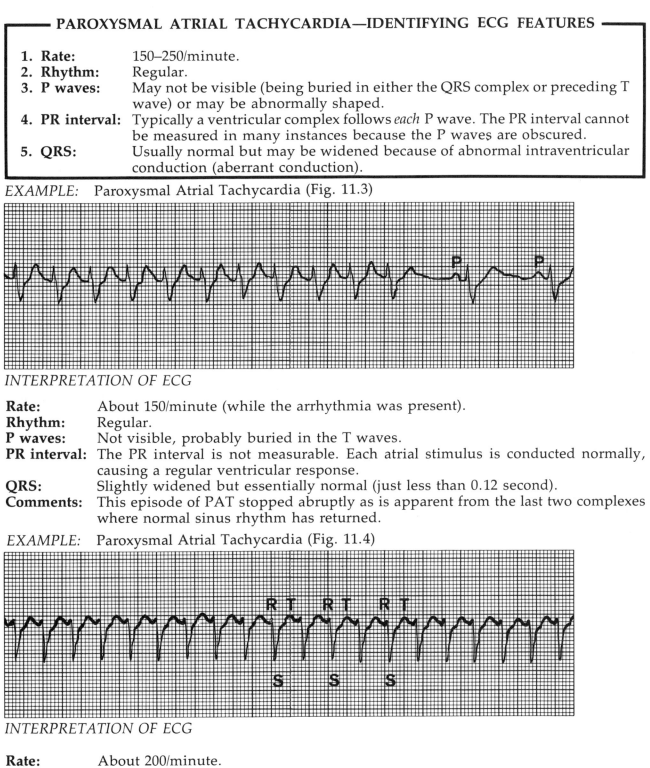

INTERPRETATION OF ECG

Rate: About 150/minute (while the arrhythmia was present).
Rhythm: Regular.
P waves: Not visible, probably buried in the T waves.
PR interval: The PR interval is not measurable. Each atrial stimulus is conducted normally, causing a regular ventricular response.
QRS: Slightly widened but essentially normal (just less than 0.12 second).
Comments: This episode of PAT stopped abruptly as is apparent from the last two complexes where normal sinus rhythm has returned.

EXAMPLE: Paroxysmal Atrial Tachycardia (Fig. 11.4)

INTERPRETATION OF ECG

Rate: About 200/minute.
Rhythm: Completely regular.
P waves: Not identified.
PR interval: Cannot be identified. Normal atrial and ventricular conduction.
QRS: Essentially normal. The small R waves and deep S waves are due to the position of the chest electrodes.
Comments: In this typical case each atrial impulse is followed by a QRS complex in a 1:1 relationship. Under certain conditions (especially digitalis toxicity) some atrial impulses may be blocked in the AV node and not conducted to the ventricles. Consequently every P wave is not followed by a QRS complex, and the 1:1 relationship is lost. The resulting arrhythmia is called PAT with block.

ATRIAL FLUTTER

Etiology

The SA node is replaced as the pacemaker by an extremely irritable focus within the walls of the atrium which stimulates the atria to contract *250–400 times/minute*. The AV node is unable to conduct all of these impulses but allows every second, third, or fourth impulse to reach the ventricle and cause depolarization and contraction. The ventricular rate is therefore determined by the degree of block in the AV node. For example, if the atrial rate is 300/minute and the AV node blocks every second impulse (2:1 block) the ventricular rate will be 150/minute.

Clinical Features

1. The occurrence of symptoms depends fundamentally on the ventricular rate. If the ventricular response is rapid (e.g., 150/minute) the patient may describe palpitations, angina, or dyspnea. If the ventricular rate is normal (e.g., with a 4:1 block) the arrhythmia may produce no signs or symptoms.
2. Atrial flutter can be identified only by means of an ECG.

Danger in Acute Myocardial Infarction

1. When atrial flutter is associated with a rapid ventricular rate, the cardiac output may be decreased and the myocardial oxygen consumption increased (as with other rapid-rate arrhythmias, e.g., PAT). This impairment predisposes left ventricular failure and additional myocardial ischemia.
2. If the ventricular rate is not increased, left ventricular performance may not be affected significantly.
3. *RISK:* Atrial flutter is a serious arrhythmia because of the potential hemodynamic consequences.

Treatment

1. Atrial flutter can be instantly terminated by precordial shock (cardioversion); very low discharge energies (less than 50 watt-seconds) are required. Because of its predictable effectiveness cardioversion should be the initial treatment, especially when the ventricular rate is rapid.
2. Drug therapy is seldom successful in restoring normal sinus rhythm. However, digitalis preparations are often used to control the ventricular rate (by increasing the degree of AV block). Other pharmacologic means for terminating atrial flutter (quinidine, propranolol) are of little use.

Nursing Role

1. When atrial flutter develops, the high-rate alarm may or may not sound, depending on the *ventricular* rate.
2. Identify the arrhythmia on the monitor and document with a rhythm strip.
3. Assess the patient's clinical status. Determine if the patient has angina or dyspnea. Record the blood pressure and pulse rate.
4. Notify the physician promptly after this arrhythmia is identified.
5. If the patient complains of angina or if there is evidence of left ventricular failure, prepare for elective cardioversion (see Chapter 17).
6. If digitalis or other drugs are used to treat atrial flutter, carefully record the heart rate and rhythm response.

Case History

   Six hours after admission to the unit, a 71-year-old man developed atrial flutter. This was noted by the nurse when the high-rate alarm sounded. The ventricular rate was 150/minute. The nurse went to the bedside and noted that the patient was apprehensive and dyspneic. She immediately notified the physician, and then recorded the blood pressure and pulse rate, and documented the arrhythmia. Anticipating that precordial shock would be used because of the circulatory impairment induced by the arrhythmia, the nurse prepared for the procedure. Cardioversion was accomplished as soon as the physician arrived, and normal sinus rhythm was restored. The patient's symptoms disappeared promptly.

ATRIAL FLUTTER—IDENTIFYING ECG FEATURES

1. Rate:	The *ventricular* rate may vary from 60 to 150, depending on the number of atrial impulses passing through the AV node.
2. Rhythm:	The ventricular rhythm is most often regular. However, as a result of changes in the degree of block in the AV node from time to time, the ventricular rhythm may become slightly irregular.
3. P waves:	There are characteristic atrial oscillations described as sawtooth waves which are easily identifiable. These waves (called F waves or flutter waves) occur regularly at a rate of 250–400/minute.
4. PR interval:	Only one-half, one-third, or one-fourth of the atrial impulses are conducted through the AV node and reach the ventricle. The resulting disparity between atrial and ventricular rates is described as atrial flutter with 2:1, 3:1, or 4:1 block. The PR interval (actually the FR interval) has no meaning and is not measured.
5. QRS:	The QRS complex is normal, indicating that conduction beyond the AV node is not disturbed.

EXAMPLE: Atrial Flutter (Fig. 11.5)

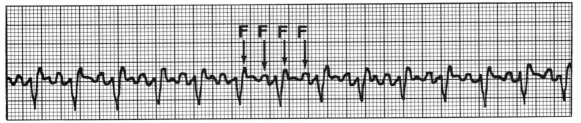

INTERPRETATION OF ECG

Rate:	About 80/minute.
Rhythm:	Regular.
P waves:	There are four F waves between each R wave (the first being buried in the T wave). Note the sawtooth appearance created by these waves.
PR interval:	Every fourth F wave is conducted to the ventricle while three are blocked in the AV node. This is designated as 4:1 block.
QRS:	Normal (0.08 second in width).
Comments:	The classical sawtooth appearance on the ECG typifies atrial flutter.

EXAMPLE: Atrial Flutter with 2:1 Block (Fig. 11.6)

INTERPRETATION OF ECG

Rate:	The *ventricular* rate is about 140/minute. The *atrial* rate is 280/minute.
Rhythm:	Regular.
P waves:	There are two F waves between ventricular complexes. These waves produce a sawtooth appearance but not as distinctively as in atrial flutter with 4:1 block (as in Fig. 11.5, above).
PR interval:	In the absence of P waves there is no PR interval. Every second atrial impulse is blocked in the AV node. This is called atrial flutter with 2:1 block.
QRS:	Normal.
Comments:	Atrial flutter with 2:1 block should always be suspected whenever a regular ventricular rate of 140–160/minute is observed.

ATRIAL FIBRILLATION

Etiology

Ectopic foci throughout the atria discharge impulses at a rate of 400–1000/minute. The atrial muscles are unable to respond or recover in a uniform way from this very rapid, irregular stimulation. Instead, the fibers comprising the atrial muscles respond individually, and as a result atrial contraction is wholly disorganized. The total effect is merely a twitching of the atrial walls rather than a true atrial contraction. In a sense the atria are no more than quivering tubes connecting the great veins with the ventricles, and they provide no assistance in filling the ventricles.

The extremely rapid impulses from the atria bombard the AV node, but the node can conduct only relatively few of these stimuli to the ventricular conduction system; the rest are blocked. The impulses that pass through the AV node do so at irregular intervals, creating an irregular ventricular rhythm.

The ventricular rate during atrial fibrillation may vary from 40–160/minute, depending on the number of impulses conducted through the AV node. When the ventricular response (rate) is more than 100/minute, atrial fibrillation is classified as rapid or uncontrolled.

Clinical Features

1. Most patients with atrial fibrillation are aware of the irregular heart action and describe palpitations or "skipping" of the heartbeat. This often disturbing sensation is usually more pronounced when the ventricular rate is rapid.
2. The grossly *irregular* rhythm is so characteristic of atrial fibrillation that this clinical finding by itself is almost diagnostic of the arrhythmia.
3. In most instances the peripheral pulse rate is slower than the heart (apical) rate. This *pulse deficit* results from variations in the volume of blood ejected with each ventricular contraction; at times the stroke volume is inadequate to produce a peripheral pulse.
4. If the ventricular rate is persistently rapid, evidence of left ventricular failure may be anticipated.

Danger in Acute Myocardial Infarction

1. The major danger of atrial fibrillation is a reduction in the pumping efficiency of the heart (decreased cardiac output). This inefficiency results not only from the rapid, irregular ventricular response but also from the loss of effective atrial contraction. (Normally the atrium serves as a booster pump for ventricular filling, and the loss of atrial contraction can cause a 20% reduction in cardiac output.) The resulting hemodynamic deficit may lead to left ventricular failure and additional myocardial ischemia.
2. During atrial fibrillation there is a propensity for clots to form within the noncontracting atria. Mural thrombi, with subsequent embolization in the circulatory system, may develop on this basis.
3. *RISK:* Atrial fibrillation is a dangerous arrhythmia from a hemodynamic standpoint, especially when the ventricular rate is rapid.

Treatment

1. Atrial fibrillation can be treated with either drug therapy or by electrical means (elective precordial shock). The choice depends on several factors: the ventricular rate, the duration of the arrhythmia, and above all the presence or absence of circulatory insufficiency as manifested by left ventricular failure or angina.
2. If a patient develops left ventricular failure or angina as a direct consequence of rapid atrial fibrillation, the arrhythmia should be terminated without delay by means of synchronized precordial shock (cardioversion) to restore normal sinus rhythm.
3. If atrial fibrillation is *not* accompanied by signs of impaired circulation, then drug therapy should be the primary method of treatment. Digitalis is the cornerstone of this program. The drug controls the rapid ventricular rate by increasing the degree of block at the AV node, but it usually does not restore normal sinus rhythm.
4. Quinidine can be used in an attempt to convert atrial fibrillation to normal sinus rhythm; although this drug is often successful, its effect may be too slow when acute left ventricular failure is present.
5. When atrial fibrillation is of longstanding duration (existing before the acute infarction) and is not associated with a rapid ventricular rate, attempts to restore normal sinus rhythm may not be indicated.

ATRIAL FIBRILLATION—IDENTIFYING ECG FEATURES

1. Rate: The ventricular rate may be normal (60–100/minute), rapid (greater than 100/minute), or slow (less than 60/minute), depending on the number of atrial impulses conducted to the ventricles.

2. Rhythm: The ventricular rhythm is totally irregular. This irregularity is the most typical finding of atrial fibrillation.

3. P waves: P waves are not present because of chaotic atrial activity. They are replaced by small, irregular, rapid oscillations called f (fibrillatory) waves.

4. PR interval: There is no PR interval. Most of the atrial impulses which bombard the AV node are blocked, but those that do pass through the node are conducted normally thereafter, although at irregular intervals. Thus the conduction pattern of atrial fibrillation is manifested by the absence of P waves and the presence of normal QRS complexes, occurring at totally irregular intervals.

5. QRS: Because conduction *below* the AV node is not affected, the QRS complexes are normal in shape and duration, but they occur irregularly.

EXAMPLE: Atrial Fibrillation (Fig. 11.7)

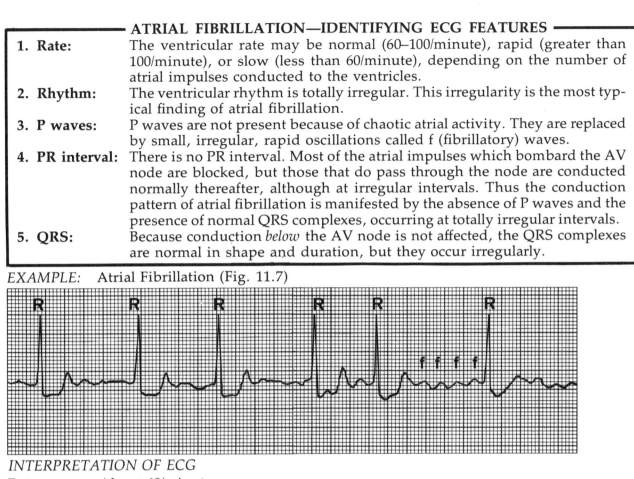

INTERPRETATION OF ECG

Rate: About 60/minute.

Rhythm: Grossly irregular.

P waves: Absent. Fibrillatory (f) waves of different sizes and shapes occur at irregular intervals.

PR interval: Absent. Most atrial impulses are blocked at the AV node, as is apparent from the ventricular rate of 60/minute.

QRS: Normal (0.04 second), indicating normal intraventricular conduction.

Comments: The most characteristic feature of atrial fibrillation is the irregular ventricular rhythm. This finding in conjunction with the absence of P waves confirms the diagnosis of atrial fibrillation.

Nursing Role

1. *If atrial fibrillation develops abruptly or is present and rapid at the time of admission:*
   a. Document the arrhythmia with a rhythm strip and notify the physician.
   b. Ascertain if the arrhythmia is compromising circulatory efficiency and inquire specifically if the patient has chest pain or dyspnea.
   c. Record the pulse rate, the extent of the pulse deficit, and the blood pressure.
   d. Prepare for elective cardioversion and have intravenous digitalis preparations at bedside.
2. *If atrial fibrillation is not rapid or if it existed before the present infarction:*
   a. Observe the patient's clinical status in a planned manner, always seeking evidence of left ventricular failure. Carefully record pulse rate, apical rate, and blood pressure.
   b. Obtain serial rhythm strips at regular intervals for comparative purposes.
   c. Advise the physician of any significant increase or decrease of the ventricular rate, or if signs or symptoms develop which suggest left ventricular failure.
3. If digitalis or quinidine is used to treat atrial fibrillation, observe the ECG for signs of drug overdosages (see Chapter 18). If the ventricular rate falls below 60/minute further administration of these drugs should be discussed with the physician.
4. Because of the possibility of embolization secondary to atrial fibrillation, this potential complication should always be considered during careful clinical assessment.

EXAMPLE: Rapid Atrial Fibrillation (Fig. 11.8)

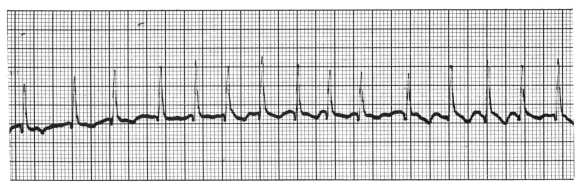

INTERPRETATION OF ECG

Rate: About 150/minute.
Rhythm: Irregular (note the differences in the R-R intervals).
P waves: Absent. The oscillations in the baseline represent f waves.
PR interval: The PR interval cannot be determined because of the absence of P waves. The AV node allows many atrial impulses to pass.
QRS: Normal (0.08 second).
Comments: The rapid ventricular response probably causes adverse hemodynamic effects and must be controlled promptly.

EXAMPLE: Rapid Atrial Fibrillation Being Controlled with Digitalis (Fig. 11.9)

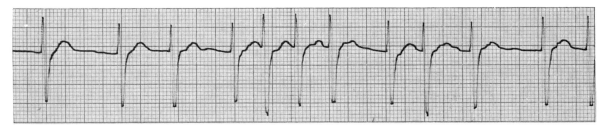

INTERPRETATION OF ECG

Rate: The average ventricular rate is about 120/minute.
Rhythm: Grossly irregular.
P waves: Absent. The f waves are of low amplitude and not clearly apparent in this lead.
PR interval: Not measurable because of absence of P waves. Atrial impulses are conducted through the AV node at varying intervals (a changing degree of AV block).
QRS: Essentially normal (0.10 second in most complexes).
Comments: Digitalis controls the ventricular rate in atrial fibrillation by increasing the degree of block at the AV node. In this instance digitalization is not complete, and the ventricular response is still rapid at times.

EXAMPLE: Atrial Fibrillation with a High Degree of AV Block (Fig. 11.10)

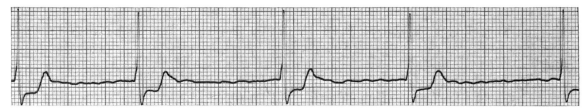

Comments: The very slow ventricular rate (about 50/minute) is the result of marked AV block. This high-degree AV block may be due to damage to the AV node or to excessive amounts of digitalis. In either case digitalis should not be used since the drug will tend to increase the block additionally and perhaps slow the rate even further.

Case History

A 68-year-old man was admitted to the CCU with acute pulmonary edema. The nurse initiated a planned treatment program which included morphine (15 mg intravenously), rotating tourniquets, the administration of oxygen, and an intravenous injection of furosemide. Although there was considerable improvement within the next hour, it was apparent that the left ventricular failure was not fully controlled. The pulse rate was 124 and irregular, and rales were heard throughout the entire chest. The ECG revealed rapid atrial fibrillation. It was felt that the decrease in cardiac output (which produced left ventricular failure) was related in part to the inefficient pumping action associated with atrial fibrillation. On this basis cardioversion was performed without additional delay. Immediately after the procedure the ventricular rate decreased to 84/minute and P waves were apparent on the ECG. There was marked improvement in the clinical course thereafter.

EXAMPLE: The Termination of Rapid Atrial Fibrillation by Means of Precordial Shock (Fig. 11.11)

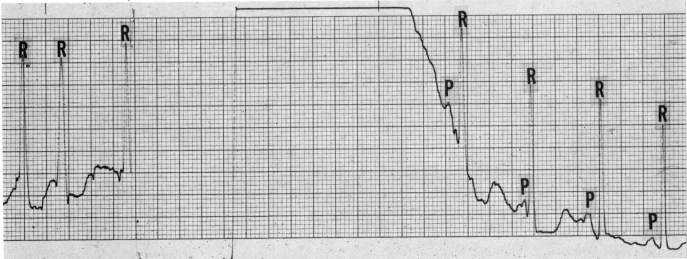

Comments: Synchronized precordial shock (cardioversion) was used to terminate the rapid atrial fibrillation. As noted on the rhythm strip, normal sinus rhythm was restored immediately after the shock (as is evident from the presence of P waves and the now regular ventricular rhythm).

EXAMPLE: Atrial Fibrillation—Flutter (Fig. 11.12)

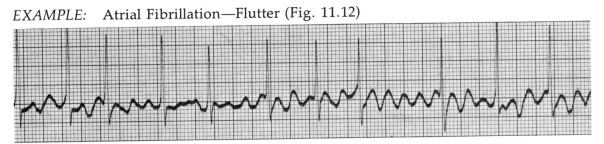

INTERPRETATION OF ECG

Rate: About 110/minute.
Rhythm: Irregular.
P waves: Absent, being replaced by sawtooth F waves of atrial flutter and irregular f waves of atrial fibrillation.
PR interval: Absent. Conduction below the AV node is normal.
QRS: Normal (0.08 second).
Comments: The atrial rhythm vacillates between atrial flutter and atrial fibrillation, reflecting the close relationship of these two arrhythmias.

ATRIAL STANDSTILL

Etiology

The SA node and the atrial muscles lose their capacity to generate any electrical impulses, and the pacemaking function is assumed by the AV nodal area or the ventricles. This failure of the atrial pacemaking centers usually develops in a progressive manner, first with loss of the SA node stimulus and then with loss of all atrial activity. When there is no longer any atrial activity, atrial standstill is said to exist. This sequence, in which the pacemaker descends progressively, is called *downward displacement of the pacemaker* and in most cases is a terminal arrhythmia associated with advanced left ventricular failure or cardiogenic shock.

Atrial standstill is seldom reversible, indicating that the atria have been severely damaged or destroyed by an ischemic process. Rarely, however, atrial standstill may develop from overdosages of digitalis or quinidine, or it may be a consequence of serious electrolyte disorders.

Clinical Features

1. Atrial standstill is seen most often in patients with severe circulatory failure. The arrhythmia itself does not produce specific signs or symptoms.
2. A sudden change in the configuration, or the disappearance, of P waves, particularly in patients with advanced circulatory failure, suggests that downward displacement of the pacemaker is occurring because of atrial damage.
3. When the pacemaker has descended to the AV nodal area, the ECG has the same characteristics of an arrhythmia originating in the AV nodal area (as described in the next chapter). However, the differences in clinical circumstances and in prognosis between the two arrhythmias make it important to consider atrial standstill and AV nodal arrhythmias as separate entities.

Danger in Acute Myocardial Infarction

1. Failure of the SA node and the atria to initiate impulses leaves the AV nodal area and the ventricles as the only remaining pacemakers. These latter centers are far less dependable than higher pacemakers, and *ventricular standstill* may occur at any time.
2. Downward displacement of the pacemaker usually indicates irreversible damage of the higher pacing centers in the heart and often heralds death.
3. *RISK:* Atrial standstill is an extremely ominous arrhythmia and usually an immediate forerunner of death due to advanced left ventricular failure.

Treatment

1. If the arrhythmia is due to extensive myocardial damage and progressive tissue ischemia, there is little hope for survival with present therapy. Treatment should be directed primarily at improving left ventricular function.
2. A transvenous pacing catheter should be inserted with the first suspicion that the SA node or atria are failing as pacemakers, and ventricular pacing should be carried out during the course of treatment for left ventricular failure.
3. If atrial standstill is a result of digitalis toxicity or severe electrolyte imbalance (rather than a reflection of progressive ischemia), measures to correct these disorders should be initiated rapidly.

Nursing Role

1. The P waves should be examined with particular care in all patients with left ventricular failure. A sudden decrease in their amplitude or shape or the abrupt disappearance of the P waves in this setting may suggest the onset of atrial standstill.
2. Notify the physician immediately and document the changing ECG pattern with a rhythm strip.
3. Verify the patient's clinical status. Death may occur despite the presence of ventricular complexes seen on the monitor. In other words, although electrical activity may continue, the myocardium is unable to respond and its pumping action ceases (power failure).
4. At the first suggestion of atrial standstill, begin to prepare for the insertion of a transvenous pacemaker.

ATRIAL STANDSTILL—IDENTIFYING ECG FEATURES

1. **Rate:**   Usually slow (40–60/minute).
2. **Rhythm:**   The ventricular rhythm is generally regular except in the dying heart where ventricular beats may be interspersed.
3. **P waves:**   There are no P waves and there is essentially a straight line between QRS complexes.
4. **PR interval:** Absent. There is no electrical conduction *above* the acting pacemaker.
5. **QRS:**   The configuration of this complex depends on the site of pacemaker function. If the ventricle is stimulated from the AV nodal area the QRS complex may be normal. However, if the impulse originates within the ventricle the QRS will be widened and distorted.

EXAMPLE: Atrial Standstill (Fig. 11.13)

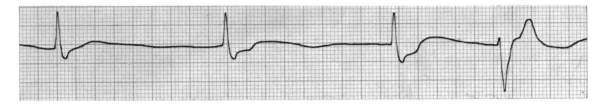

INTERPRETATION OF ECG

Rate: About 40/minute.
Rhythm: Slow and regular (except for the last complex).
P waves: Absent (no atrial activity).
PR interval: The pacemaker has descended to the AV node.
QRS: Widened (0.12 second), reflecting a delay in ventricular conduction.
Comments: The last complex is ventricular in origin, indicating further downward displacement of the pacemaker.

Case History

A 71-year-old man with an acute anteroseptal myocardial infarction was admitted with obvious signs of left ventricular failure. The treatment program included digitalis and a rapid-acting diuretic. The response to therapy was poor, and the patient remained in heart failure. About 8 hours after admission the nurse noted a change in the previously existing sinus tachycardia. There was a loss of upright P waves along with a decrease in cardiac rate from 128 to 96. The physician was notified immediately. Before his arrival 10 minutes later, the nurse documented a further change in the ECG in the form of inverted P waves (indicating that an atrial pacemaker was now operative). While a transvenous pacemaker was being inserted, the rate decreased to 58 and the ECG revealed that all SA and atrial activity had ceased and that the AV nodal area was now the pacemaker. Death occurred despite pacemaking attempts.

The electrocardiographic change from sinus tachycardia to atrial standstill is shown in the following examples (Fig. 11.14(A) and (B)):

Figure 11.14(A).   Sinus Tachycardia.

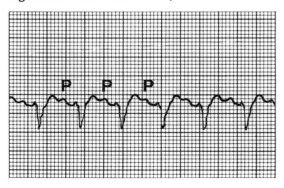

Figure 11.14(B).   Atrial Standstill.

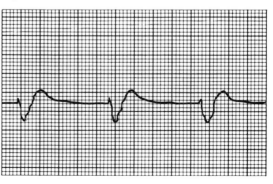

12

Arrhythmias Originating in the AV Nodal Area (Junctional Arrhythmias)

Premature Junctional Contractions
Passive Junctional Rhythm
Paroxysmal Junctional Tachycardia
Nonparoxysmal Junctional Tachycardia

Recent studies have shown that the AV node itself does not initiate impulses and that the site of origin of what had been called nodal rhythms is actually in the junctional tissue surrounding the AV node. In deference to this anatomic fact, disturbances previously classified as nodal arrhythmias are now properly termed junctional arrhythmias.

There are three types of junctional rhythms, each with a different etiology and a different prognosis. In addition, junctional tissue may give rise to premature contractions (premature junctional contractions).

Of the three classes of junctional arrhythmias, one is characterized by slow impulse formation in the junctional tissue (passive junctional rhythm) and the other two are due to accelerated impulse activity (paroxysmal junctional tachycardia and nonparoxysmal junctional tachycardia).

The presence of a junctional arrhythmia indicates that the SA node and atria have been replaced as pacemakers by the AV junctional tissue. This condition may develop because of failure of the SA node or atria to discharge impulses after injury or because the junctional tissue fires at a rate faster than that of the higher centers (and therefore assumes the role of pacemaker). Junctional arrhythmias (except junctional premature contractions) must be regarded as major arrhythmias; they demand prompt treatment.

PREMATURE JUNCTIONAL (NODAL) CONTRACTIONS

Etiology

An ectopic focus in the *AV nodal area* discharges before the onset of the next impulse from the SA node. This stimulus is transmitted downward through the His-Purkinje system and produces a ventricular beat designated as a premature *junctional* (or nodal) contraction (PJC)—in contrast to a premature *ventricular* contraction, which originates in the ventricle itself. The impulse may at the same time be transmitted upward to the atria, causing atrial stimulation (P waves) just before or after the QRS complex. These ectopic beats are believed to result from irritability of the junctional tissue secondary to ischemia.

Clinical Features

1. Patients are rarely aware of PJCs, and symptoms are infrequent.
2. Although PJCs produce some irregularity of the heartbeat, it is not possible to identify specifically PJCs by clinical examination, and the diagnosis can be established only by ECG.

Danger in Acute Myocardial Infarction

1. Although it has been speculated that junctional premature contractions may give rise to junctional tachycardia in the same sense that atrial premature beats may trigger atrial fibrillation, this sequence has not been proved. Consequently PJCs cannot be regarded as a distinct forerunner of junctional tachycardia.
2. Infrequent or isolated PJCs have no significant effect on circulatory efficiency.
3. PJCs probably represent a sign of irritability in the junctional tissue, and an increase in the frequency of these ectopic beats may reflect ischemic injury to the nodal or His bundle area.
4. *RISK:* Premature junctional contractions are not serious in their own right and can be classified as a minor arrhythmia.

Treatment

1. If PJCs occur infrequently, treatment is unnecessary.
2. If their frequency increases, these ectopic beats can usually be terminated by administering lidocaine or procainamide intravenously.

Nursing Role

1. Identify premature *junctional* contractions and distinguish them from the more serious premature *ventricular* contractions.
2. If the relative frequency of PJCs increases, notify the physician.
3. If PJCs are treated with an intravenous infusion of lidocaine or procainamide, adjust the rate of flow to control the ectopic beats.

Case History

 A 58-year-old man with an acute inferior myocardial infarction developed infrequent ectopic beats during the second day of hospitalization. From the monitor lead alone, the nurse was unable to decide whether these beats were premature junctional contractions or premature ventricular contractions. When the frequency of these ectopic beats increased gradually over the next 3 hours, a 12-lead ECG was taken to identify their specific origin. Premature junctional contractions were evident. The physician was notified, and it was decided that no therapy was necessary.

```
┌─────────────────────────────────────────────────────────────────────────┐
│      ── PREMATURE JUNCTIONAL (AV NODAL) CONTRACTIONS ──                   │
│                 IDENTIFYING ECG FEATURES                                  │
```

1. Rate: Normal.

2. Rhythm: Regular, except for the premature beat and the pause that follows.

3. P waves: Because the atria are stimulated in a *retrograde* manner by impulses originating in the junctional tissue, the shape and position of the P waves vary with the conduction time to the atria. Usually the P waves are *inverted* and occur either immediately before or after the QRS complex. Sometimes P waves cannot be identified at all (being buried in the QRS complex).

4. PR interval: There is retrograde conduction to the atria. When a P wave precedes the QRS complex, the PR interval is usually shortened (less than 0.12 second).

5. QRS: Usually normal because conduction from the AV nodal area to the Purkinje network is not disturbed. (Occasionally the impulse may be transmitted slowly or abnormally, producing a wide QRS complex. This is called aberrant conduction.)

EXAMPLE: Premature Junctional (Nodal) Contractions (Fig. 12.1)

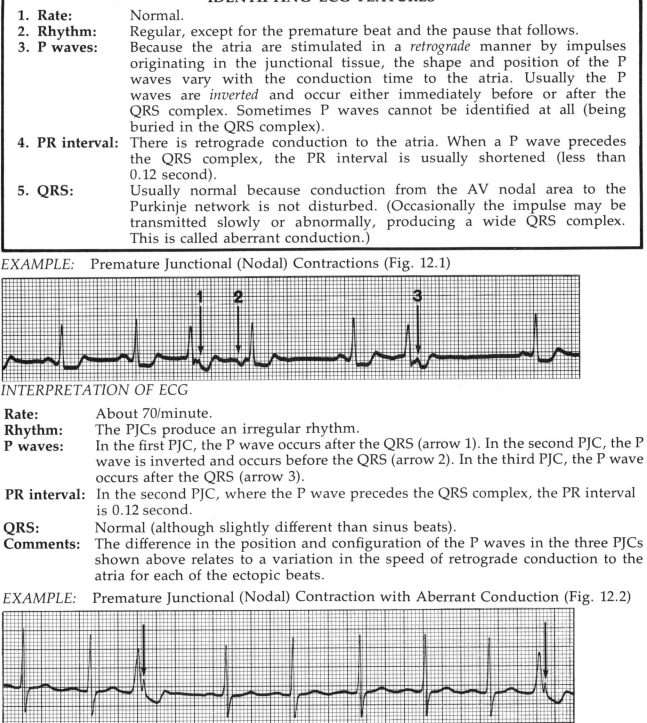

INTERPRETATION OF ECG

Rate: About 70/minute.

Rhythm: The PJCs produce an irregular rhythm.

P waves: In the first PJC, the P wave occurs after the QRS (arrow 1). In the second PJC, the P wave is inverted and occurs before the QRS (arrow 2). In the third PJC, the P wave occurs after the QRS (arrow 3).

PR interval: In the second PJC, where the P wave precedes the QRS complex, the PR interval is 0.12 second.

QRS: Normal (although slightly different than sinus beats).

Comments: The difference in the position and configuration of the P waves in the three PJCs shown above relates to a variation in the speed of retrograde conduction to the atria for each of the ectopic beats.

EXAMPLE: Premature Junctional (Nodal) Contraction with Aberrant Conduction (Fig. 12.2)

INTERPRETATION OF ECG

Rate: About 90/minute.

Rhythm: Essentially regular except for the two premature complexes.

P waves: The P waves in the PJCs occur after the QRS complexes (arrows).

PR interval: Except for the PJCs, where the P waves follow the QRS complexes, the PR intervals are normal.

QRS: The QRS complexes of the PJCs are wide and aberrant in shape because conduction to the ventricles is abnormal.

Comments: PJCs with aberrant, wide QRS complexes may be difficult to distinguish from premature *ventricular* contractions (PVCs), and multiple leads may be needed for proper interpretation.

PASSIVE JUNCTIONAL RHYTHM

Etiology

A focus in the *AV nodal area* replaces the SA node as the cardiac pacemaker. This displacement results from depression of SA node activity, permitting the AV node to assume command. (The inherent rhythmicity of the junctional tissue is normally slower than that of the SA node, and the AV nodal area does not serve as pacemaker unless the rate of the SA node is markedly depressed.)

Junctional impulses spread both *downward* to the ventricles and *upward* to the atria. Thus with a passive junctional rhythm the AV nodal area controls both atrial and ventricular activity. The depression of the SA node which permits a junctional rhythm to develop is usually the result of excessive vagal activity. Ischemic damage of the SA node or digitalis toxicity are other causative factors.

Clinical Features

1. This arrhythmia seldom produces symptoms, unless the rate is very slow.
2. The only clinical finding suggesting passive junctional rhythm is a slow, *regular* rate, usually 40–60 beats/minute.
3. A junctional rhythm cannot be distinguished with certainty from other bradycardias except by ECG.
4. Passive junctional rhythm is often temporary, and the SA node may regain its normal role spontaneously.

Danger in Acute Myocardial Infarction

1. Because of the inherently slow rate of junctional impulses (40–60/minute), ectopic foci with more rapid rates may take over the pacemaking function. Such foci may cause either junctional or ventricular tachycardia, especially in the presence of myocardial ischemia.
2. A passive junctional pacemaker is not dependable and there is a danger of downward displacement of impulse formation to the ventricle.
3. As with other slow-rate arrhythmias, cardiac output may decrease significantly and produce cerebral or myocardial ischemia.
4. *RISK:* Although most patients can tolerate a junctional rhythm without difficulty, this arrhythmia is nevertheless dangerous because it indicates a less dependable pacemaker than the SA node is in command and that there is a potential threat of serious ectopic rhythms developing.

Treatment

1. There is no specific drug therapy for passive junctional rhythm, but atropine is sometimes successful in accelerating the heart rate.
2. If the slow heart rate compromises the circulation, a transvenous pacemaker can be used to increase the ventricular rate (and, in turn, cardiac output).
3. If ventricular ectopic beats develop in the presence of junctional rhythm, they are best controlled by rate acceleration (cardiac pacing). For some reason lidocaine is not usually effective in terminating ventricular ectopic beats that develop during slow heart rates (in contrast to its great effectiveness in controlling premature ventricular beats that occur during normal or fast heart rates).
4. If the arrhythmia is secondary to digitalis or quinidine overdosages the offending drug should be withdrawn promptly.

Nursing Role

1. Identify the arrhythmia as a passive junctional rhythm. Rule out the possibility that the slow heart rate is due to sinus bradycardia or advanced heart block.
2. Observe the monitor carefully for premature ventricular beats, which are likely to develop in the presence of this bradycardia. Notify the physician if such ectopic activity is noted.
3. Be alert for signs and symptoms of cerebral or myocardial insufficiency, particularly when the rate is below 50/minute.
4. If a junctional rhythm develops *suddenly*, notify the physician.
5. If the patient is receiving digitalis or quinidine, discuss the further use of these drugs with the physician before administering the next dose.

Case History

A 56-year-old man was admitted to the CCU with a heart rate of 48/minute. He was in no distress, and there was no evidence of left ventricular failure. On a rhythm strip the nurse noted that the P waves were inverted and followed the QRS complexes, from which she concluded that the bradycardia was due to a junctional rhythm. Two hours later the patient developed premature ventricular contractions at a rate of 4–6/minute. Lidocaine was administered but was not effective in controlling these ectopic beats. After an unsuccessful attempt at increasing the heart rate with intravenous atropine, a transvenous pacemaker was inserted and the ventricle paced at a rate of 80/minute. The ectopic beats disappeared promptly.

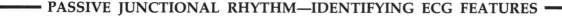

PASSIVE JUNCTIONAL RHYTHM—IDENTIFYING ECG FEATURES

1. **Rate:**   Slow, generally 40–60/minute.
2. **Rhythm:**   Regular.
3. **P waves:**   Abnormal (because the atria are stimulated in a retrograde manner). The P waves may occur a) before the QRS, b) after the QRS, or c) may not be visible, being buried with the QRS complex. When present, the P waves are usually inverted.
4. **PR interval:** The PR interval is shortened (less than 0.12 second), reflecting stimulation of the atria by a pacemaker in the AV nodal area.
5. **QRS:**   Normal, indicating that conduction downward through the ventricular pathways is not disturbed.

EXAMPLE: Passive Junctional Rhythm (Fig. 12.3)

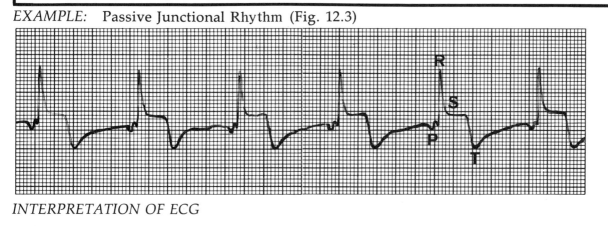

INTERPRETATION OF ECG

Rate: About 60/minute.
Rhythm: Regular.
P waves: Inverted, and occurring immediately before the QRS complex—characteristic of early retrograde conduction to the atria.
PR interval: Shortened (0.06 second), indicating rapid atrial stimulation from the AV nodal area.
QRS: Normal.
Comments: The ST segment elevations and T wave inversions are characteristic of injury and ischemia of myocardial tissue.

EXAMPLE: Passive Junctional Rhythm (Fig. 12.4)

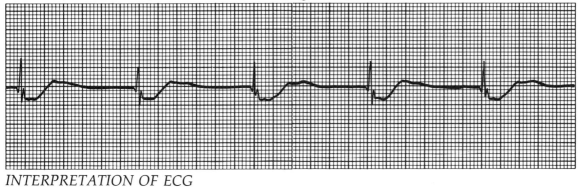

INTERPRETATION OF ECG

Rate: About 50/minute.
Rhythm: Regular.
P waves: Not specifically identified, being buried within the QRS complexes.
PR interval: Not measurable.
QRS: Normal.
Comments: The slow, regular rate is characteristic of a junctional pacemaker.

PAROXYSMAL JUNCTIONAL TACHYCARDIA

Etiology

An irritable center in the *junctional* tissue repeatedly discharges impulses more rapidly than the SA node and assumes the pacemaking role. The impulse spreads downward through the ventricle causing a rapid ventricular response. Paroxysmal junctional tachycardia (PJT) may develop secondary to ischemia of the AV nodal area, but metabolic disturbances or increased catecholamine secretion are probably more common causes. Digitalis intoxication is occasionally the underlying mechanism of this arrhythmia.

Clinical Features

1. The arrhythmia usually begins *abruptly* and may terminate with the same suddenness. (This paroxysmal action is similar to that found in paroxysmal atrial tachycardia or ventricular tachycardia.)
2. The symptoms are those anticipated with a rapid ventricular rate: Dyspnea is common and ischemic pain may occur, particularly if the tachycardia is sustained.
3. Paroxysmal junctional tachycardia cannot be distinguished from other regular, rapid-rate arrhythmias (e.g., PAT) by clinical examination. The diagnosis can be established only by ECG.

Danger in Acute Myocardial Infarction

1. The rapid ventricular rate frequently results in a decrease in the cardiac output and predisposes to left ventricular failure as well as myocardial and cerebral ischemia. This threat is related directly to the duration of the tachycardia.
2. Junctional tachycardia may deteriorate into ventricular tachycardia or even ventricular fibrillation (indicating that a ventricular focus has replaced the junctional pacemaker).
3. *RISK:* Paroxysmal junctional tachycardia is a very dangerous arrhythmia in terms of hemodynamic consequences and is a warning of impending lethal ventricular arrhythmias.

Treatment

1. If junctional tachycardia is *sustained* and results in obvious evidence of circulatory inefficiency (i.e., signs of left ventricular failure, angina, or cerebral ischemia), the arrhythmia should be terminated *immediately* by means of synchronized precordial shock.
2. If the arrhythmia produces no overt symptoms and the patient is not in distress, drug therapy can be attempted initially. Lidocaine, given intravenously, is the preferred agent.
3. Even if the paroxysm of junctional tachycardia is of short duration and subsides spontaneously without therapy, antiarrhythmic treatment (lidocaine) should nevertheless be instituted to prevent recurrent episodes.
4. If digitalis is suspected as an etiologic factor, the drug should be discontinued. Propranolol or diphenylhydantoin (Dilantin), given intravenously, can be used to treat digitalis toxicity.
5. Junctional tachycardia should not be allowed to persist under any circumstances and vigorous therapy is indicated to control this arrhythmia.

Nursing Role

1. Paroxysmal junctional tachycardia will trigger the high-rate alarm system. Identify the presence of this rapid-rate arrhythmia and document it with an ECG strip.
2. Go to the bedside and examine the patient. Assess the clinical condition, including respiration, pulse rate, blood pressure, and the presence of symptoms (angina or dyspnea).
3. Notify the physician immediately.
4. Start oxygen therapy.
5. Prepare a syringe containing 100 mg lidocaine; also prepare an infusion of lidocaine (3000 mg lidocaine in 500 cc fluid) for continuous intravenous drip.
6. If the arrhythmia persists and there are signs of circulatory failure, prepare for elective precordial shock.

Case History

A 50-year-old male with an acute inferior myocardial infarction showed no complications during the first 12 hours after admission. Ten minutes after his lunch, the high-rate alarm sounded. The nurse noted a rate of 180/minute. The monitor showed regular QRS complexes followed by inverted P waves. At the bedside the nurse observed that the respirations were rapid and that the patient was apprehensive. The blood pressure was 90/60. Oxygen was started and the physician notified. Physical examination showed signs of early left ventricular failure. An intravenous injection of 100 mg lidocaine was given rapidly, and within 1 minute normal sinus rhythm had returned. A continuous intravenous infusion of lidocaine was then administered (2 mg/minute) to prevent recurrence of the arrhythmia.

```
━━━━━ PAROXYSMAL JUNCTIONAL TACHYCARDIA ━━━━━
              IDENTIFYING ECG FEATURES

  1. Rate:         Usually 140-220/minute.
  2. Rhythm:       Regular.
  3. P waves:      The shape and position of P waves vary according to the site of impulse
                   formation within the junctional tissue and the manner of retrograde trans-
                   mission to the atria. The most common pattern is an inverted P wave occur-
                   ring immediately before or after the QRS complex.
  4. PR interval:  Atrial stimulation may occur immediately before, during, or immediately
                   after the QRS complex, and therefore the PR interval is either very short or
                   absent.
  5. QRS:          Normal; conduction through the intraventricular tracts is not disturbed.
```

EXAMPLE: Paroxysmal Junctional Tachycardia (Fig. 12.5)

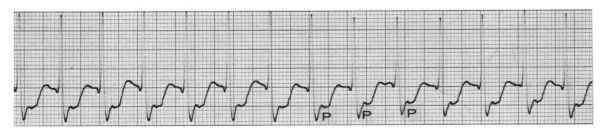

INTERPRETATION OF ECG

Rate: About 140/minute.
Rhythm: Regular.
P waves: Occur after the QRS complexes.
PR interval: Absent. The AV junctional tissue is the pacemaker for both the atria and ventri-
                 cles.
QRS: Normal.
Comments: It is often difficult to distinguish paroxysmal junctional tachycardia from paroxys-
                 mal atrial tachycardia from a single monitor lead. A 12-lead ECG is necessary to
                 identify the position of the P waves.

EXAMPLE: Paroxysmal Junctional Tachycardia (Fig. 12.6)

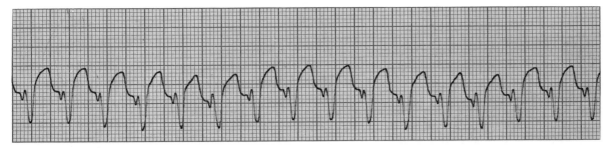

INTERPRETATION OF ECG

Rate: About 160/minute.
Rhythm: Regular.
P waves: Inverted, and immediately precede the QRS complexes.
PR interval: Shortened (0.06 second).
QRS: Normal (0.08 second).
Comments: This arrhythmia began abruptly and terminated spontaneously 3 minutes later in
                 typical paroxysmal fashion.

NONPAROXYSMAL JUNCTIONAL TACHYCARDIA

Etiology

A focus in the *junctional tissue* replaces the SA node as pacemaker. The rate of junctional impulses is between 70 and 130/minute (in contrast to paroxysmal junctional tachycardia in which the rate ranges from 140 to 220/minute). (When the heart rate is less than 100/minute, as it often is in nonparoxysmal junctional tachycardia, it would seem contradictory to describe the arrhythmia as a tachycardia. The reason for this seemingly improper terminology is that the inherent rate of impulses originating in the AV nodal area is 40–60/minute; therefore any rate above 60/minute is, in effect, a junctional tachycardia.)

Nonparoxysmal junctional tachycardia, which is more common than paroxysmal junctional tachycardia, often develops in the presence of advanced congestive failure or cardiogenic shock and in this circumstance probably represents a stage of downward displacement of the pacemaker in a severely damaged heart. However, nonparoxysmal junctional tachycardia may occur in the absence of circulatory failure. The arrhythmia may also be produced by digitalis toxicity.

Clinical Features

1. Unlike paroxysmal junctional tachycardia, nonparoxysmal junctional tachycardia develops and terminates *gradually*, rather than abruptly; this is the most distinguishing characteristic of the arrhythmia.
2. When the arrhythmia accompanies advanced left ventricular failure the signs and symptoms of the failing heart dominate the clinical picture.
3. In the absence of circulatory failure the arrhythmia seldom produces symptoms or physical findings.
4. Nonparoxysmal junctional tachycardia can be identified only by ECG.

Danger in Acute Myocardial Infarction

1. The arrhythmia often indicates that extensive myocardial damage has occurred and that further downward displacement of the pacemaker (to the ventricles) may develop.
2. In its own right, nonparoxysmal junctional tachycardia may contribute to a reduction in cardiac output because the atrial component of ventricular filling is lost with a junctional pacemaker.
3. *RISK:* Nonparoxsymal junctional tachycardia is often associated with a high mortality and should be regarded as a serious complication. Death, however, is not due to the arrhythmic disturbance but to underlying myocardial damage.

Treatment

1. There is no specific treatment for this arrhythmia. When circulatory failure is present, the treatment program is aimed at combating this complication with the hope that the arrhythmia will subside once circulatory efficiency is improved.
2. Because of the threat that the junctional pacemaker may be replaced by a ventricular pacemaker, a transvenous pacemaker may be inserted.
3. If there is any possibility that the arrhythmia is a consequence of digitalis toxicity, the drug should be discontinued and potassium administered intravenously.

Nursing Role

1. Because the arrhythmia develops gradually and its rate is between 70 and 130/minute, the monitor alarm system will *not* be activated and therefore the identification of nonparoxsymal tachycardia depends on careful monitor observation.
2. Ascertain that the arrhythmia is nonparoxysmal junctional tachycardia and document it with a rhythm strip.
3. Be especially alert for this arrhythmia among patients with advanced circulatory failure or cardiogenic shock and notify the physician immediately once identification has been made.
4. Prepare for the insertion of a transvenous pacemaker, which may be utilized in the treatment program.
5. When the arrhythmia develops in the absence of circulatory failure, the possibility of digitalis intoxication should be considered and the physician consulted prior to further administration of the drug.

Case History

A 74-year-old man was admitted to CCU with severe chest pain and signs of marked left ventricular failure. The ECG revealed an acute anterior wall myocardial infarction and the presence of sinus tachycardia. The patient was treated with furosemide and digoxin but showed little improvement during the next 2 hours. The nurse noted that the heart rate gradually decreased from 130 to 80/minute. She suspected at first that the rate slowing was due only to digitalis, but on examining a rhythm strip she noted a change in the P waves, which were now inverted and followed the QRS complexes. It was apparent that the patient had developed nonparoxysmal junctional tachycardia, and she called the physician immediately.

```
┌─────────────────────────────────────────────────────────────────────┐
│  ━━━━━ NONPAROXYSMAL JUNCTIONAL TACHYCARDIA ━━━━━                     │
│              IDENTIFYING ECG FEATURES                                  │
│                                                                       │
│  1. Rate:        70-130/minute. Slower rates usually indicate passive│
│                  junctional rhythm, and faster rates suggest          │
│                  paroxysmal junctional tachycardia.                   │
│  2. Rhythm:      Regular.                                             │
│  3. P waves:     May occur before or after the QRS complex or may not │
│                  be present.                                          │
│  4. PR interval: Retrograde conduction to the atria may or may not    │
│                  occur. When a PR interval is identifiable the        │
│                  interval is usually less than 0.12 second.           │
│  5. QRS:         Normal, because conduction from the junctional tissue│
│                  to the ventricles is not affected.                   │
└─────────────────────────────────────────────────────────────────────┘
```

EXAMPLE: Nonparoxysmal Junctional Tachycardia (Fig. 12.7)

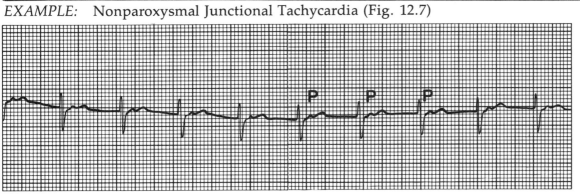

INTERPRETATION OF ECG

Rate: About 100/minute.
Rhythm: Regular.
P waves: Occur immediately after QRS complexes.
PR interval: Absent because of retrograde conduction to atria.
QRS: Normal.
Comments: In contrast to paroxysmal junctional tachycardia, which develops suddenly, this arrhythmia developed gradually. Also, the rate never exceeded 100/minute.

EXAMPLE: Nonparoxysmal Junctional Tachycardia (Fig. 12.8)

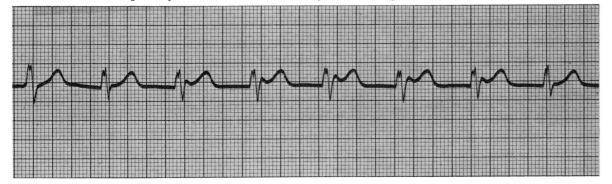

INTERPRETATION OF ECG

Rate: About 80/minute.
Rhythm: Regular.
P waves: Not definitely identified, probably incorporated in the QRS complex.
PR interval: There is no PR interval. The atria are stimulated (by the junctional tissue) after ventricular activation has started.
QRS: Essentially normal (0.10-0.11 second).
Comments: This arrhythmia is distinguished from a passive junctional rhythm on the basis of rate (80/minute). With passive junctional rhythm the rate would not be faster than 40-60/minute.

13

Arrhythmias Originating in the Ventricles

Premature Ventricular Contractions
Ventricular Tachycardia

Disturbances in the heartbeat that originate in the SA node, the atria, or the AV nodal area are jointly classified as *supraventricular* arrhythmias. If the impulse begins in the ventricles, below the level of the AV nodal area, the resulting disorder is termed a *ventricular* arrhythmia.

The most common ventricular arrhythmia (in fact, the most common of *all* arrhythmias) is the premature ventricular contraction. Practically all patients with acute myocardial infarction exhibit ventricular ectopic beats during the first few days after the attack. Premature ventricular beats result from the discharge of an ectopic focus within the ventricular walls (or the conduction pathway) before the expected arrival of the next impulse from a supraventricular center. These ectopic beats represent a sign of myocardial irritability secondary to ischemia, and the frequency of their occurrence is probably a fair index of the degree of ischemic irritation.

There is good evidence that ventricular fibrillation is a direct consequence of myocardial irritability, and that this lethal arrhythmia usually begins with a premature ventricular contraction. The scale of irritability leading to ventricular fibrillation can be viewed as follows:

1. occasional premature ventricular contractions
2. premature ventricular contractions occurring more than 6 times/minute or originating from more than one ventricular focus (multifocal premature beats)
3. a series of four or more *consecutive* premature contractions (ventricular tachycardia)
4. ventricular fibrillation

Although the relationship between premature ventricular contractions and ventricular fibrillation is clearly established, it should not be assumed that all ventricular ectopic beats are potentially dangerous. *It is only in the presence of myocardial ischemia that premature ventricular contractions are likely to provoke ventricular fibrillation*. Many normal individuals without evidence of heart disease display premature ventricular beats which pose no threat.

Ventricular tachycardia is an immediate forerunner of ventricular fibrillation in many instances. In addition to this extreme threat, ventricular tachycardia, when sustained, seriously endangers the circulation by markedly reducing cardiac output. For these reasons the arrhythmia must never be allowed to persist.

Because of its supreme importance *ventricular fibrillation* is considered separately in the next chapter.

PREMATURE VENTRICULAR CONTRACTIONS

Etiology

An irritable focus within the *ventricle* discharges before the arrival of the next anticipated impulse from the SA node. This ectopic focus stimulates the ventricle directly and causes a *premature ventricular contraction* (PVC). Premature ventricular beats are the most common of all arrhythmias associated with acute myocardial infarction and represent a sign of ventricular irritability.

Clinical Features

1. Many patients are aware of PVCs and describe the sensation as "palpitations" or "my heart is skipping." The greater the frequency of these ectopic beats, the more likely the patient is to notice them.
2. When listening to the heart or taking the pulse, a longer-than-normal pause is noted immediately after the premature beats. This delay (called the compensatory pause) is characteristic of PVCs and is practically diagnostic of the arrhythmia.

Danger in Acute Myocardial Infarction

1. PVCs indicate myocardial irritability and are of critical importance because they may initiate repetitive ventricular firing in the form of ventricular tachycardia or ventricular fibrillation. This sequence PVCs → ventricular tachycardia → ventricular fibrillation is most apt to occur when PVCs exist in any of the five following forms:

   a. when PVCs occur frequently, especially six or more times per minute
   b. when every second beat is a PVC (bigeminy)
   c. when the PVC strikes on the T wave of the preceding complex (the "R on T" pattern)
   d. when PVCs originate from more than one irritable focus in the ventricle (multifocal PVCs)
   e. when PVCs occur sequentially for two or three beats (short runs of PVCs)

2. PVCs develop in at least 90% of all patients with acute myocardial infarction. Therefore the mere presence of PVCs is far less significant than an increase in frequency or the development of one of the five dangerous forms of PVCs listed above.

3. Overdosages of digitalis often cause PVCs. This relationship is suggested especially when PVCs occur as bigeminy.

4. Premature ventricular beats commonly develop in the presence of hypokalemia. Depletion of potassium levels often occurs among patients treated with diuretic agents.

5. *RISK:* If PVCs appear infrequently, the threat of provoking serious ventricular arrhythmias is not great. However, if these ectopic beats occur with increasing frequency or are of a dangerous type, they should be considered as a serious warning of impending ventricular tachycardia or ventricular fibrillation.

PREMATURE VENTRICULAR CONTRACTIONS
IDENTIFYING ECG FEATURES

1. **Rate:** Usually normal, but PVCs can occur at any rate.
2. **Rhythm:** The premature beat and the compensatory pause that follows it create a momentary irregularity in the rhythm. Characteristically, the interval between the beat preceding and the beat following a PVC is equal to two normal beats (as shown in Fig. 13.1, below).
3. **P waves:** Not identifiable in the ectopic beat because the impulse originates in the *ventricle*, not in the SA node or atrium.
4. **PR interval:** A PVC does not have a PR interval because the ventricle is stimulated directly and there is no conduction from the atrium to the ventricles.
5. **QRS:** The QRS complex is *always* widened and distorted in shape. The particular configuration of the QRS complex depends on the site of the ventricular stimulus. However, the T wave is oppositely directed from the QRS complex.

EXAMPLE: Isolated Premature Ventricular Contraction (Fig. 13.1)

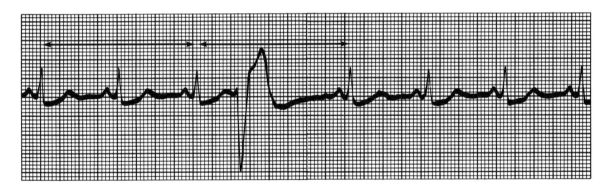

INTERPRETATION OF ECG

Rate: About 80/minute.
Rhythm: Regular except for one PVC.
P waves: Absent in premature contraction; normal in the other cardiac cycles.
PR interval: Absent in the PVC because the impulse originates in the ventricle. (Conduction of the remaining beats is normal.)
QRS: The ectopic complex is widened and bizarre in configuration, and the T wave is *oppositely* directed from the QRS complex.
Comments: The interval between the beat preceding the PVC and the beat following the PVC is equal to the time of two normal beats (arrows).

Treatment

1. Lidocaine is the primary agent used to control PVCs. Suppression of the irritable ventricular focus can be achieved promptly in most instances by administering 50–100 mg lidocaine as a rapid intravenous injection ("push dose"). This should be followed by a continuous infusion of lidocaine given at a rate of 1–3 mg/minute (10–30 microdrops/minute of a solution containing 3000 mg lidocaine in 500 cc glucose solution) in order to control further myocardial irritability. Alternatively procainamide (Pronestyl) can be given intravenously to inhibit PVCs, but this drug has the disadvantage of often producing hypotension and for this reason is a less desirable choice than lidocaine. (See Chapter 18 regarding antiarrhythmic drugs.)
2. If lidocaine (or procainamide) in customary doses fails to suppress PVCs, it is unwise to continue to increase the amount given since overdosages of both drugs produce toxic effects. In this situation an intravenous infusion of potassium (40 mEq KCl in 500 cc dextrose solution) is very often effective in controlling ectopic activity, particularly if there is evidence of hypokalemia.
3. Premature ventricular beats can sometimes be abolished with antiarrhythmic agents administered orally. Procainamide (500 mg every 6 hours) and quinidine (400 mg every 6 hours) are the most effective of the oral agents. Because of their slow action these drugs should not be used for immediate, or primary, control.
4. If PVCs develop during treatment with digitalis or with the use of diuretics, the possibility of drug-induced ectopic beats should always be considered: In this circumstance the drugs may have to be discontinued and potassium administered.

Nursing Role

1. Identify PVCs and distinguish these ectopic beats from atrial or junctional premature contractions.
2. Carefully assess the relative frequency of PVCs during successive time intervals to ascertain any change. Also identify the type of PVC noted.
3. If PVCs occur in any of the most threatening forms, the physician should be notified and lidocaine should be administered immediately.
4. If an infusion of lidocaine is used to control PVCs, adjust the rate of flow to continuously suppress ectopic activity.
5. If lidocaine is given repeatedly or in large quantities, seek signs of overdosage as manifested by petit mal or grand mal seizures. If procainamide is being used instead of lidocaine, the possibility of drug-induced hypotension should be recognized.
6. In the event PVCs develop during digitalis therapy, advise the physician before administering the next dose of digitalis.

Case History

A 51-year-old woman with an acute myocardial infarction showed evidence of PVCs from the time of her admission to the unit. These ectopic beats occurred at a rate of 1–2/minute. During the next several hours the nurse noted that the PVCs gradually increased in frequency and that bigeminy had developed. The physician was advised of this change and a push dose of lidocaine (75 mg) was given. The PVCs disappeared within a minute of the injection. An intravenous infusion of lidocaine was then started. Two hours later the PVCs reappeared and the nurse increased the rate of infusion from 1 mg to 2 mg/minute after which the PVCs disappeared.

FIVE DANGEROUS FORMS OF PREMATURE VENTRICULAR CONTRACTIONS

EXAMPLE 1: Frequent PVCs occurring more than six/minute (Fig. 13.2)

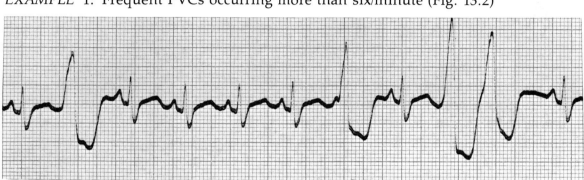

INTERPRETATION OF ECG

Rate: About 110/minute.
Rhythm: Irregular because of premature beats.
P waves: Not identified in ectopic beats.
PR interval: Absent in PVCs. The remaining beats are conducted normally from the SA node (PR interval is 0.14 second).
QRS: The ectopic beats are very wide (about 0.18 second) and distorted in shape.
Comments: There are four PVCs within this 6-second strip; two of them are consecutive. This high frequency of PVCs indicates marked ventricular irritability.

EXAMPLE 2: Bigeminy (alternate PVCs or coupled rhythm) (Fig. 13.3)

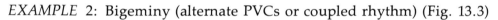
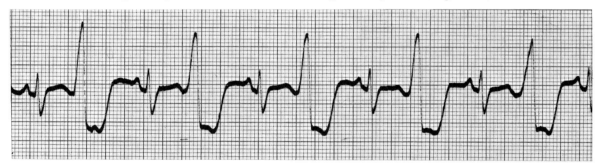

INTERPRETATION OF ECG

Rate: About 100/minute.
Rhythm: Irregular due to coupled beats.
P waves: Absent in the PVCs.
PR interval: In every other complex the ventricle is stimulated directly by an ectopic focus within the ventricular wall. There is no PR interval in these ectopic beats.
QRS: Grossly distorted in PVCs and obviously different from the beats originating in the SA node.
Comments: Bigeminy is often an immediate forerunner of ventricular tachycardia and warns of this more dangerous arrhythmia.

EXAMPLE 3: The R on T Pattern (Fig. 13.4)

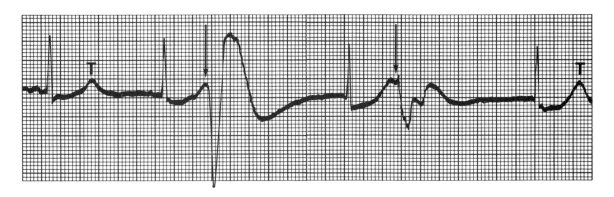

INTERPRETATION OF ECG

Rate: About 60/minute.
Rhythm: The ectopic beats create an irregularity in the basic rhythm.
P waves: Absent in premature ventricular contractions.
PR interval: Absent. The ectopic beats arise in the ventricle. There is no conduction from the atrium and hence no PR interval.
QRS: The two ectopic beats are distorted but have different configurations. This difference in their shape indicates that more than one irritable focus is present in the ventricle (multifocal PVCs).
Comments: Both PVCs strike directly on the T waves of the preceding complexes (arrows). When a PVC occurs at the time of the T wave (the R on T pattern) there is a high risk of precipitating ventricular fibrillation. This sequence is shown below. Note the onset of ventricular fibrillation when an isolated PVC (arrow) strikes the T wave of the preceding beat.

EXAMPLE: Onset of Ventricular Fibrillation of PVC Striking T Wave of Preceding Beat (Fig. 13.5)

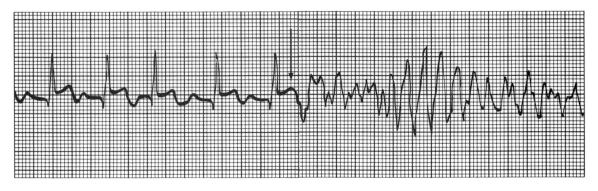

EXAMPLE 4: Multifocal PVCs (Fig. 13.6)

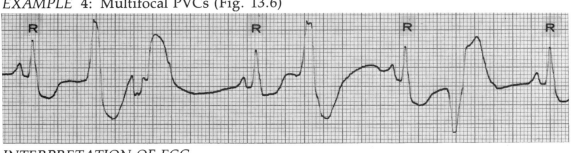

INTERPRETATION OF ECG

Rate: About 80/minute.

Rhythm: Irregular.

P waves: There are no P waves with the PVCs.

PR interval: There is no conduction from the atria to the ventricles in the premature beats.

QRS: All of the premature beats have widened and distorted QRS complexes, but these vary from one another in contour since they originate from separate ventricular foci (multifocal PVCs).

Comments: Multifocal PVCs reflect advanced ventricular irritability, and vigorous antiarrhythmic treatment must be used to terminate this ectopic activity.

EXAMPLE 5: Sequential PVCs (Fig. 13.7)

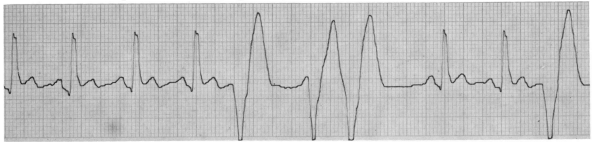

INTERPRETATION OF ECG

Rate: About 100/minute.

Rhythm: Irregular because of frequent PVCs.

P waves: Not visible with PVCs.

PR interval: Absent in the PVCs; there is no conduction from a supraventricular center.

QRS: Typically widened and distorted. Note that the T waves are directed oppositely from the QRS complexes in the ectopic beats.

Comments: After the first PVC, two other PVCs occur in a row. This sequence may lead to repetitive ventricular firing in the form of ventricular tachycardia or ventricular fibrillation.

VENTRICULAR TACHYCARDIA

Etiology

Ventricular tachycardia may be defined as a series of four or more *consecutive* premature ventricular contractions occurring at a rapid rate. These repetitive premature beats reflect advanced myocardial irritability and indicate that an ectopic focus in the ventricle commands the heart rate.

Occasionally ventricular tachycardia may develop spontaneously without warning, but usually the arrhythmia is preceded by signs of myocardial irritability in the form of premature ventricular contractions. When the ectopic ventricular focus discharges repetitively, ventricular tachycardia is said to exist. Ventricular tachycardia is often an immediate forerunner of *ventricular fibrillation*.

Clinical Features

1. Most patients are immediately aware of the sudden onset of rapid heart action, and describe palpitations and dyspnea. When the latter symptoms are associated with chest pain (a common situation) the patient often suspects that a catastrophic event has occurred and marked apprehension is immediately evident.
2. The blood pressure generally falls after the onset of this arrhythmia, and findings of left ventricular failure may develop with surprising rapidity if the tachycardia is sustained. These adverse hemodynamic effects are due to decreased cardiac output resulting from decreased ventricular filling time.
3. The pulse rate is usually accelerated to 140–220 beats/minute. The high-rate monitor alarm will be triggered by the onset of ventricular tachycardia.
4. On many occasions ventricular tachycardia occurs in short runs, or bursts, and then stops spontaneously within a few seconds; symptoms may not be impressive in this circumstance.

Danger in Acute Myocardial Infarction

1. If ventricular tachycardia is sustained and becomes an established rhythm (rather than terminating spontaneously within seconds), the rapid ventricular rate can be expected to produce adverse hemodynamic effects. These are manifested by signs of decreased cardiac output, producing heart failure, cardiogenic shock, or cerebral insufficiency. Sudden death may occur during ventricular tachycardia.
2. At any time during the course of ventricular tachycardia, the arrhythmia may *abruptly* change into ventricular fibrillation. For this reason ventricular tachycardia must be considered in the same life-threatening category as ventricular fibrillation.
3. *RISK:* Ventricular tachycardia represents an extreme danger—an absolute emergency.

VENTRICULAR TACHYCARDIA—IDENTIFYING ECG FEATURES

1. **Rate:** Usually 140–220 beats/minute, but may be faster.
2. **Rhythm:** The ventricular rhythm is essentially regular, but there may be a slight irregularity.
3. **P waves:** The SA node continues to discharge *independently* during ventricular tachycardia, but the P waves bear no relationship to the QRS complexes. However, the P waves can seldom be identified specifically, being buried in the QRS complexes.
4. **PR interval:** The ventricles are stimulated directly by an ectopic focus within their walls and beat independently of the atria. There is no conduction from atria to the ventricles and therefore no PR interval.
5. **QRS:** Wide, slurred complexes typical of repetitive PVCs.

EXAMPLE: Sustained Ventricular Tachycardia (Fig. 13.8)

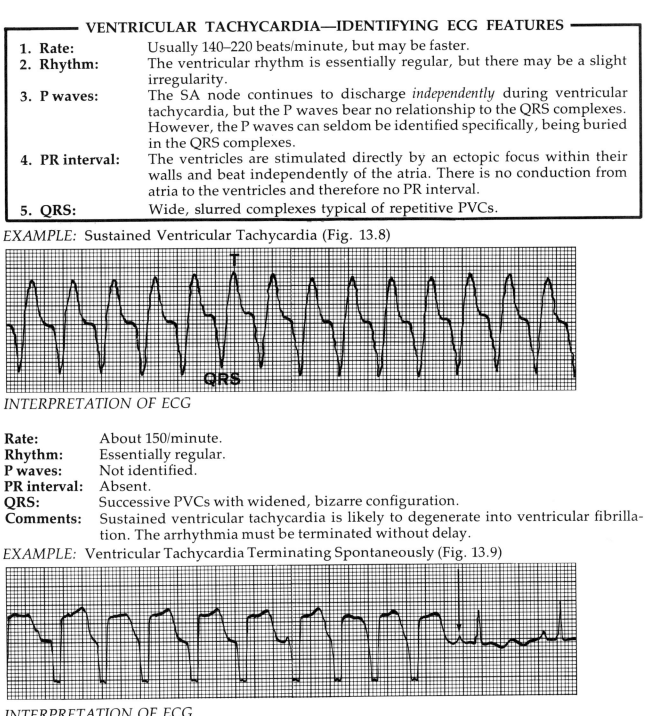

INTERPRETATION OF ECG

Rate: About 150/minute.
Rhythm: Essentially regular.
P waves: Not identified.
PR interval: Absent.
QRS: Successive PVCs with widened, bizarre configuration.
Comments: Sustained ventricular tachycardia is likely to degenerate into ventricular fibrillation. The arrhythmia must be terminated without delay.

EXAMPLE: Ventricular Tachycardia Terminating Spontaneously (Fig. 13.9)

INTERPRETATION OF ECG

Rate: About 150/minute (during ventricular tachycardia).
Rhythm: Almost regular.
P waves: Not identified until normal sinus rhythm returns.
PR interval: Absent. A series of PVCs comprise the rhythm.
QRS: Widened and slurred, indicating their ventricular origin.
Comments: This episode of ventricular tachycardia stopped spontaneously without treatment and was followed by normal sinus rhythm (arrow). Short runs of this type are the most common form of ventricular tachycardia.

Treatment

1. About 50% of all episodes of ventricular tachycardia end as abruptly as they began, even without treatment. The transiency of these attacks should not afford comfort since there is a high risk of further episodes of ventricular tachycardia or the sudden onset of ventricular fibrillation. Even if ventricular tachycardia is of brief duration and stops spontaneously, vigorous antiarrhythmic therapy is nevertheless indicated. In this latter circumstance, an infusion containing 3000 mg of lidocaine in 500 cc glucose solution should be started promptly to prevent recurrence of this serious arrhythmia. The flow should be set initially at 1 mg (10 microdrops)/minute and then adjusted subsequently to suppress premature beats.
2. If ventricular tachycardia is *not* self-limited and continues, lidocaine should be administered as a rapid injection intravenously in a dosage of 100 mg. After the arrhythmia is controlled with this push dose, further amounts of lidocaine should be given according to the regimen described in the previous paragraph.
3. Failure to convert ventricular tachycardia to normal sinus rhythm with lidocaine should be considered an indication for *immediate precordial shock*. Additional attempts with drug therapy are ill-advised; as a general rule, if ventricular tachycardia persists by the time the push dose of lidocaine is completed, the next step should be precordial shock.
4. Procainamide is sometimes as effective as lidocaine in terminating ventricular tachycardia and can be used in this situation. Other antiarrhythmic agents are seldom valuable.
5. If ventricular tachycardia recurs despite a continuous infusion of lidocaine or procainamide, hypokalemia should be suspected and an intravenous infusion containing 40 mEq KCl in 1000 cc glucose solution can be given, even empirically.
6. If, for any reason, ventricular tachycardia persists for 5 minutes or longer, lactic acidosis can develop and sodium bicarbonate may be needed to combat this problem.

Nursing Role

1. When the high-rate alarm sounds, observe the oscilloscope immediately to identify the cause of the rapid-rate arrhythmia. If ventricular tachycardia is present, an emergency situation exists and the planned program of treatment must be instituted at once.
2. Go to the bedside and examine the patient. If he is *unconscious*, proceed immediately with precordial shock (see Chapter 17). If the patient is *conscious*, assess his clinical state, including the presence of dyspnea and chest pain.
3. Call the physician *at once*.
4. Prepare a syringe containing 100 mg lidocaine and administer this drug intravenously without delay.
5. Prepare an infusion containing 3000 mg lidocaine in 500 cc glucose solution for use after the push dose.
6. Allow the write-out system of the monitor (or the electrocardiograph) to run continuously until the arrhythmia is terminated.
7. Bring the defibrillator to the bedside and prepare for precordial shock.
8. *Remember that ventricular fibrillation may develop at any time during the course of ventricular tachycardia.*

Case History

A 47-year-old man with an acute myocardial infarction was admitted to the CCU in no distress. Just after the monitor electrodes had been attached and an intravenous infusion of dextrose solution started, the high-rate alarm sounded. The nurse recognized immediately that ventricular tachycardia had developed. She examined the patient who complained of recurrent chest pain. In accordance with the standing orders of the unit, the nurse prepared a syringe containing 50 mg lidocaine, which she injected rapidly into the existing intravenous line. The ventricular tachycardia stopped within 30 seconds. The physician was notified of this event and instructions were given regarding a continuous lidocaine infusion.

EXAMPLE: Rapid Ventricular Tachycardia (Fig. 13.10)

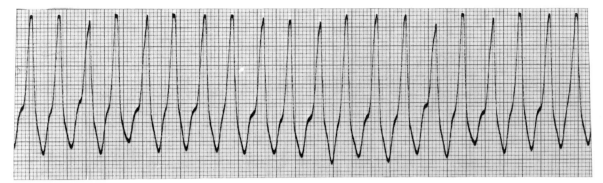

INTERPRETATION OF ECG

Rate: About 200/minute.
Rhythm: Slightly irregular.
P waves: Not identified.
PR interval: Absent. The ventricles are stimulated directly by an ectopic focus at a rate of 200/minute. There is no atrioventricular conduction.
QRS: The complexes are widened and distorted in shape.
Comments: This very rapid ventricular rate is extremely detrimental to the pumping efficiency of the heart; it must be terminated immediately.

EXAMPLE: Extreme Ventricular Tachycardia (Ventricular Flutter) (Fig. 13.11)

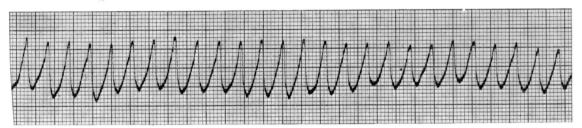

INTERPRETATION OF ECG

Rate: About 270/minute.
Rhythm: Slightly irregular.
P waves: Not visible.
PR interval: Absent. A persistent irritable focus in the ventricle serves as the pacemaker and supersedes the supraventricular centers.
QRS: The very rapidly occurring complexes resemble a helix (similar to a stretched, coiled spring).
Comments: This extreme form of ventricular tachycardia is sometimes designated *ventricular flutter*. In many instances it is an immediate forerunner of ventricular fibrillation and must be treated with the same urgency as ventricular fibrillation—by means of precordial shock (defibrillation).

14

Ventricular Fibrillation:

A Death-Producing Arrhythmia

Ventricular fibrillation is the most common cause of *sudden* death in patients with coronary heart disease. As noted, this lethal arrhythmia is triggered in most instances by PVCs or ventricular tachycardia. However, ventricular fibrillation can arise *spontaneously* without preceding signs of ventricular irritability, and therefore there is always a threat of sudden death in patients with acute myocardial infarction. Once ventricular fibrillation develops, the only hope for survival is the instant application of resuscitative techniques.

Within the CCU the program to resuscitate the "dead" patient is distinctly different from that utilized elsewhere in the hospital.* *In the CCU the first step in resuscitation is to terminate ventricular fibrillation by precordial shock (defibrillation).* This means that external cardiac compression, mouth-to-mouth ventilation, the administration of oxygen, and other cardiopulmonary resuscitative measures are deliberately bypassed in favor of immediate defibrillation. It is sometimes difficult for nurses and physicians to realize that there is no reason to initiate external cardiac compression and mouth-to-mouth ventilation when ventricular fibrillation occurs in the CCU. These techniques are only interim measures used in other settings to sustain the circulation until ventricular fibrillation can be terminated electrically. In the CCU, where everything is in readiness to halt the arrhythmia immediately, supportive measures have little importance and in fact do no more than waste precious time. *When a patient develops ventricular fibrillation in the CCU, precordial shock must be given without delay by the first person reaching the bedside and should precede any and all other steps!*

This reversal of the customary management of cardiac arrest (as practiced in the CCU) in no way minimizes the value of cardiopulmonary resuscitation as a lifesaving measure. The ability to sustain an adequate circulation by means of external cardiac compression and mouth-to-mouth ventilation has been of inestimable help in combating sudden death outside the prepared setting of a specialized unit. The greatest usefulness of these methods is in sustaining vital organ perfusion until resuscitative equipment can be brought to the patient. All medical and paramedical personnel should be thoroughly competent in performing cardiopulmonary resuscitation.

---

*The previously accepted definition of death, namely the cessation of the heartbeat, peripheral pulses, and respiration, has become obsolete, since many patients have been restored to useful life despite these signs of circulatory arrest. A more meaningful definition must include irreversible damage to the brain as the ultimate criterion of death. The need to define death more precisely has assumed great importance since the advent of organ and heart transplantation where death of the donor must be clearly delineated for legal and moral purposes.

VENTRICULAR FIBRILLATION

Etiology

The individual muscle fibers which jointly comprise the ventricular wall normally are stimulated simultaneously and contract in unison. The fibers then recover together and rest until the next impulse causes another contraction. In ventricular fibrillation an *extraordinary* electrical force arising within the ventricle repeatedly stimulates these muscles at a rate so extremely rapid that the recovery period disappears and the individual muscle fibers merely twitch continuously but do not contract. Since the muscular twitching (ventricular fibrillation) is completely ineffective in propelling blood from the ventricles, the circulation stops abruptly and *death follows within minutes*. Immediately after the onset of ventricular fibrillation, the patient becomes unconscious (and convulsions frequently occur) because of inadequate cerebral oxygenation.

The exact mechanism that triggers ventricular fibrillation is not known. Although this lethal arrhythmia may develop spontaneously, there is usually evidence of myocardial irritability in the form of PVCs before the onset of this catastrophic event. It is generally believed that following myocardial infarction the injured myocardium is sensitized so that a minimal electrical stimulus can initiate ventricular fibrillation. The usual electrical stimulus responsible for this chain reaction appears to be a PVC which strikes during the vulnerable phase of the cardiac cycle (at the time of the T wave).

Ventricular fibrillation can develop in patients with acute myocardial infarction who have no obvious complications at the time. This form of ventricular fibrillation is defined as *primary ventricular fibrillation*. In contrast, if this lethal arrhythmia occurs as a terminal rhythm in a patient dying of advanced left ventricular failure, it is classified as *secondary ventricular fibrillation*. This distinction is very important because death can be predictably prevented by prompt defibrillation in all instances of *primary* ventricular fibrillation, while the secondary form is seldom responsive to resuscitation because of the underlying heart failure. Primary ventricular fibrillation reaches its peak incidence within the first few hours of myocardial infarction and then decreases thereafter.

Clinical Features

1. The patient loses consciousness almost instantly after the onset of ventricular fibrillation. *It is safe to assume that a conscious patient does not have ventricular fibrillation.*

2. Peripheral pulses cannot be detected, and no heart sounds are audible; the blood pressure is unobtainable.

3. The pupils dilate rapidly, and convulsions may occur as a result of immediate cerebral anoxia.

4. Cyanosis develops quickly and total *cessation of circulation* is evident.

Danger in Acute Myocardial Infarction

1. Death occurs within a few minutes after the onset of ventricular fibrillation unless the arrhythmia is terminated. The exact duration of life with primary ventricular fibrillation depends on several factors, probably the most important of which is the patient's age. For example, an 80-year-old man may die within less than a minute after the onset of ventricular fibrillation, whereas a much younger patient may survive 3 minutes or more before death becomes irreversible. For this reason the precise time available for successful resuscitation cannot be defined. *The average time is probably 2 minutes.*

2. Although ventricular fibrillation can still be terminated after this critical 2-minute period, irreversible brain damage may have developed.

3. *RISK: SUPREME DANGER! Death is inevitable unless resuscitation is accomplished immediately.*

VENTRICULAR FIBRILLATION—IDENTIFYING ECG FEATURES

The ECG pattern is characterized by a rapid, repetitive series of *chaotic* waves originating in the ventricles; the waves have no uniformity and are bizarre in configuration. PQRST waves cannot specifically be identified. The complexes differ from each other and occur in completely irregular fashion. A typical example of ventricular fibrillation is seen in Figure 14.1.

This gross irregularity can hardly be mistaken for any other arrhythmia. The only other possibility to account for such gross distortion is a disorder of the monitor or the electrocardiograph machine.

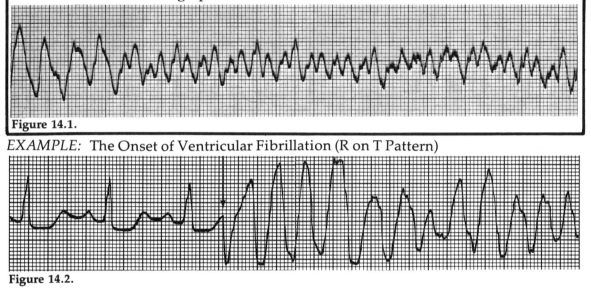

Figure 14.1.

EXAMPLE: The Onset of Ventricular Fibrillation (R on T Pattern)

Figure 14.2.

Comments: A premature ventricular contraction striking the T wave of the preceding complex (arrow) precipitates ventricular fibrillation.

Case History

Note: The following case history describes the first instance of lifesaving defibrillation performed by a nurse in the absence of a physician. This event took place in 1963 and became the precedent for the now established practice of defibrillation by nurses.

A 72-year-old male was admitted to the CCU of the Presbyterian-University of Pennsylvania Medical Center with a history of chest pain that had subsided by the time of his arrival. He had no complaints; in fact, he wanted to go home. An ECG showed an acute myocardial infarction. Physical examination was normal, and there was no evidence of complications. He remained in normal sinus rhythm with a rate ranging from 60 to 74 beats/minute. Occasional premature ventricular beats were noted.

Some 60 hours after admission, in the middle of the night, the monitor alarm sounded. The nurse instantly recognized ventricular fibrillation on the oscilloscope and ran to the bedside where the patient was found to be unconscious. She immediately called the physician and set a timing device for 2 minutes. She turned on the defibrillator, set the energy level at 400 watt-seconds, and applied electrode paste to the defibrillator paddles. The 2-minute-interval timer sounded, but the physician had not arrived. (The practice at that time was for the nurse to proceed with defibrillation herself only if a physician had not arrived within 2 minutes.) The nurse then defibrillated the patient without further delay. Normal sinus rhythm was established almost immediately (Fig. 14.3). The patient survived and was still alive 10 years later.

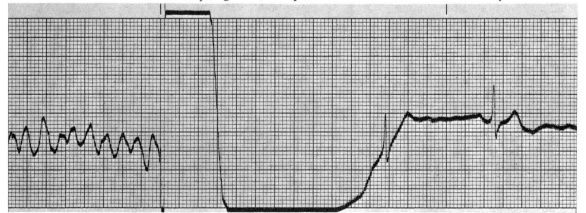

Figure 14.3.

Treatment

The treatment program for primary ventricular fibrillation has four phases.

1. *Recognition.* The initial step in the treatment of ventricular fibrillation is immediate identification of the arrhythmia. When ventricular fibrillation occurs, the alarm system of the monitor is triggered. The electrocardiographic pattern of ventricular fibrillation is readily distinguished by a series of chaotic waves which have no uniformity and are bizarre in their configuration (Fig. 14.4). If the arrhythmia cannot be identified instantly, no further time should be wasted in monitor observation. Instead, the observer should proceed immediately to the bedside and ascertain if the patient is unconscious as a result of circulatory arrest. If the patient is *unconscious* and peripheral pulses are not detectable, the planned treatment program should be initiated instantly.

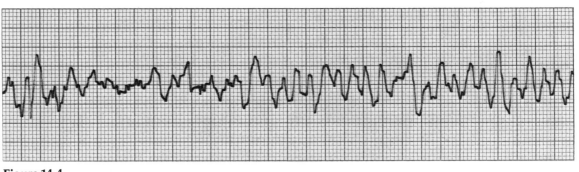

Figure 14.4.

2. *Termination of ventricular fibrillation.* Precordial shock (defibrillation) is the first and only treatment for ventricular fibrillation. *This shock should be administered by the first person to reach the bedside, whether a nurse or physician.* Defibrillation must be accomplished within 2 minutes; the sooner the shock is delivered, the greater is the chance for recovery.

   It is essential to realize that precordial shock must always be the initial step in treatment, and that time should never be wasted with customary cardiopulmonary resuscitation techniques.

   Regardless of the machine used to perform defibrillation, the maximal energy setting (400 watt-seconds) should always be used.

3. *Correction of lactic acidosis.* Every patient who develops ventricular fibrillation can be expected to have some degree of lactic acidosis as a result of the cessation of circulation regardless of the brevity of the arrest. (The etiology of lactic acidosis was discussed in the section on cardiogenic shock.) Therefore sodium bicarbonate should be administered immediately after the arrhythmia is terminated.

4. *Prevention of recurrence of ventricular fibrillation.* The myocardial irritability which led to ventricular fibrillation in the first place represents a potential threat for subsequent episodes. In other words, the source of the original problem is still present and must be treated vigorously if further episodes of this lethal arrhythmia are to be prevented. This prevention is best accomplished by the use of a continuous infusion of lidocaine (3000 mg in 500 cc glucose) at a rate designed to control or at least minimize PVCs.

Nursing Role

1. Ventricular fibrillation will trigger the alarm system of the monitor. (Either the high- or low-rate alarm may sound.)

2. Identify the bizarre irregular pattern of ventricular fibrillation. Even if in doubt, do not waste time with further monitor observation. Allow the electrocardiographic record to run continuously to document the event.

3. Go to the bedside and examine the patient. If he is conscious and responds to your call, ventricular fibrillation is *not* the problem. If the patient is unconscious, ascertain the absence of peripheral pulses and heart sounds.

4. If assistance is available, ask that the emergency system call be sounded and that an automatic timer be activated.

5. Turn on the power switch of the defibrillator and set the instrument dial at the maximum energy (400 watt-seconds). If a DC defibrillator is used, make certain the synchronizer switch is in the *off* position (see Chapter 17).

6. *Perform defibrillation immediately. Do not wait for the arrival of a physician or other personnel before proceeding.*

   The steps in defibrillation are as follows:
   a. Make certain the machine is *on*; that the energy level is maximum; and that the synchronizer is *off*.
   b. Apply a generous amount of electrode paste to the defibrillator paddles and spread the jelly evenly by approximating the surfaces of the paddles.
   c. Hold the paddles tightly against the chest wall. The exact position of the paddles is not important as long as the current will traverse the axis of the heart.
   d. Trigger the discharge mechanism of the defibrillator.
   Remember that survival after ventricular fibrillation is directly dependent on the rapidity with which the shock is delivered.

7. Immediately after the shock is delivered, observe the monitor to see if the fibrillation has terminated. (If an oscilloscope is not visible from the bedside, the prompt return of peripheral pulses or the return of consciousness indicates successful defibrillation.)

8. If ventricular fibrillation persists after the initial attempt, a second or third shock should be given promptly.

9. If precordial shock has not been successful after three attempts (an unlikely situation with the use of proper technique), additional shocks are probably unwarranted at this time. Instead, external cardiac compression and mouth-to-mouth ventilation should be started without further delay. During the period of cardiopulmonary resuscitation, sodium bicarbonate (40 mEq) should be injected rapidly and then defibrillation attempted again. An intracardiac injection of epinephrine may sometimes be used before precordial shock is tried again.

10. Unsuccessful defibrillation after all of these measures usually implies that ventricular fibrillation is *secondary* to advanced left ventricular failure. Survival in this circumstance is unlikely. (Failure to terminate *primary* ventricular fibrillation indicates that the resuscitation attempt was started too late—a situation that should *never* occur in a CCU.)

15

Disorders of Conduction

As described previously, impulses normally arise in the SA node; travel by way of the internodal tracts to the atrioventricular (AV) node; pass through the AV node to the bundle of His, the left and right bundle branches, and their divisions (fascicles) to the Purkinje network; and terminate in the myocardial cells. Any interference or abnormal delay in the passage of impulses from the SA node through the Purkinje-myocardial junction is described as a *heart block*. Heart blocks can occur at any level of the conduction system, but it is customary to categorize these disorders into three classes according to the main anatomic sites of involvement (Fig. 15.1):

1. Blocks in the SA node or atria
2. Blocks in the AV node or the surrounding junctional area (atrioventricular or junctional blocks)
3. Blocks in the His-Purkinje system (intraventricular or subjunctional blocks)

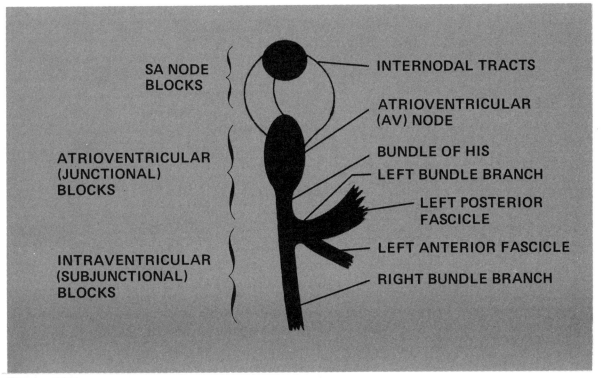

Figure 15.1

Blocks in the SA Node or Atria

When an impulse is blocked within the SA node or in the internodal tracts the electrical stimulus does not reach the atria or the ventricles. As a result, the entire PQRST complex is absent. Blocks in the SA node or internodal tracts cannot be specifically distinguished electrocardiographically or clinically from sinoatrial (SA) arrest, a disorder of impulse formation discussed previously (see Chapter 10). Consequently blocks involving the SA node are not considered separately in this section.

Atrioventricular (Junctional) Blocks*

Blocks interfering with conduction of impulses between the atria and ventricles usually develop because of ischemic injury to the AV node or AV junctional tissue. Less commonly, increased parasympathetic (vagal) activity or drugs (especially digitalis) produce these disturbances.

Atrioventricular blocks are categorized into first-degree, second-degree, and third-degree (complete) AV block, a classification based on the extent of the conduction defect between the atria and the ventricles. In first-degree block the AV node merely delays impulses before they enter the intraventricular conduction system, but each impulse is conducted to the ventricles. In second-degree AV block, where nodal involvement is greater, some atrial impulses are actually blocked in the AV node and are not conducted beyond this point. In third-degree (complete) AV block the more seriously affected AV node prevents transmission of *all* impulses from the atria to the ventricles. (In this circumstance the inherent automaticity of the ventricles produces ventricular contractions in the absence of stimulation from supraventricular centers.) These three forms of atrioventricular block are discussed individually in this chapter.

Intraventricular (Subjunctional) Blocks

Disturbances in conduction occurring *below* the level of bifurcation of the bundle of His are categorized as intraventricular or subjunctional blocks.

When these blocks develop during the acute phase of acute myocardial infarction they generally reflect ischemic damage to the conduction pathways (particularly in the interventricular septal area). However, intraventricular blocks may exist before acute myocardial infarction. In this circumstance the block is a consequence of chronic degeneration or fibrotic scarring of the bundle branches and intraventricular network.

Until recently it was believed that the bundle of His divided into two branches, the left bundle branch and the right bundle branch. Histological studies have shown, however, that the left bundle branch consists of two parts, an anterior and a posterior fascicle. For this reason the bundle of His is considered to have three branches (or fascicles), any of which can be blocked individually or in combination. Several types of intraventricular block may develop in this trifascicular system:

1. Block of the right bundle branch (RBBB)
2. Block of the *main* left bundle branch (LBBB)
3. Block of the *anterior* fascicle of the left bundle branch (called left anterior hemiblock or LAH)
4. Block of the *posterior* fascicle of the left bundle branch (called left posterior hemiblock or LPH)
5. Block involving the right bundle branch and one of the fascicles of the left bundle branch (called bifascicular block since two of the three branches are involved)
6. Blocks involving all three branches of the bundle of His (called trifascicular blocks)

---

*As shown in Figure 15.1, the AV junctional area extends from the level at which the internodal tracts enter the AV node to the point where the His bundle divides into its left and right bundle branches. In this discussion the term AV block includes blocks in the AV junctional area as well as in the AV node itself.

The diagnosis and differentiation of these various forms of intraventricular block require a 12-lead ECG (and sometimes even more sophisticated studies of electrical conduction called His-Bundle electrograms). Consequently it is not possible to ascertain the precise type of intraventricular block from a single monitor lead used in the CCU. Because interpretation of 12-lead ECGs is outside the customary nursing role, no attempt will be made here to discuss the diagnostic features of each type of intraventricular block. However, intraventricular blocks are characterized by wide QRS complexes (greater than 0.12 second); and this one electrocardiographic finding, readily detectable on a cardiac monitor, should indicate to the nurse that a bundle branch block is present.

Intraventricular blocks developing as the result of acute myocardial infarction are more dangerous than atrioventricular blocks, particularly when more than one fascicle is involved. Bifascicular or trifascicular blocks often lead to complete heart block and ventricular standstill. Moreover, acute intraventricular blocks generally reflect extensive myocardial infarction involving the interventricular septum.

FIRST-DEGREE AV HEART BLOCK

Etiology

The impulse arises in the SA node and is conducted normally to the AV node. Within the AV node or the junctional tissue the impulse is abnormally delayed before its passage to the intraventricular conduction system. This delay, manifested by a prolonged PR interval, usually results from ischemia of the AV node, but antiarrhythmic drugs and vagal overactivity may also produce this type of AV heart block.

Clinical Features

1. There are no symptoms or physical findings characteristic of first-degree AV block.
2. The diagnosis can be made only by ECG.

Danger in Acute Myocardial Infarction

1. First-degree AV block is not a serious arrhythmia in its own right. It does not reduce hemodynamic efficiency nor does it affect the rate or rhythm of the heart.
2. The arrhythmia is important because it usually indicates injury to the AV nodal area and may warn of impending second- or third-degree heart blocks. The latter blocks, which reflect *advanced* stages of AV nodal involvement, are far more dangerous and may lead to ventricular standstill.
3. *RISK:* First-degree AV block is often an early warning of more advanced heart block but is not a dangerous arrhythmia in itself.

Treatment

1. If there is only a slight delay in conduction (e.g., PR interval of 0.21–0.25 second), and the block does not increase, treatment is unnecessary.
2. If the conduction delay is greater than 0.26 second or, more significantly, if the block progresses, atropine (0.5 mg–1.0 mg intravenously) can be used in an attempt to accelerate AV conduction. Isoproterenol may be used in the event atropine fails (see Chapter 18).
3. If drug therapy is unsuccessful in controlling a *progressive* first-degree block, insertion of a transvenous pacing catheter may be indicated. This prophylactic approach reduces the risk of further unpredictable progression of first-degree block to complete block.
4. If first-degree heart block develops during the course of treatment with digitalis or any antiarrhythmic agent, the further use of these drugs should be carefully considered in view of their known ability to depress AV nodal conduction.

Nursing Role

1. When first-degree heart block is identified, record a rhythm strip and carefully measure the PR interval. If the PR interval is greater than 0.26 second or if it shows progressive lengthening subsequently, advise the physician.
2. Carefully observe the monitor for the sudden appearance of second- or third-degree block. If these advanced forms of heart block develop, notify the physician immediately.
3. In patients with evidence of first-degree block who are receiving digitalis or other antiarrhythmic agents, discuss the further administration of these drugs with the physician.

Case History

A 50-year-old man with an acute inferior myocardial infarction showed ECG evidence of a first-degree heart block at the time of admission. The PR interval was 0.24 second. Six hours later the nurse noted that the PR interval had increased to 0.30 second. She notified the physician, who ordered atropine (0.5 mg intravenously). The PR interval remained constant thereafter, and no further treatment was given.

```
┌─────────────────── FIRST-DEGREE AV HEART BLOCK ───────────────────┐
│                        IDENTIFYING ECG FEATURES                    │
│                                                                    │
│  1. Rate:          Normal.                                         │
│  2. Rhythm:        Regular.                                        │
│  3. P waves:       Normal, originating in the SA node.             │
│  4. PR interval:   Prolonged beyond 0.20 second. This prolongation │
│                    is due to a delay in the passage of the impulse │
│                    through the AV node.                            │
│  5. QRS:           Normal. Intraventricular conduction is not      │
│                    disturbed.                                      │
└────────────────────────────────────────────────────────────────────┘
```

EXAMPLE: First-Degree AV Block (Fig. 15.2)

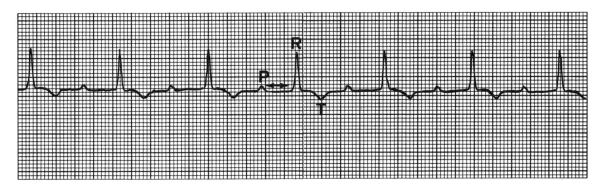

INTERPRETATION OF ECG

Rate: About 70/minute.
Rhythm: Regular.
P waves: Normal.
PR interval: The PR interval is almost 0.40 second, indicating a conduction delay through the AV node.
QRS: Normal (0.08 second).
Comments: Marked first-degree block may progress to more advanced AV block.

EXAMPLE: First-Degree AV Block (Fig. 15.3)

INTERPRETATION OF ECG

Rate: About 80/minute.
Rhythm: Regular.
P waves: Normal.
PR interval: Prolonged (0.32 second).
QRS: Normal (0.06 second).
Comments: Atropine will sometimes accelerate atrioventricular conduction, and the PR interval may become normal after such therapy.

SECOND-DEGREE AV HEART BLOCK

Etiology

Impulses originate in the SA node, activate the atria to produce P waves, and reach the AV node in normal fashion. In the AV junction (or sometimes below this area) some of these impulses are blocked and do not reach the ventricles. When this block occurs a P wave is *not* followed by a QRS complex and a ventricular beat is absent (dropped). Consequently in second-degree AV block the number of P waves always exceeds the number of QRS complexes.

Impulses may be blocked at regular or irregular intervals. When the block occurs regularly (for example, after every second, third, or fourth P wave), the conduction disturbance is known as 2:1, 3:1, or 4:1 second-degree block, respectively. In this circumstance the PR interval of all conducted beats is constant, and does not vary. Irregular second-degree block is known as Wenckebach-type block. It occurs when conduction through the AV node becomes progressively more difficult with each successive impulse until finally a ventricular beat is dropped. The ECG pattern of Wenckebach-type block is characterized by *progressive* prolongation of the PR interval until an atrial impulse is completely blocked and a QRS complex fails to appear. After the blocked beat the entire sequence is repeated. This intermittent failure of conduction to the ventricles produces an irregular rhythm.

Second-degree heart block results most often from ischemic damage to the conduction system. In Wenckebach second-degree block the injury is almost always confined to the AV node itself, whereas in constant 2:1, 3:1, or 4:1 block either the AV node, the AV junction, or the His-Purkinje system may be involved. Digitalis or increased vagal activity may also cause second-degree block.

Because the clinical features, prognosis, and treatment of these two forms of second-degree heart block (i.e., Wenckebach-type block with a varying PR interval and 2:1 type block with a constant PR interval) differ in several respects they will be considered side by side in the following discussion.†

Clinical Features

Wenckebach-Type Second-Degree Block

1. Symptoms depend primarily on the ventricular rate. Unless the rate is markedly slow the patient is usually unaware of the presence of this conduction disorder.

2. Although Wenckebach block produces an irregular rhythm (when a ventricular beat is dropped) the diagnosis can be established only by ECG findings, not by physical examination.

2:1-Type Second-Degree Block

1. As with Wenckebach-type block, symptoms are related to the ventricular rate. With rates under 50/minute the patient may experience angina, dyspnea, or cerebral insufficiency.

2. The diagnosis of 2:1, 3:1, or 4:1 AV block is made from ECG findings.

Danger in Acute Myocardial Infarction

Wenckebach-Type Second-Degree Block

1. This form of second-degree block is usually the result of ischemic injury to the AV node; and although the block may progress to third-degree (complete) heart block, it seldom advances to ventricular standstill.

2:1-Type Second-Degree Block

1. Second-degree block with a constant PR interval can develop because of injury to the AV node, the AV junctional area, or the His-Purkinje system. When the block occurs *below* the AV node (subjunctional block) there is great danger of progression to complete block and ventricular standstill. As a general rule, the width of the QRS complex reflects the location of the block. Blocks occurring in the AV node or junctional area are usually associated with *narrow* QRS complexes (less than 0.10 second). In contrast, subjunctional blocks are manifested by *wide* QRS complexes (0.12 second or greater). Thus the wider the QRS complex, the more serious the block.

---

†Wenckebach-type block is also called Mobitz I block, whereas second-degree block with a constant PR interval is described as Mobitz II block. The term Mobitz II block has more than one meaning, however, and for this reason we avoided the Mobitz classification in this discussion.

2. Wenckebach block is most often a *temporary* disturbance associated with inferior wall myocardial infarction, and it generally subsides spontaneously within 72–96 hours.
3. Circulatory efficiency is rarely affected by Wenckebach block, and this conduction disorder is usually well tolerated.
4. *RISK:* Wenckebach second-degree block is an important and potentially dangerous disorder of conduction. It may lead to complete block but seldom to ventricular standstill and sudden death.

2. Like Wenckebach blocks, 2:1 blocks are usually temporary disorders and generally disappear after a few days.
3. Circulatory efficiency may be affected in the higher degrees of block (3:1, 4:1) because of the slow ventricular heart rate.
4. *RISK:* 2:1-type second-degree block must be considered a serious warning arrhythmia which may lead to complete heart block and ventricular standstill. The risk of developing these lethal complications is greater when the QRS complexes are wide, but any form of 2:1 block is potentially dangerous.

Treatment

Wenckebach-Type Second-Degree Block

1. Since Wenckebach blocks seldom progress to ventricular standstill, many physicians believe that treatment is unnecessary. Others, however, adopt a more cautious approach and prefer to insert a temporary transvenous pacemaker catheter in the right ventricle when this conduction disturbance is identified (see Chapter 17).
2. If the ventricular rate is less than 50/minute, isoproterenol (Isuprel) can be used in an attempt to increase conduction through the AV node. An intravenous infusion of this drug (1 mg in 250 cc 5% glucose solution) may be administered. Atropine (1 mg intravenously) sometimes decreases the degree of AV block but is less dependable than isoproterenol.
3. With the slim hope that Wenckebach block has been caused by digitalis or quinidine, these drugs should be withheld if the block persists.

2:1-Type Second-Degree Block

1. Because of the unpredictable course of this form of second-degree block and the ever present threat of sudden development of complete block or ventricular standstill, it is a sound practice to insert a temporary transvenous pacemaker as soon as second-degree block with a constant PR interval is identified.
2. Treatment with isoproterenol or atropine may be attempted if the block is associated with narrow QRS complexes, but drug therapy should not be relied on when wide QRS complexes are present.
3. Antiarrhythmic drugs and digitalis should be withdrawn in the presence of second-degree block.

Nursing Role

1. Identify the slow-rate arrhythmia as second-degree block and document this conduction disorder on a rhythm strip. Second-degree block must be distinguished from sinus bradycardia and complete AV heart block.
2. Measure the PR intervals throughout the rhythm strip and determine if they vary in duration (Wenckebach block) or if they are constant (2:1 block).
3. Ascertain if the QRS complexes are narrow (0.10 second or less) or wide. Wide QRS complexes should alert the nurse to the possibility that complete heart block or ventricular standstill may develop.
4. Notify the physician promptly once second-degree block has been identified.
5. With Wenckebach block the physician may elect either to treat the block with drugs (atropine or isoproterenol) or to insert a temporary transvenous pacemaker. (Some physicians choose to observe the arrhythmia without treatment.)
6. Second-degree heart block with constant PR intervals is likely to be treated with temporary cardiac pacing. Therefore the nurse should prepare for the insertion of a transvenous pacemaker (see Chapter 17).
7. If second-degree heart block is observed, withhold further doses of digitalis and antiarrhythmic agents until the physician has assessed the problem.
8. Observe the monitor carefully for progression of the degree of block. Remember that complete heart block or ventricular standstill may be only a step behind, especially with second-degree heart block associated with constant PR intervals and wide QRS complexes.

```
┌─────────────────────────────────────────────────────────────────┐
│          SECOND-DEGREE AV BLOCK (WENCKEBACH TYPE)                 │
│                  IDENTIFYING ECG FEATURES                         │
│                                                                   │
│  1. Rate:        The ventricular rate is usually slow but may be  │
│                  normal.                                          │
│  2. Rhythm:      Irregular because of the dropped beats.          │
│  3. P waves:     Because some impulses from the atria are blocked │
│                  in the AV nodal area, there are always more P    │
│                  waves than QRS complexes.                        │
│  4. PR interval: The PR interval lengthens *progressively* until  │
│                  an atrial impulse is blocked completely in the   │
│                  AV node and a QRS complex fails to appear (a     │
│                  dropped beat). Following the dropped beat the PR  │
│                  interval shortens, and then the entire sequence  │
│                  is repeated.                                     │
│  5. QRS:         Usually normal.                                  │
└─────────────────────────────────────────────────────────────────┘
```

EXAMPLE: Second-Degree AV Block (Wenckebach Type) (Fig. 15.4)

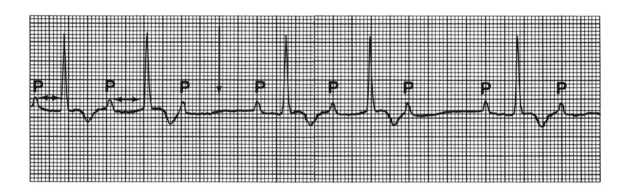

INTERPRETATION OF ECG

Rate:	The ventricular rate is about 50/minute. The atrial rate is 80/minute.
Rhythm:	Every third atrial impulse is blocked, creating an irregular ventricular rhythm.
P waves:	Normal in configuration, and occur at regular intervals. The number of P waves exceeds the number of QRS complexes.
PR interval:	The PR interval progressively increases in the first two beats. Then, the third atrial impulse (P wave) is blocked, and a QRS complex does not appear (arrow). The entire sequence is then repeated in the cardiac cycles that follow.
QRS:	Normal (0.08 second).
Comments:	The repeated sequence of progressive lengthening of the PR intervals until a ventricular beat is dropped is the key diagnostic feature of Wenckebach block.

SECOND-DEGREE AV BLOCK (2:1 TYPE)
IDENTIFYING ECG FEATURES

1. **Rate:** The ventricular rate is usually slow and is one-half, one-third, or one-fourth the atrial rate (i.e., 2:1, 3:1, 4:1 block).
2. **Rhythm:** Regular, because the block occurs at constant intervals.
3. **P waves:** There are two, three, or four times as many P waves as QRS complexes.
4. **PR interval:** Every second, third, or fourth atrial impulse is conducted to the ventricle producing a QRS complex. The remaining atrial impulses are blocked. In the conducted beats the PR interval is constant.
5. **QRS:** Usually normal when the block is in the AV junctional area; usually widened when the block is below this area (subjunctional block).

EXAMPLE: Second-Degree AV Block (2:1 Type) (Fig. 15.5)

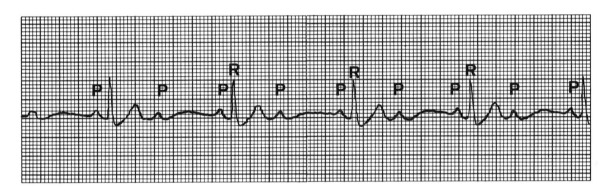

INTERPRETATION OF ECG

Rate: The ventricular rate is 50/minute. The atrial rate is 100/minute.
Rhythm: Regular.
P waves: There are two normal P waves between ventricular complexes.
PR interval: Every second P wave is blocked. The PR interval of the conducted beats is constant. The impulses that pass through the junctional area are conducted normally to the ventricles.
QRS: Normal (0.08 second).
Comments: The ventricular rate is one-half the atrial rate (2:1 block).

Case History

A 64-year-old man was admitted to the CCU because of an acute anterior wall myocardial infarction. The original rhythm strip revealed normal sinus rhythm, but the PR interval was 0.24 second (first-degree AV block). About 1 hour later the slow-rate alarm sounded, and the nurse noted the heart rate had suddenly decreased from 90 to 45/minute. On examining the rhythm strip it was apparent that there were two P waves for each QRS complex and that a 2:1-type second-degree heart block had developed. It was also noted that the QRS complex was widened (0.12 second). The nurse advised the physician of these findings, and it was decided that a temporary transvenous pacemaker should be inserted, particularly in light of the widened QRS complexes and the potential threat of progression to complete heart block (or ventricular standstill).

THIRD-DEGREE (COMPLETE) AV BLOCK

Etiology

Impulses from the SA node are *completely* blocked and do not reach the ventricles. The block may occur in the AV node, the junctional area, or the His-Purkinje system. Regardless of the site of the block the atria and ventricles beat *independently* of each other. The SA node serves as the pacemaker for the atria; the ventricles beat because of the inherent automaticity of ventricular muscle, at a rate of 30–40 beats/minute. The most common cause of complete heart block is ischemic damage to the AV junction or to the conduction system below it. Rarely, extreme vagal hyperactivity or digitalis toxicity may be responsible for the block.

Clinical Features

1. The presence of complete heart block can be suspected from clinical examination. The key finding is a very slow, regular heart rate (usually less than 40 beats/minute) which remains constant and does not fluctuate (a fixed heart rate).
2. Episodes of syncope and convulsions may occur with complete heart block. These attacks (Stokes-Adams attacks) are caused by cerebral ischemia resulting from a marked reduction in cardiac output that accompanies the slow, fixed heart rate.
3. Signs and symptoms of left ventricular failure are frequently present.

Danger in Acute Myocardial Infarction

1. The *independent* ventricular pacemaker is not dependable and may cease abruptly (causing ventricular standstill) or may be replaced by a faster ectopic focus in the ventricle (leading to ventricular tachycardia or ventricular fibrillation).
2. Because the ventricular rate is constant at 30–40 beats/minute and cannot increase, the cardiac output is insufficient in most instances to meet circulatory demands; consequently myocardial ischemia and left ventricular failure often develop.
3. Grossly reduced blood flow to the brain may cause fainting and convulsions (Stokes-Adams syndrome). Cerebral blood flow impairment of a lesser degree is manifested by mental confusion, vertigo, and lightheadedness.
4. *RISK:* Complete heart block is an *extremely dangerous* arrhythmia representing a clear warning of impending ventricular standstill or ventricular fibrillation.

Treatment

1. The most dependable and predictably effective method of treating complete heart block is transvenous cardiac pacing. A catheter electrode should be inserted as soon as third-degree block is identified.
2. While preparing for the insertion of the pacemaker, an intravenous infusion of isoproterenol (Isuprel), 1 mg in 250 cc glucose solution, should be given slowly. Occasionally isoproterenol may reduce the degree of AV block and increase the heart rate. Despite this seeming effectiveness of drug therapy, sudden recurrence of complete block often occurs, and therefore it is a wise practice to insert a transvenous pacemaker in *all* patients who develop complete heart block.
3. Cardiac pacing should be continued until normal sinus rhythm returns, and the pacing catheter should remain in place for at least 5 days thereafter.
4. Rarely, complete heart block persists because of *irreversible* damage to the conduction system. In this circumstance a permanent pacemaker is required.
5. Because complete heart block is often preceded by lesser degrees of AV block the treatment of this arrhythmia should begin ideally when *progressive* heart block is first identified (as explained in the description of second-degree block).

THIRD-DEGREE (COMPLETE) AV BLOCK
IDENTIFYING ECG FEATURES

1. **Rate:** The ventricular rate is usually 30–40/minute. The atrial rate, which is independent of the ventricular rate, is always faster (generally in the range of 60–120/minute).

2. **Rhythm:** Both atrial and ventricular rhythms are regular but independent of each other.

3. **P waves:** There are more P waves than QRS complexes. Because atrial stimulation is unaffected, the size and shape of the P waves are normal.

4. **PR interval:** Because the atria and ventricles have independent pacemakers there is no relationship between atrial (P waves) and ventricular (QRS) rhythms. As a result, the PR interval is never constant.

5. **QRS:** Configuration of the complex depends on the site of the block and the location of the ectopic ventricular pacemaker. If the block and the ectopic pacemaker are near the AV node the QRS complex may be normal. In contrast, when the block and the pacemaker are subjunctional the QRS complexes are usually widened and distorted.

EXAMPLE: Complete Heart Block (Third-Degree Block) (Fig. 15.6)

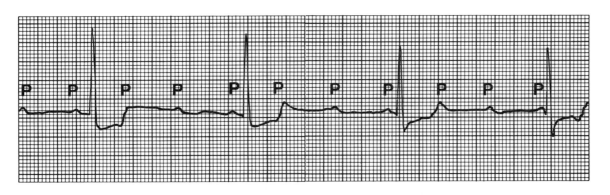

INTERPRETATION OF ECG

Rate: The ventricular rate is about 40/minute. The atrial rate is 110/minute.

Rhythm: The atrial and ventricular rhythms are regular but bear no relationship to each other.

P waves: Occur regularly but independently of the QRS complexes.

PR interval: Inconstant throughout because there is no conduction between the atria and ventricles, each functioning under the control of its own pacemaker.

QRS: Normal, suggesting that the ventricular pacemaker is probably in the nodal (junctional) area rather than subjunctional.

Comments: A heart rate of 40/minute or less associated with an inconstant PR interval offers an immediate clue to the diagnosis of complete heart block.

Nursing Role

1. Identify this slow-rate arrhythmia and distinguish it from marked sinus bradycardia, junctional rhythm, and second-degree AV block. Document the disorder with a rhythm strip.
2. Notify the physician immediately after this arrhythmia is recognized.
3. Prepare an infusion containing 1 mg isoproterenol in 250 cc dextrose solution.
4. Because of the threat of ventricular fibrillation developing in the presence of the slow ventricular rate, a defibrillator should be brought to the bedside and made ready for use.
5. Keep a syringe containing 100 mg lidocaine at the bedside.
6. Prepare for the insertion of a transvenous pacemaker (see Chapter 17).
7. Assess the patient's clinical condition repeatedly, with particular emphasis on signs or symptoms that indicate left ventricular failure.
8. Diligently observe the monitor for premature ventricular contractions; these ectopic beats may forewarn of ventricular tachycardia or fibrillation.
9. If a transvenous pacemaker has been inserted previously for prophylactic reasons (because of second-degree AV block or block in the His-Purkinje system), verify that the pacemaker is functioning properly.
10. If ventricular standstill develops, initiate cardiopulmonary resuscitation (CPR) immediately. Sound an emergency alarm.

Case History

A 56-year-old man was admitted to the CCU in acute distress. He complained of substernal pain, shortness of breath, and a feeling of faintness. On examining the patient the nurse found that the blood pressure was 96/68, and that the pulse rate was only 36/minute. A rhythm strip confirmed the nurse's clinical suspicion of complete heart block. The physician was notified promptly of these findings, and it was decided that a temporary transvenous pacemaker should be inserted without delay to increase the heart rate. The physician requested that an intravenous infusion of isoproterenol be given while preparations were being made to insert a pacing catheter. When the heart was paced at a rate of 70/minute there was marked clinical improvement, reflecting increased cardiac output. A rhythm strip recorded during the course of cardiac pacing is shown in Figure 15.7.

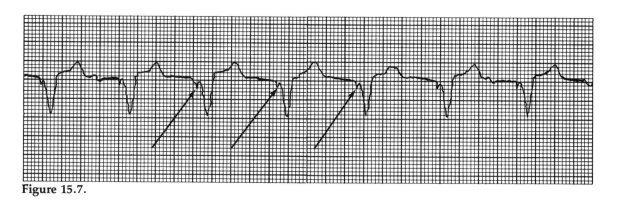

Figure 15.7.

Although the complete heart block still exists (as evidenced by the random position of the P waves), the ventricular rate is now controlled by the pacemaker. The pacing stimuli (arrows) occur 80 times/minute, creating a ventricular response at this rate.

EXAMPLE: Complete Heart Block with Wide QRS Complexes (Fig. 15.8)

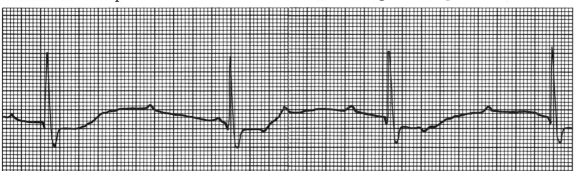

INTERPRETATION OF ECG

Rate: The ventricular rate is about 40/minute (the inherent rate of ventricular muscle).

Rhythm: Regular.

P waves: Occur at regular intervals at a rate of more than 80/minute.

PR interval: The PR interval is inconstant. All impulses from the SA node are blocked.

QRS: The ventricular complexes are wide (greater than 0.12 second); wide complexes of this type usually reflect a subjunctional ventricular pacemaker.

Comments: Because subjunctional pacemakers are unreliable and may fail abruptly, complete heart block associated with wide QRS complexes carries a high risk.

EXAMPLE: Complete Heart Block Leading to Ventricular Tachycardia and Fibrillation (Figure 15.9 was a continuous rhythm strip but has been divided and reduced in scale for purposes of full reproduction.)

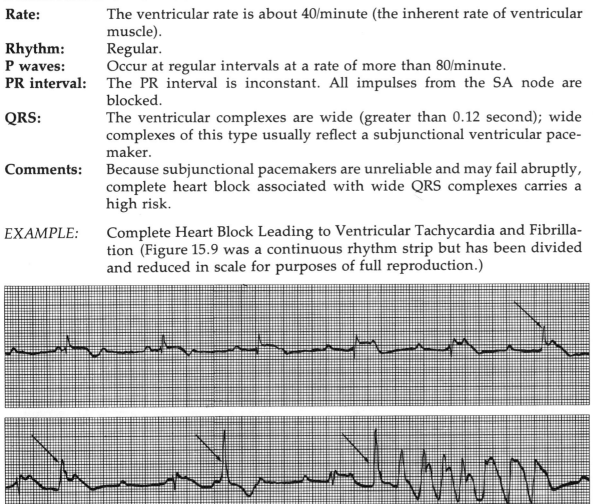

Figure 15.9. A continuous rhythm strip divided and reduced in scale for purposes of full reproduction.

Comments: The electrocardiographic sequence seen above demonstrates one of the greatest dangers of complete heart block: the development of *ventricular fibrillation*. In the presence of the very slow ventricular rate associated with complete heart block, PVCs developed (arrows). These ectopic beats caused repetitive ventricular firing and ventricular fibrillation (lower strip).

INTRAVENTRICULAR (SUBJUNCTIONAL) BLOCKS
BUNDLE BRANCH BLOCKS

Etiology

All blocks occurring below the AV junctional area are categorized as intraventricular (or subjunctional) blocks. The cardiac impulse originates normally in the SA node and passes through the AV node to the bundle of His without difficulty. The impulse is then blocked in the right or left bundle branches (or their networks) because of injury to these areas. As a consequence of obstruction to conduction involving the right bundle branch or the left bundle branch, the respective ventricles are activated abnormally. The ventricle affected by the bundle branch block is finally activated by impulses which reach it through the interventricular septum from the normally stimulated side. This circuitous route for complete ventricular activation (i.e., both ventricles) requires additional time and causes a wide QRS complex, the characteristic feature of bundle branch block.

Bundle branch block is usually the result of chronic degeneration or fibrotic scarring of the intraventricular conduction system and is often present before the acute infarction. However, bundle branch block may develop as a complication of acute myocardial infarction. The prognosis in the latter circumstance is usually more ominous than it is in chronic bundle branch block.

This discussion focuses on blocks of the main bundle branches, and does not consider the various types of fascicular blocks mentioned in the introduction of this chapter.

Clinical Features

1. Bundle branch block causes no specific symptoms and produces no definite diagnostic physical findings.
2. Although right bundle branch block (RBBB), left bundle branch block (LBBB), and blocks involving the individual fascicles of the left bundle branch can be readily distinguished from each other by their electrocardiographic patterns, the single lead used in cardiac monitoring is insufficient for this purpose and localization of the block can be made only by means of a 12-lead electrocardiogram.

Danger in Acute Myocardial Infarction

1. Intraventricular blocks that develop acutely as a result of myocardial infarction (in contrast to chronic, preexisting blocks) usually reflect extensive damage to the myocardium and are associated with a high mortality. Death may be due to electrical failure (ventricular standstill) or to circulatory (power) failure.
2. Blocks involving more than one of the three intraventricular conduction pathways (the right bundle branch, the left anterior bundle branch, and the left posterior bundle branch) are especially dangerous because they may abruptly cause ventricular standstill.
3. Left bundle branch block obscures the characteristic ECG findings of acute myocardial infarction; therefore diagnosis of infarction is difficult in its presence.
4. *RISK:* Bundle branch block is a very serious disorder when the block is a consequence of the acute myocardial infarction, since it is usually indicative of extensive myocardial damage with involvement of the interventricular septal area.

Treatment

1. There is no drug therapy for intraventricular blocks.
2. A temporary transvenous cardiac pacemaker should be inserted prophylactically whenever intraventricular block develops acutely after myocardial infarction in an attempt to combat sudden ventricular standstill. Many clinicians believe that a pacemaker should also be inserted even with chronic heart block when more than one fascicle is affected (e.g., right bundle branch block and left anterior hemiblock). However, the benefit of this technique is still uncertain.
3. Rarely, intraventricular block may reflect overdosage of digitalis or an antiarrhythmic agent (particularly quinidine). In this circumstance the block may disappear after the drug is withdrawn.

Nursing Role

1. If an intraventricular block (manifested on the monitor by a widened QRS complex) develops acutely, document the conduction disturbance with an ECG strip and notify the physician of this change.
2. Obtain a 12-lead ECG at this time so that the physician can localize the site of the block and the number of fascicles involved. (As noted, these facts *cannot* be ascertained from the monitor strip alone.)
3. Because it is likely that a temporary transvenous pacemaker will be inserted, prepare for this procedure.
4. Carefully observe the patient's clinical condition. This observation is particularly important since intraventricular blocks are usually associated with extensive infarctions and the risk of multiple complications is great.
5. If the patient develops an intraventricular block during the course of drug therapy, discuss the problem with the physician before the next dose is administered.

BUNDLE BRANCH BLOCK—IDENTIFYING ECG FEATURES

1. **Rate:** Usually normal but sometimes bundle branch block is rate related, appearing and disappearing with changes in the heart rate.
2. **Rhythm:** Regular.
3. **P waves:** Normal.
4. **PR interval:** Normal, because impulses reach the *uninvolved* ventricle without delay.
5. **QRS:** *Always* widened to 0.12 second or more, and the configuration of the complex is distorted. After the uninvolved ventricle is stimulated the impulses must then be transmitted through the interventricular septum to activate the blocked side. This delay in activation causes the QRS complexes to be wide and notched.

EXAMPLE: Bundle Branch Block (Fig. 15.10)

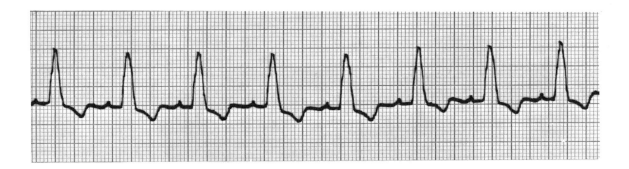

INTERPRETATION OF ECG

Rate: About 80/minute.
Rhythm: Regular.
P waves: Normal.
PR interval: Normal (0.18 second) since the impulse from the SA node passes through the uninvolved bundle without delay and activates one ventricle normally.
QRS: The complex is abnormally widened (more than 0.12 second), indicating that the time for *total* ventricular activation is prolonged. (The impulse must pass through the interventricular septum to stimulate the blocked ventricle.)
Comments: With a single monitor lead it is usually not possible to distinguish which of the bundle branches is blocked. This localization, which has prognostic importance, is made with a 12-lead ECG, from which the respective patterns can be readily identified. The monitor lead indicates only that an intraventricular conduction defect is present.

Case History

A 70-year-old woman was admitted to the CCU with a history of severe substernal pain of 2 hours' duration. The nurse noted a widened QRS complex on the initial rhythm strip. A 12-lead ECG demonstrated a left bundle branch block. The admitting physician stated that this pattern had been present for at least 3 years. Because of the LBBB the diagnosis of acute myocardial infarction could not be made definitely at the time. Despite this uncertainty, the patient was treated as if an acute infarction had occurred. The question was resolved within a few days when enzyme studies confirmed the diagnosis of acute myocardial infarction.

16

Ventricular Standstill:

A Death-Producing Arrhythmia

If the electrical stimulus to the ventricles becomes inadequate or ceases entirely, the ventricles will not contract effectively; this state is designated *ventricular standstill.** The end result of this catastrophe is the same as with ventricular fibrillation: sudden death!

Ventricular standstill may develop in two ways: as a primary arrhythmia *(primary ventricular standstill)* or as a terminal arrhythmia during advanced left ventricular failure *(secondary ventricular standstill)*. The latter mechanism is far more common.

In primary ventricular standstill atrial impulses are discharged normally and produce P waves. However, the impulses are completely blocked and never reach the ventricles. The block may occur in the AV junction or, more often, in the intraventricular conduction system. Despite the seeming suddenness of ventricular standstill, the catastrophe is preceded in practically all instances by some form of heart block. When ventricular stimulation ceases, unconsciousness develops immediately and death occurs unless effective ventricular contractions can be restored instantly. On some occasions ventricular standstill is only a transient phenomenon, and conduction and ventricular stimulation return spontaneously. These intermittent episodes are characterized by syncope and are described as *Stokes-Adams attacks*.

In contrast to primary ventricular standstill, secondary ventricular standstill is always associated with circulatory failure and is a terminal event in patients dying of cardiogenic shock or advanced left ventricular failure. In these conditions inadequate tissue perfusion results in hypoxia, acidosis, and electrolyte imbalance, all of which depress electrical conductivity. At a critical point the heart's electrical activity becomes insufficient to stimulate the myocardium and ventricular standstill develops. This secondary type of standstill seldom yields to resuscitative techniques (including cardiac pacing) because the oxygen-deprived myocardium is unable to respond to any stimulation. In other words, the basic circulatory deficit that affected electrical conductivity in the first place is still present. Death from secondary ventricular standstill usually occurs gradually; electrical activity may continue, but muscle contractions are weak and ineffective in propelling blood from the ventricles. This state is designated as mechanical or power failure—in contrast to failure of electrical stimulation and conduction.

---

*There is some confusion regarding the proper terminology of this catastrophe. The terms ventricular standstill, ventricular asystole, cardiac standstill, and cardiac arrest are used interchangeably to designate cessation of heart action.

At the bedside, without an ECG, one cannot distinguish ventricular standstill from ventricular fibrillation since both arrhythmias are characterized by the absence of audible heart sounds. It is common practice, therefore, to classify cessation of the circulation as *cardiac arrest* even though ventricular fibrillation may actually be at fault. In the CCU, where the lethal arrhythmia can be specifically identified, it is poor practice to use the general term cardiac arrest when the arrhythmia is in fact either ventricular standstill or ventricular fibrillation.

VENTRICULAR STANDSTILL

Etiology

Ventricular contraction depends on adequate ventricular stimulation. Thus if impulses fail to reach the ventricles or if impulse formation ceases, ventricular standstill occurs. In primary ventricular standstill the problem originates in the conduction system. All impulses generated by the SA node (or atria) are blocked and therefore the ventricles are totally dependent on an inherent ventricular pacemaker. When this ventricular focus stops discharging, the ventricles are left without any source of electrical stimulation. The underlying cause of secondary ventricular standstill is hypoxia, which depresses conduction, impulse formation, and myocardial responsiveness to stimulation.

Clinical Features

1. When ventricular standstill develops there is complete cessation of circulation. No heartbeat can be heard, no peripheral pulses can be felt, the blood pressure is unobtainable, and signs of cerebral anoxia (unconsciousness and dilatation of the pupils) are evident. *Death occurs within minutes.* The clinical picture is therefore identical to that of ventricular fibrillation.
2. Electrocardiographically, ventricular standstill is readily distinguishable from ventricular fibrillation. It is essential to identify which of these lethal arrhythmias is present because of the totally different approaches to resuscitation.

Danger in Acute Myocardial Infarction

1. Primary ventricular standstill is an immediate and direct cause of death unless resuscitation can be accomplished within a minute or two. This death-producing arrhythmia is much less common than primary ventricular fibrillation.
2. Secondary ventricular standstill is almost inevitably fatal with current means of treatment.
3. *RISK: Ventricular standstill is undoubtedly the most dreaded and the most dangerous of all arrhythmias.* Even with primary ventricular standstill the results with resuscitation are distressingly poor (and certainly less successful) than with resuscitation from ventricular fibrillation. For this reason, *prevention* of ventricular standstill is of supreme importance.

Treatment

The treatment and resuscitation program has four phases:
1. *Recognition.* When primary ventricular standstill occurs, the low-rate alarm of the monitoring system will be activated. The electrocardiographic pattern is characterized by the absence of ventricular (QRS) complexes while atrial activity (P waves) persists (Fig. 16.1). If the ECG pattern cannot be identified instantly, no further time should be spent in observing the monitor. The nurse should proceed immediately to the bedside to see if the patient is unconscious.

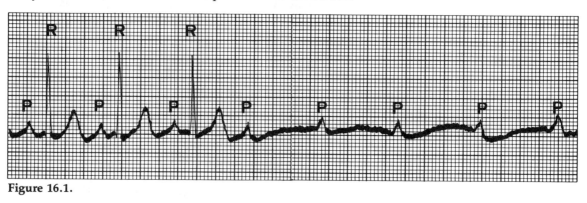

Figure 16.1.

2. *Termination of ventricular standstill.* If the patient is unconscious and there is no evidence of circulation, the nurse or physician who reaches the bedside first should strike the patient's chest with a forceful blow directly over the sternum. Occasionally this simple step, if performed within seconds of the onset of ventricular standstill, will cause resumption of the heartbeat.

   If the blow to the chest is ineffective, external cardiac compression and mouth-to-mouth ventilation should be initiated instantly and continued while the following measures are carried out.

   a. An emergency alarm should be sounded to summon the personnel to assist in the resuscitative attempt.

   b. After an airway has been established to administer oxygen and while effective external cardiac compression is being performed in an effort to maintain cerebral circulation, cardiac pacing should be attempted. The technique of cardiac pacing is described in the following chapter.

   c. Epinephrine (5 cc of a 1:10,000 solution) may be injected directly into the heart in an effort to stimulate electrical activity.

3. *Correction of lactic acidosis.* Lactic acidosis must be anticipated in every patient who develops ventricular standstill. Sodium bicarbonate should be administered intravenously as soon as possible and an infusion continued while cardiopulmonary resuscitation is in progress. Unless the acidosis is corrected, the heart will not respond to pacing or other measures.

4. *Prevention of recurrence.* If resuscitation is successful, cardiac pacing should be continued until signs of heart block or bradycardia have disappeared. A transvenous pacemaker should be left in place for at least 1 week after sinus rhythm has been reestablished.

Nursing Role

When a Transvenous Pacemaker Has NOT Been Inserted Prophylactically

1. When the low-rate alarm sounds, attempt to identify the ECG pattern on the monitor. Is the arrhythmia ventricular fibrillation or ventricular standstill?
2. Go to the bedside at once and examine the patient. If the patient is awake and conscious it is quite certain that a false alarm has occurred.
3. If the patient is unconscious and has no peripheral pulses or heartbeat, sound the emergency alarm system.
4. Deliver a sharp blow to the chest wall directly over the sternum. This simple procedure may sometimes reestablish the heartbeat and is always worth trying.
5. If the heartbeat does not return immediately after the blow to the chest, begin the planned program of cardiopulmonary resuscitation (CPR).
6. Continue external cardiac compression and mouth-to-mouth ventilation until other personnel provide assistance.
7. While CPR is in progress, one member of the team should prepare a syringe containing 40 mEq sodium bicarbonate for immediate intravenous injection. Start an infusion containing 400 mEq sodium bicarbonate after the initial injection.
8. Bring all necessary equipment for cardiac pacing to the bedside for immediate use by the physician.
9. In the event of failure with other measures, the physician may inject 5 cc of 1:10,000 epinephrine directly into the heart. Prepare a syringe with an intracardiac needle for this purpose.

When a Transvenous Pacemaker Has Been Inserted Prophylactically

1. As noted previously, ventricular standstill is usually preceded by some form of heart block or extreme bradycardia. Thus the development of ventricular standstill cannot actually be considered as unexpected; only the onset is sudden. By recognizing the warning arrhythmias and inserting a transvenous pacemaker prophylactically, it should be possible to prevent the occurrence of primary ventricular standstill. As soon as a QRS complex fails to appear, a demand pacemaker automatically begins to discharge impulses and stimulates the ventricles to contract.
2. The nursing role in cardiac pacing is described in the next chapter.

Case History

   A 78-year-old man was admitted to the CCU with signs of advanced left ventricular failure. The ECG revealed an anteroseptal myocardial infarction, and a rhythm strip showed sinus tachycardia with a rate of 124/minute. He was treated with furosemide (Lasix), rotating tourniquets, oxygen, and intravenous digoxin. The response to therapy was poor, and the patient continued to exhibit marked dyspnea. During the course of treatment the heart rate slowed abruptly to 58/minute, and a junctional rhythm was recognized on a monitor strip. A transvenous pacemaker was inserted, but pacing was ineffective and the ventricles did not respond to stimulation (because of severe hypoxia). About 5 minutes later the patient lost consciousness. The nurse was unable to record a blood pressure, and no peripheral pulses were palpable. The monitor now showed isolated, broad, distorted QRS complexes occurring about 10 times/minute. Resuscitation attempts were unsuccessful. The cause of death was advanced left ventricular failure. The terminal rhythm was secondary ventricular standstill.

PRIMARY VENTRICULAR STANDSTILL
IDENTIFYING ECG FEATURES

1. **Rate:**   At the onset of ventricular standstill the ventricles cease to contract.
2. **Rhythm:**   There is no heartbeat when asystole develops.
3. **P waves:**   Usually normal; they continue independently despite the cessation of ventricular activity.
4. **PR interval:** Atrial activity may persist, but the impulses are not conducted to the ventricle and there is no ventricular stimulation.
5. **QRS:**   None.

EXAMPLE: Primary Ventricular Standstill (Fig. 16.2)

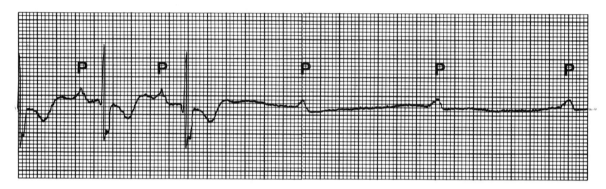

INTERPRETATION OF ECG

Rate: After the third QRS complex, ventricular activation ceases and there is no heartbeat.
Rhythm: There is no cardiac rhythm because of total cessation of ventricular contractions.
P waves: Atrial activity continues after ventricular standstill.
PR interval: Although the atria are stimulated, no impulses reach the ventricles.
QRS: Absent when the ventricular stimulation ceases.
Comments: In this case, ventricular standstill developed in the presence of an intraventricular conduction defect. A 12-lead ECG showed a right bundle branch block as well as a block of the anterior subdivision of the left bundle branch (bilateral bundle branch block). A first-degree heart block is also apparent in the single-lead tracing shown above.

——— SECONDARY VENTRICULAR STANDSTILL ———
IDENTIFYING ECG FEATURES

1. **Rate:**   Electrical activity in the ventricles may continue, producing infrequent QRS complexes (rate 10–30/minute).
2. **Rhythm:**   The isolated electrical activity in the ventricle is insufficient to stimulate ventricular contraction, and so there is no heartbeat or peripheral pulses.
3. **P waves:**   Absent, since atrial death has occurred (downward displacement of pacemaker).
4. **PR interval:** There is no conduction through the heart. The QRS complexes arise from the ventricles.
5. **QRS:**   Wide, slurred complexes at a very slow rate.

EXAMPLE: Secondary Ventricular Standstill (Fig. 16.3)

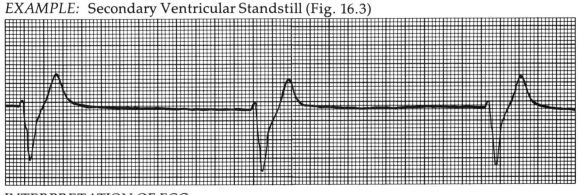

INTERPRETATION OF ECG

Rate: Isolated ventricular electrical activity at a rate of less than 30/minute.
Rhythm: The occasional ventricular complexes do not actually constitute a cardiac rhythm. They represent isolated electrical activity but are not associated with effective ventricular contractions.
P waves: Absent.
PR interval: Absent. There is no conduction through the heart.
QRS: Very wide and distorted.
Comments: Cardiac pacing is seldom effective in secondary ventricular standstill. The myocardium is unable to respond to the electrical stimulus because of hypoxia.

EXAMPLE: Dying Heart (Fig. 16.4)

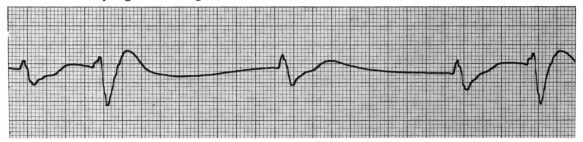

Comments: Although there is occasional electrical activity in the ventricle, true stimulation of the myocardium does not occur. The bizarre, distorted complexes may continue for several minutes even though the patient is clinically dead. This ECG pattern is common among patients dying of advanced left ventricular failure (secondary ventricular standstill).

17

The Electrical Treatment of Arrhythmias:

Cardiac Pacing and Precordial Shock

CARDIAC PACING

If for some reason the inherent electrical system of the heart does not generate impulses or fails to conduct impulses to the ventricles, it is possible to stimulate the myocardium and induce ventricular contraction by means of electrical impulses from an external source. This stimulation is achieved by using a battery-powered device called a pacemaker, which discharges repetitive electrical impulses so that an effective heart rate can be maintained and life preserved. The impulses are delivered to the heart by way of a catheter electrode, which is passed through the venous system into the right ventricular cavity; the technique is known as transvenous pacing.*

Conduction disturbances resulting from acute myocardial infarction are almost always transient in nature and usually disappear during the healing phase of the attack; therefore cardiac pacing is used only as a temporary measure in this circumstance. By contrast, in patients with chronic, irreversible heart block (unrelated to myocardial infarction) permanent cardiac pacing is required. Permanent pacing, which involves surgical implantation of a pacemaker under the skin, has no application in the treatment of the acute phase of myocardial infarction and therefore is not discussed further here. The following description focuses on temporary transvenous pacing.

---

*Before the introduction of transvenous pacing in the early 1960's pacing was accomplished by means of a large electrode placed on the chest wall. This method of stimulation (called external pacing) is no longer used because it was not predictably effective. Furthermore the magnitude of electrical current required to effect ventricular contractions through the closed chest wall is so great that the stimulus causes local pain, intense spasms of the skeletal muscles, and (with prolonged use) skin burns. Another technique that has all but been abandoned is transthoracic pacing. In this form of pacing the myocardium is stimulated by a thin wire electrode inserted directly into the ventricular wall by way of a needle introduced through the rib cage. The advantage of this method is the rapidity with which pacing can be initiated in catastrophic situations. However with the ability to prevent primary ventricular standstill by prophylactic pacemaker insertion (in patients with advanced heart block), transthoracic pacing is rarely required, except perhaps as a desperation measure during cardiopulmonary resuscitation.

Transvenous Pacing

The heart can be safely and effectively stimulated by delivering electrical impulses through a small electrode positioned in the right ventricular cavity. The transvenous pacing electrode is introduced into a peripheral vein and then advanced through the venous system to the vena cava, the right atrium, and finally is lodged against the endocardial surface of the right ventricle. The electrical stimuli are furnished by a small battery-powered generator (pacemaker). This technique is called transvenous pacing.

The prime purpose of transvenous pacing is to *prevent* primary ventricular standstill. This lethal arrhythmia seldom develops spontaneously (see Chapter 16); in most instances it is preceded by second- or third-degree heart block, or by bundle branch block involving more than one fascicle. By inserting a transvenous pacemaker when these advanced forms of heart block are detected, ventricular standstill can be avoided.

In addition to this fundamental indication, transvenous pacing is also employed in the treatment of persistent bradyarrhythmias. It is a common practice to accelerate the heart rate deliberately by transvenous pacing when marked sinus bradycardia or passive junctional rhythm are refractory to customary drug therapy and compromise the cardiac output.

Temporary pacing is also used to control resistant ectopic rhythms (for example, frequent premature ventricular contractions or recurrent ventricular tachycardia) which are rate related. By pacing the heart at a rate faster than its existing rate, premature beats can often be suppressed. This principle of arrhythmia control is called *overdriving* the heart.

Equipment for Transvenous Pacing

A transvenous pacing system consists of two basic components:

1. A *pulse generator* (battery operated) serves as the source of electrical impulses. Both the rate and the intensity of these impulses can be regulated by control mechanisms.
2. An insulated wire *catheter* that carries the current from the pulse generator (pacemaker) to one or two small electrodes situated in the distal end of the catheter. The electrodes are in contact with the endocardial surface of the myocardium and permit the ventricle to be stimulated directly.

The Pulse Generator.   There are two types of pacemakers: set rate and demand. The differences between these pacing systems and their respective functions are discussed in the following paragraphs.

The set-rate pulse generator.   This device, the first available for cardiac pacing, is seldom used in most CCUs at the present time. Nevertheless it is important to consider the design and operation of set-rate pacemakers to understand the newer pacemakers now in use. Very simply, these pulse generators initiate impulses at a fixed or set rate. For example, if the rate dial of the pacemaker is positioned at 60/minute, an impulse is fired every second (60 impulses/minute). Each pacing impulse (manifested on the ECG as a "pacing spike") stimulates the myocardium to produce a QRS complex as shown in Figure 17.1. The resulting QRS complexes are widened and have the configuration of a left bundle branch block pattern. (This is understandable since the electrode delivering the stimulus to the myocardium is in the right ventricle and the impulse must be transmitted from this site to the left ventricle, creating a delay in complete ventricular activation.)

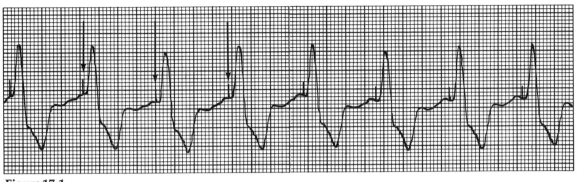

Figure 17.1.

Although set-rate pacing is a dependable method for myocardial stimulation, it has one serious drawback that limits its usefulness in elective cardiac pacing: The instrument disregards the existing electrical activity of the heart and continues to discharge impulses at a fixed rate. Thus a natural beat from the heart and an artificial pacing stimulus may occur at the same time, as demonstrated in Figure 17.2. This phenomenon is called *competition*. Note that after two paced beats, three natural beats arise from the SA node. The set-rate pacemaker nevertheless continues to discharge impulses during this period (arrows).

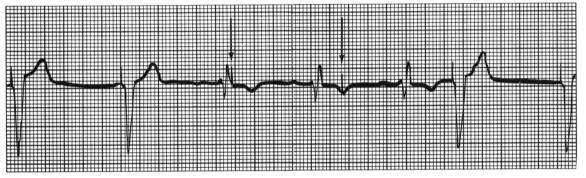

Figure 17.2.

When the natural and paced rhythms compete in this way there is a potential threat of inducing serious arrhythmias. This is particularly true when the pacing stimulus happens to hit on the T wave of the preceding natural beat. The arrival of the pacing stimulus during the period of the T wave, the *vulnerable period*, may create repetitive firing in the form of ventricular tachycardia or, worse, ventricular fibrillation. In other words, set-rate pacing has the same theoretical danger of inducing ventricular fibrillation as does a premature contraction striking a T wave. An example of ventricular fibrillation developing as the result of a set-rate pacing stimulus striking the T wave of a preceding natural beat is depicted in Figure 17.3.

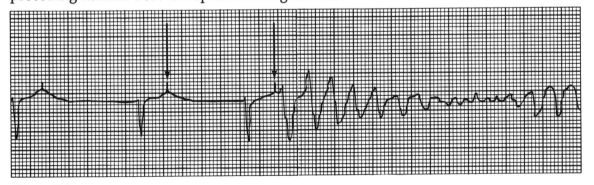

Figure 17.3.

Although competition certainly does not result in ventricular arrhythmias in all or even most instances (as evident in Figure 17.4, where the pacing stimulus hits the T wave of a premature ventricular contraction without provoking repetitive firing), this potential danger nevertheless exists. The risk of inducing ventricular fibrillation is distinctly increased in the presence of myocardial ischemia, and it is for this reason that set-rate pacing is undesirable in the treatment of acute myocardial infarction. This form of cardiac pacing should be reserved for slow, regular-rate arrhythmias (e.g., chronic complete heart block).

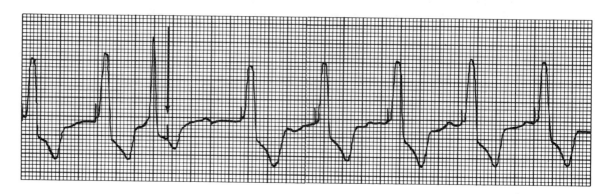

Figure 17.4.

The demand pulse generator.   To avoid the potential risk of competition associated with fixed-rate pacing, a more sophisticated pulse generator was developed. Instead of discharging impulses at a fixed rate, irrespective of the heart's inherent electrical activity, the newer pacemakers are designed to be noncompetitive and to discharge only on *demand*.

The principle of demand pacemaking is as follows: The pacemaker fires an impulse only if a QRS complex does *not* occur within a preset time interval. If a heartbeat does occur within this designated period the pacemaker recognizes this electrical activity and deliberately withholds the pacing impulse. On this basis a pacing impulse cannot strike the T wave of a premature ventricular contraction since the pacemaker will sense the ectopic beat (which occurs within the preset time interval) and accordingly will not discharge an impulse. On the other hand, if the pacemaker does *not* sense a natural or ectopic beat, it discharges impulses at a preset rate. An example of how a demand pacemaker functions is shown in Figure 17.5. Note that the pacemaker stops discharging impulses when a series of natural beats occurs (all of which fall within the preset time interval). However, when the interval is again exceeded because a natural beat did not occur the pacemaker begins to discharge again.

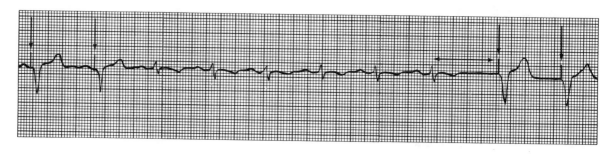

Figure 17.5.

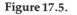

For a pacemaker to function on demand it must receive an electrocardiographic signal indicating that a natural or ectopic beat has occurred; it is this signal that inhibits the pacemaker from discharging unwanted impulses. This information is obtained by having the catheter tip (which is in contact with the endocardial surface of the right ventricle) serve as an exploring electrode to detect each QRS complex. The electrical activity of the heart is transmitted back through the catheter to a sensing device within the pacemaker. The pacing catheter thus serves to relay electrocardiographic signals to the pacemaker as well as to send pacing impulses from the instrument to the myocardium (Figure 17.6).

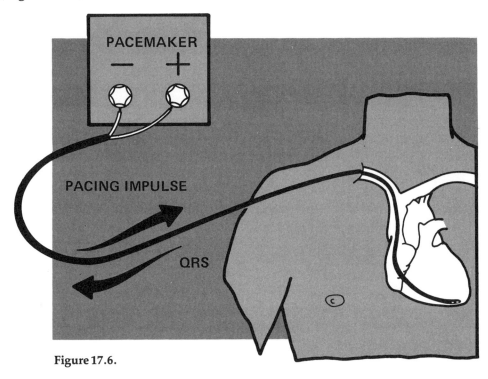

Figure 17.6.

Catheter Electrodes.   There are two basic types of catheter electrodes: those with a single electrode incorporated in the tip of the catheter (unipolar electrode) and those with two electrodes positioned about 1 cm apart at the distal end of the catheter (bipolar electrode), as shown in Figure 17.7. As with any electrical circuit the electrical impulse must flow between two poles (or electrodes) in order to stimulate the heart. With

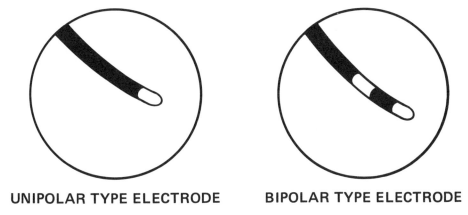

UNIPOLAR TYPE ELECTRODE   BIPOLAR TYPE ELECTRODE

Figure 17.7.

a unipolar catheter only one electrode (the negative pole) is within the heart, and a second electrode (the positive pole) is required to complete the circuit. This latter electrode usually consists of a wire suture placed in the skin of the chest wall.

The bipolar catheter electrode, which is used far more commonly than the unipolar system, obviates the need for a secondary skin electrode since both electrodes are incorporated into the catheter itself. Because of this dual electrode system bipolar catheters are of greater diameter (larger gauge) than unipolar catheters and therefore may be more difficult to insert. Nonetheless bipolar catheters are preferable to unipolar types because the presence of two adjacent electrodes within the heart enhances the likelihood of direct contact with the endocardial surface of the right ventricle, a requirement for successful pacing. With the unipolar catheter the electrode may easily become displaced from the ventricular wall and thus interrupt effective pacing.

Technique of Transvenous Pacing

Catheter Insertion.   The pacing electrode can be introduced into the venous system through an antecubital, femoral, jugular, or subclavian vein. Selecting the vein to be used for this purpose is essentially a matter of individual preference; there are advocates for each approach. Although an arm vein is usually the easiest to enter percutaneously, the route to the heart is long and tortuous, often making it difficult to advance the catheter into the ventricle. Furthermore, any movement of the arm may result in displacement of the catheter after it has been properly positioned. The jugular and subclavian veins, being closer to the superior vena cava, are shorter, more direct routes to the right ventricle. For this reason and because displacement of the catheter is less likely, these latter sites are generally preferred.

Introduction of the catheter electrode.   Once a particular vein has been selected, the surrounding skin area must be scrupulously prepared as for any surgical procedure. The area is draped to prevent contamination.

Several specially designed needles are available for catheter insertion. Most of these placement units consist of a large-bore needle (with a stylus) and a thin plastic sheath which fits over this cannula (Figure 17.8). After the skin is infiltrated with a local anes-

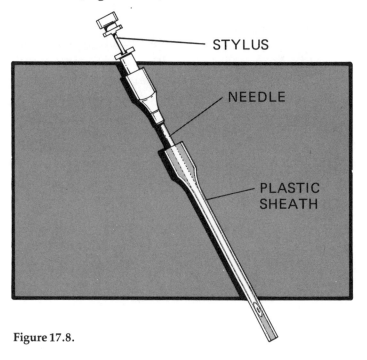

Figure 17.8.

thetic, the unit is inserted into the vein; the needle (and stylus) is then removed, leaving the plastic sheath positioned in the vein.

The catheter electrode is introduced through this plastic sheath into the vein and advanced to the right ventricle. After the electrode is in proper position within the ventricle, the plastic conduit is removed so that the catheter extends directly through the skin opening. In instances where needle penetration of the skin or vein is difficult, a small surgical "cut-down" incision can be made to facilitate entry to the vein.

Passage of the catheter electrode.   Regardless of the site of introduction, the catheter is advanced slowly to the superior vena cava, into the right atrium, through the tricuspid valve, and to the right ventricle where it is positioned against the endocardial surface. The pathway of the catheter (as shown on a chest x ray) is noted in Figure 17.9. Two methods are available to guide the catheter to its ultimate position in the ventricle. The first involves fluoroscopy where the radiopaque catheter is directly visualized during its passage. Although this technique is very desirable, most CCUs are not equipped with the expensive apparatus needed for this purpose (i.e., a portable fluoroscope with an image intensifier). Therefore when a catheter is to be positioned with this technique, patients have to be moved to either an x-ray department or a cardiac catheterization laboratory. This separation of the patient from the prepared setting of the CCU poses obvious risks and is hardly ideal.

The catheter can also be guided to the right ventricle by electrocardiographic means. This method can be performed in.the CCU and avoids the danger of moving the

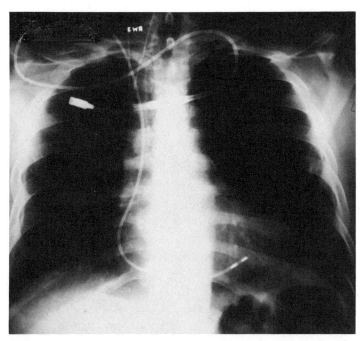

Figure 17.9.   Transvenous pacing catheter in right ventricle. Note that this is a bipolar catheter.

patient. The principle of this "blind" technique of insertion is as follows: As the electrode is being advanced to the heart an electrocardiogram can be recorded *through* the catheter by attaching its free end to the chest lead (V lead) terminal of the ECG machine. In other words, the catheter tip serves as an exploring electrode from within the heart. The resulting tracing is called an *intracavitary* electrocardiogram. Because the ECG patterns from the vena cava, the atrium, and the right ventricle have different configurations, it is possible to identify the position of the electrode in this way. Typical ECG patterns from these various locations are shown in Figure 17.10 (A–F). Note the large distinctive complexes recorded when the catheter enters the ventricle (17.10D). When this method of electrocardiographic guidance is used it is necessary to connect all of the limb leads to the patient just as if a customary electrocardiogram were to be recorded. The only difference is that the chest (V) lead, rather than being used as a skin electrode, is joined to the free end of the catheter with an alligator clamp.

Attachment of the Catheter Electrode to the Pacemaking Device.   As shown in Figure 17.11, the pacemaker has two terminals for connection of the electrodes; these are clearly marked as positive (+) and negative (−). When a unipolar electrode is used, the free end of the catheter is attached to the negative (−) terminal of the pacemaker, and the wire from the skin electrode (suture) to the positive (+) terminal. With a bipolar catheter electrode the two wires extending from the catheter can be connected to the terminals without concern about positive or negative poles.

Rate of Pacing.   The pacing rate is governed by several principles. First, the number of pacing stimuli per minute must always exceed the existing heart rate. In complete heart block, for example, where the inherent cardiac rate may be 30–40/minute, the pacing rate would be set at 60–70/minute. Second, it is undesirable to pace the heart at an overly fast rate since the oxygen demand of the myocardium is increased with rapid pacing and patients may experience angina. Furthermore, when the heart is paced rapidly the time for ventricular filling is decreased and cardiac output may be adversely affected. Therefore the pacing rate must be adjusted for each patient so that pumping efficiency is not reduced while the underlying arrhythmia is being controlled.

Energy of Pacing.   In determining the energy or intensity of the stimulus required for cardiac pacing it is necessary to consider a fundamental characteristic of myocardial contractility: When the heart is stimulated by an electrical impulse it responds (contracts) either completely or not at all (the "all-or-none" law). The lowest electrical energy that will cause myocardial contraction is called the *threshold level*. If the intensity of a pacing stimulus is less than the threshold level contraction will *not* occur. Conversely, a pacing stimulus greater than the threshold level will not produce a stronger contraction since the muscle already contracts to its fullest extent at the threshold point. In other words, there is a critical level of electrical energy below which contraction will not occur and above which it is not augmented.

Therefore, in setting the intensity of the pacing impulse it is necessary to first determine the threshold level. This is accomplished as follows: After the catheter has been positioned correctly and attached to the pacemaker, the energy control dial is increased gradually from the lowest milliampere setting to a point where a QRS complex is noted with each stimulus. This setting is the threshold level.

ECG PATTERNS DURING PACEMAKER INSERTION

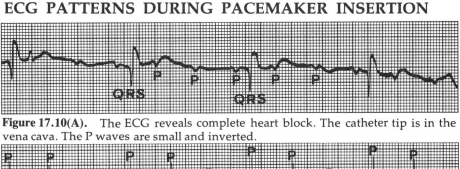

Figure 17.10(A).   The ECG reveals complete heart block. The catheter tip is in the vena cava. The P waves are small and inverted.

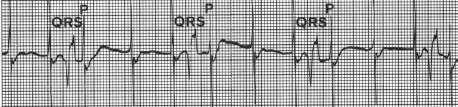

Figure 17.10(B).   The catheter tip is now in the right atrium. Note the very tall, biphasic P waves recorded from this intra-atrial position.

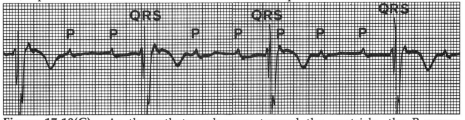

Figure 17.10(C).   As the catheter advances toward the ventricle, the P waves diminish in size while the QRS complexes become larger.

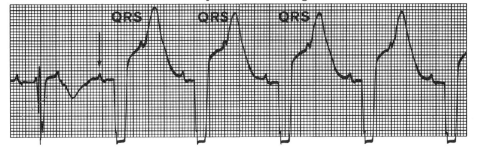

Figure 17.10(D).   The catheter tip passes from the right atrium to the right ventricle (arrow), as indicated by the sudden appearance of very large QRS complexes.

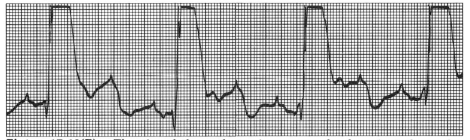

Figure 17.10(E).   The tip of the catheter is now wedged against the endocardial wall of the right ventricle. In this position the ST segment is markedly elevated.

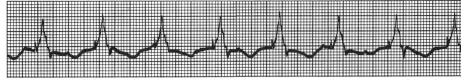

Figure 17.10(F).   After the catheter has been properly positioned and the pacemaker turned on, a standard ECG reveals effective pacing.

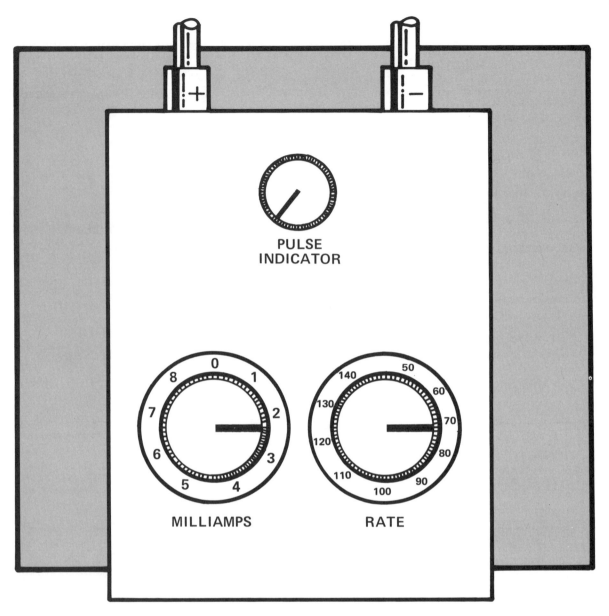

Figure 17.11.

When a catheter electrode is properly positioned and the electrode is in good contact with the endocardium, the threshold level in most patients is usually less than 2 milliamperes. If the threshold is much higher, for example 6 or 8 milliamperes, it is likely that the catheter is poorly situated in the ventricle and that repositioning of the tip is required. Because the threshold is not constant at all times, and varies with the contact of the electrode tip and the endocardium (as well as other factors), it is customary to set the initial energy level for pacing at twice the threshold value to overcome this variation. For example, if the threshold is found to be 1 milliampere, the final setting for the pacing stimulus should be 2 milliamperes.

Duration of Pacing. As already noted, transvenous pacing is employed fundamentally as a prophylactic measure when advanced forms of heart block or bradyarrhythmias (refractory to drugs) exist. Because these particular arrhythmic disturbances are almost always of a transient nature in acute myocardial infarction, cardiac pacing is required only on a temporary basis until a normal rate and rhythm have returned.

While the exact duration of these rhythm disturbances varies with the site of infarction and the rate of healing (among other factors), most of these disorders last less than 10 days and pacing is seldom necessary beyond this period. After normal sinus rhythm has returned, it is customary to leave the pacing catheter in place for another week in case the arrhythmia returns. Following this additional period, the pacing catheter is removed.

Problems with Temporary Transvenous Pacing

Several difficulties may be encountered during the course of temporary pacing. The most common of these are as follows.

Displacement of the Catheter Tip.   For pacing to be effective the catheter electrode must remain proximate to the inner wall of the right ventricle. Displacement of the tip of the catheter is a frequent event during temporary pacing and is undoubtedly the most common cause of pacing failure. Displacement occurs with greater frequency when the catheter has been introduced via an arm vein (motion of the arm tends to move the entire catheter), but dislodgement of the tip may result from a change of body position regardless of the insertion site.

Displacement of the pacing electrode may be suspected when each pacing stimulus fails to produce a QRS complex. This means that the pacing impulse is ineffective and is not *capturing* the heartbeat. An example of *loss of capture* is shown in the ECG in Figure 17.12. It is apparent that none of the pacing spikes (arrows) stimulate the ventricle to produce QRS complexes. Once displacement has occurred the catheter usually has to be repositioned in the ventricle to achieve effective pacing, although occasionally changing the position of the patient in bed will restore the catheter to its proper position.

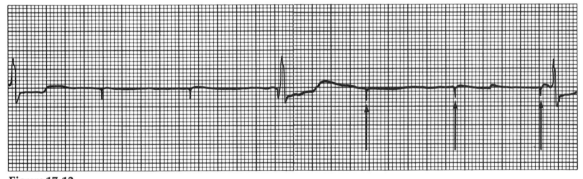

Figure 17.12.

Development of Competition.   As discussed previously, competition of rhythms can be expected when fixed-rate pacemakers are used. The problem is particularly common when the heart is being paced because of temporary heart block or other slow-rate arrhythmias, and normal sinus rhythm returns suddenly. In this circumstance the natural and paced rhythms (which may now be of similar rates) compete with each other. Although theoretically competition should not develop during demand pacing, the problem can in fact occur. This competition usually results from failure of the sensing mechanism of the pacemaker to recognize spontaneous heartbeats. Unless the R wave transmitted back to the sensing mechanism is of sufficient amplitude (voltage), the pacemaker will not sense the beat and will discharge an impulse; this results in competition. When competition is caused by inadequate sensing the catheter tip must be moved to a different location in the right ventricle to obtain a better R wave signal for the sensing mechanism.

Loss of Pacing Artifact.   If the pacing stimulus does not produce an artifact (spike) on the ECG it can be presumed that one of the components of the pacing system has failed. The source of the problem is usually not difficult to identify. If the pulse indicator (on the face of the pacemaker) shows no movement it implies that either the batteries are exhausted or the pulse generator is broken. If, on the other hand, the pulse indicator dial shows that the pacemaker is functioning, it can be reasoned that impulses, while originating normally, are not reaching the heart. This condition may develop because of a broken wire within the catheter or, more simply, because the catheter terminal has become disconnected from the pulse generator.

Perforation of the Ventricular Wall by the Catheter Tip.   Since the catheter electrode is deliberately placed against the inner surface of the ventricular wall it is understandable that the catheter tip may embed itself in the myocardium, particularly when the catheter remains in the heart for many days. In some patients the catheter actually burrows through the full thickness of the myocardium and finally perforates the right ventricular wall. However, this untoward event produces surprisingly few effects. Because the blood pressure within the right ventricle is normally quite low (unlike the high pressure within the left ventricle), perforation of the right ventricular chamber seldom produces any hemodynamic consequences. Moreover, if there is bleeding into the pericardium the amount of blood is generally trivial and does not produce cardiac tamponade.

That perforation of the ventricular wall has occurred can be suspected by noting a sudden loss of capture after a period of successful pacing. On some occasions the catheter perforation is recognized by the appearance of contractions of the diaphragm or the chest wall. This muscle twitching (which is usually obvious to the patient) signifies that the catheter electrode has perforated the right ventricle and has traveled to the diaphragm or the intercostal muscles. The diagnosis can often be confirmed by means of a chest x ray, which shows the catheter tip outside the right ventricle. In the event of perforation it is necessary to withdraw the catheter gently and reposition it in the right ventricle.

Thrombophlebitis and Skin Infection.   Since pacing catheters must often remain in the venous system for prolonged periods there is always the possibility that thrombophlebitis may develop from mechanical irritation of the vein wall. The likelihood of this inflammatory reaction is perhaps greater when smaller veins are used as insertion sites (e.g., arm veins); however other factors undoubtedly contribute to this complication. If thrombophlebitis is marked, the catheter must be removed and another one inserted in a different vein.

Because the skin puncture site is in effect an open wound, local infection may occur. The risk can be minimized (almost excluded) by adherence to strict surgical asepsis at the time of catheter placement and by the routine use of antibiotic (neomycin) ointment subsequently.

The Nursing Role in Cardiac Pacing

Preparation for Catheter Insertion

1. When a decision has been made to pace the heart temporarily it is important to explain to the patient why the procedure is necessary and how it will be performed. The emphasis of the explanation should be on the preventive benefit derived from being able to control the heart rate as desired with pacing.

2. If cardiac pacing is to be performed on an elective basis (e.g., in a patient with second-degree heart block) it is customary to have an operative permit signed by the patient. In emergency situations this measure can be disregarded.

3. When the catheter is to be positioned by electrocardiographic (rather than fluoroscopic) means, the limb lead electrodes should be attached to all of the extremities and a separate ECG machine brought to the bedside. After the catheter has been inserted into the venous system, the chest (V) lead terminal is connected to the free end of the pacing catheter by means of an alligator clamp. This exploring electrode records an intracavitary tracing from which the position of the catheter electrode can be determined. It is essential that *all of the equipment used be grounded properly* to prevent the threat of electrocution by extraneous electrical current passing through the catheter to the heart. Some institutions use battery-powered electrocardiographic machines to reduce this danger.

4. A syringe containing 100 mg lidocaine should be prepared and placed at the bedside. In addition, the nurse should verify the patency of the preexisting "keep-open" intravenous line. This preparedness is essential to combat any ventricular irritability that may develop suddenly while the catheter is being positioned within the heart.

5. A defibrillator should be available for immediate use in the event (even though unlikely) that the catheter may induce ventricular fibrillation.

Catheter Insertion

1. The skin surrounding the intended site of catheter insertion is prepared with soap, alcohol, and a skin antiseptic, as with any surgical procedure. An "eye sheet" is used to drape the area, leaving only the operative site exposed. In addition, the patient's face is covered with a loose drape to prevent breath contamination. (Pathogens from the mouth and nose are a far greater source of wound infection than bacteria found on the skin.)

2. The needle placement set and the appropriate catheter should be sterile and ready for use. Sterilization can be accomplished by the use of bactericidal solutions or preferably a gas technique; autoclaving should not be used because of the plastic materials contained in the catheter and needle sheath.

3. A local anesthetic (procaine or lidocaine) is used to infiltrate the skin before the large-bore needle is inserted into the vein.

4. As the catheter is advanced into the heart the ECG must be monitored with great care to detect premature ventricular beats that may develop. Consequently the ECG must be observed *continuously* during the insertion procedure. This is accomplished with usual cardiac monitoring equipment (when the catheter is placed by fluoroscopy) or with an ECG machine (when placement is guided by an intracavitary electrode).

5. After the physician has placed the catheter in a proper position and effective capture of the heartbeat has been achieved, the catheter must be secured to the skin. This may be accomplished by placing a suture around the catheter and through the skin or, more simply, by adhesive tape. An antibiotic ointment (neomycin or bacitracin) is then applied to the skin entry site and a dry dressing firmly affixed.

Subsequent Care

During the course of cardiac pacing the major responsibility of the nurse is to verify that the pacemaker system is functioning properly and effectively. As noted, several problems may arise during temporary pacing, and careful observation of the patient and the monitor is essential to detect these disturbances as soon as they occur.

Loss of Capture. If there is loss of capture the nurse should notify the physician immediately because the pacing stimulus is wholly ineffective in this situation. Depending on the underlying arrhythmia for which pacing is being used, loss of capture can be associated with serious consequences. For example, if pacing fails during complete heart block, ventricular standstill may result (Fig. 17.13).

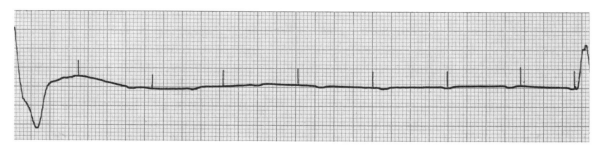

Figure 17.13.

Absence of Pacing Artifacts. A second situation demanding emergency action is the sudden disappearance of pacing artifacts on the ECG (Fig. 17.14). In many instances the cause of this crisis can be promptly identified and corrected by the nurse. The first step in solving the problem is to make certain the catheter terminals have not become disconnected from the pacemaker device. If these connections are found to be secure, the next thing to do is to ascertain that an adequate stimulus is being generated by the battery. If there is no movement of the pulse indicator, the pacemaker batteries may be exhausted and a different pacemaker should be attached. (To prevent the catastrophe of battery failure a careful record should be kept of the number of hours each pacemaker is actually used. While the effective battery life of most pulse generators is presumably 800 hours, it is good practice to change batteries routinely after 600 hours of use.) If pacemaker malfunction cannot be corrected instantly, cardiopulmonary resuscitation should be initiated without delay.

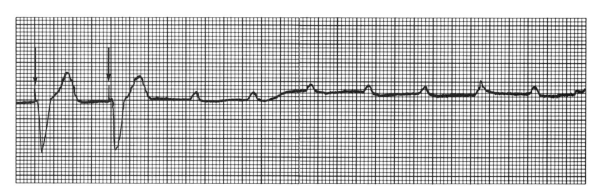

Figure 17.14.

Competition. Of less importance than loss of capture or pacemaker failure is the development of competition between the paced and natural cardiac rhythms. If competition occurs during fixed-rate pacing it may indicate that normal sinus rhythm has returned. The presence of competition during demand pacing suggests difficulty with the sensing system of the pacemaker unit. In either instance the nurse should apprise the physician of this undesirable rhythm.

Perforation of Ventricle.   That the catheter tip has perforated the right ventricle may be suspected when there is a sudden loss of capture. However, this finding is not diagnostic since loss of capture is most often the result of simple displacement of the catheter tip within the ventricular cavity. A more important finding is the appearance of contractions of the diaphragm or muscles of the chest wall which occur synchronously with pacing impulses. This complication should be reported to the physician immediately.

Thrombophlebitis and Skin Infection.   The nurse should carefully examine the catheter insertion site for signs of local infection. An antibiotic ointment should be applied daily. In changing the dressing care must be taken not to move the catheter. In addition to skin infections, signs of thrombophlebitis should be sought, particularly when the catheter has been introduced through an arm vein or has been in place several days.

PRECORDIAL SHOCK

Precordial shock is used either as a lifesaving emergency method for terminating ventricular fibrillation (defibrillation) or an elective procedure to convert certain atrial and ventricular tachyarrhythmias to normal rhythm (cardioversion). The principle of precordial shock in treating ventricular fibrillation is straightforward: A high-voltage shock of very brief duration (only a few thousandths of a second) delivered through the chest wall is capable of abruptly stopping the chaotic electrical activity within the heart that produced the lethal arrhythmia. Once the bizarre fibrillatory rhythm is terminated in this way, the heart's natural pacemaker regains command and an effective beat is reestablished. This same principle is utilized in elective cardioversion where brief depolarization of the entire heart (at a particular time in the cardiac cycle) halts the ectopic pacemaker and allows the SA node to assume control again.

While enormous electrical energy (about 7000 volts) is required to defibrillate the heart through the chest wall, this electrical force is so very short in duration the current does not injure the myocardium.

Equipment for Precordial Shock

Precordial shock to terminate ventricular fibrillation can be delivered by an alternating current (AC) or a direct current (DC) defibrillator. Although both types of defibrillators are equally effective for this particular purpose, the DC defibrillator can also be used for elective precordial shock. Because of this greater versatility, DC machines are now used routinely in CCUs.

A DC defibrillator builds and stores thousands of volts in a capacitator within seconds and discharges this energy on demand in less than 5 milliseconds. The stored energy is delivered to the heart through a circuit consisting of two electrodes (or paddles, as they are commonly called) which are held against the chest wall. The paddles are large in diameter (usually 3–4 inches), allowing the electrical discharge to pass through a wide area of skin to prevent electrical burns. To facilitate passage of current through the skin, a thick layer of conductive paste is applied to the skin and electrode surfaces before the energy is discharged. The handles of the paddles are insulated to protect the operator from leakage of current.

The electrical energy is discharged by pressing a button switch incorporated in the handles of the electrodes. The amount of current delivered by the defibrillator can be adjusted according to need by a dial setting on the machine. This electrical force is measured in *watt-seconds* (w/s); the scale ranges from 1–400 w/s.

Synchronized and Nonsynchronized Precordial Shock

When precordial shock is used electively to convert atrial and ventricular tachyarrhythmias (cardioversion), it is important that the electrical discharge be synchronized with the cardiac cycle. This need can be appreciated on the following basis: When any electrical impulse, even a premature ventricular contraction, strikes during the vulnerable period of the cardiac cycle (i.e., during the time of the T wave, as shown in Fig. 17.15) there is a potential danger of inducing *ventricular fibrillation*. The same threat may exist if a precordial shock (or a pacemaker impulse) arrives during the critical interval of the vulnerable period. To avoid this hazard, precordial shock is deliberately synchronized so that the electrical force is delivered at a point in the cardiac cycle when the

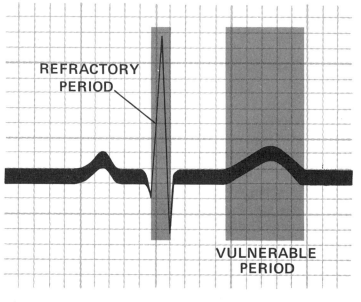

Figure 17.15.

heart is refractory to stimulation; this nonvulnerable (refractory) period corresponds to the time of the QRS complex. The equipment for precordial shock is so designed that the discharge energy can be synchronized with the safe (refractory) period of the cardiac cycle. When the synchronizer switch is *on* and the discharge button is triggered, the instrument waits until the next R wave before delivering its energy. On the other hand, if the synchronizer is *off*, discharge occurs at the instant the machine is triggered, without reference to the cardiac cycle.

It is essential to understand clearly just when precordial shock should or should not be synchronized. *In terminating ventricular fibrillation with precordial shock (defibrillation), the synchronizer switch must be in the* off *position*. If the synchronizer switch is on in this circumstance, the machine will *not* fire because it waits for a QRS complex, which of course is nonexistent during ventricular fibrillation.

Conversely, when precordial shock is employed *electively* to convert other arrhythmias (e.g., atrial fibrillation) the synchronizer must be *on* to avoid the possibility of the discharge striking during the vulnerable period and inducing ventricular fibrillation.

Energy of Discharge

As indicated, the level of discharge energy is adjustable and must be set for the particular arrhythmias being treated. *For ventricular fibrillation the maximum energy (400 watt-*

seconds) should always be used. For elective cardioversion the precise energy setting varies with several factors. First, it is known that certain arrhythmias are more responsive to precordial shock than others and require lesser energies for conversion. For example, atrial flutter can generally be terminated with minimal electrical force (e.g., 10–30 w/s) whereas atrial fibrillation is often more resistant and demands a higher energy setting. Second, cardioversion may provoke ventricular arrhythmias among patients receiving digitalis, and for this reason high energies are usually avoided in this circumstance. Third, factors such as the patient's body build, weight, and the presence of emphysema may increase the voltage demands. Many physicians prefer to attempt cardioversion using very low energies at first (e.g., 20 w/s or less) and if the trial is unsuccessful to increase the level on successive attempts until cardioversion is finally accomplished; others employ higher energies (e.g., 200 w/s or more) initially.

Technique of Elective Cardioversion and the Nursing Role

Preparation for Procedure

1. The procedure should be explained to the patient by a member of the nurse-physician team. Because the word shock has frightening connotations, it is wise to avoid this term when describing the treatment.
2. In many institutions it is customary to have an operative permit signed by the patient when elective cardioversion is to be performed.
3. All necessary equipment and materials should be at the bedside. This includes the machine which delivers the synchronized shock along with syringes, antiarrhythmic drugs, and anesthetic agents.
4. Although elective cardioversion is a remarkably safe procedure when properly performed, it is theoretically possible that the shock might induce ventricular fibrillation. For this reason emergency equipment for cardiopulmonary resuscitation should be in readiness. A syringe containing 100 mg lidocaine should always be at the bedside for immediate use to combat premature ventricular contractions that may develop after cardioversion.
5. Prior to the procedure an intravenous pathway must be established and its patency verified. This conduit is used to administer the anesthetic agent and any antiarrhythmic drugs that may be necessary.
6. In order for the electrical shock to be properly synchronized with the R wave of the cardiac cycle, it is necessary to use electrocardiographic electrodes for sensing R waves. These electrodes should be placed on all four extremities. (With some equipment the ECG electrodes are unnecessary because the customary monitoring electrodes serve this purpose.)

Setting the Machine for Cardioversion

1. The synchronizer switch is turned *on* so that the discharge of energy will coincide with the R wave of the cardiac cycle.
2. Because synchronization cannot be achieved unless the ventricular complexes are of sufficient amplitude to trigger the discharge, the "gain" dial may have to be adjusted to obtain R waves of adequate size (as evidenced by a flashing light or other signal). If complexes of sufficient height cannot be obtained by increasing the gain, a different lead must be used to obtain taller waves (e.g., changing from a lead II to a lead I position).
3. For safety it is wise to verify that proper synchronization will occur when the machine is fired. This is accomplished by a test mechanism within the machine

which indicates where the discharge will fall in the cardiac cycle when the shock is actually delivered.

4. The energy (watt-seconds) to be used for the cardioversion attempt is set at the desired level by the physician.

Anesthesia

Although precordial shock itself creates little actual pain because of the extremely short duration of the stimulus, the sensation (and the associated generalized muscle contraction) is nevertheless frightening and unpleasant for most patients. Because an analgesic effect is required for only a few seconds, very short-acting agents—e.g., sodium methohexital (Brevital) or diazepam (Valium)—are given intravenously just before the shock is delivered.

Paddle Electrodes: Preparation and Placement

1. Prior to the procedure the paddles should be carefully cleaned with scouring powder to remove metallic oxides that form on the surface of the electrodes and interfere with the flow of current.

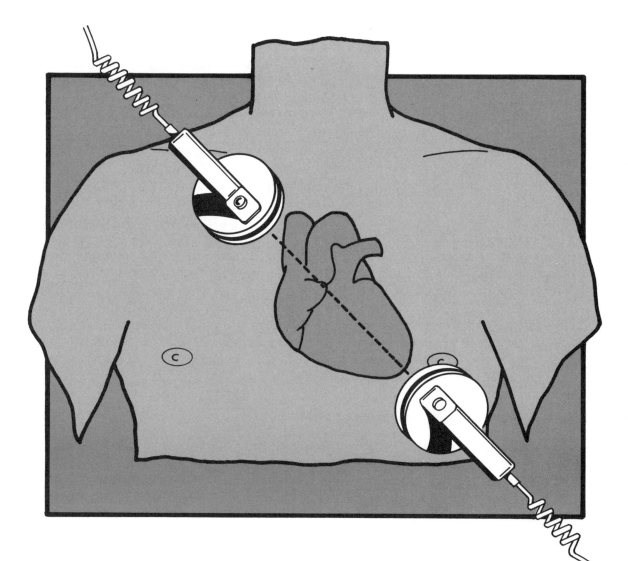

Figure 17.16.   Placement of paddles. One is in the right sternal area and the other on the left lateral chest wall.

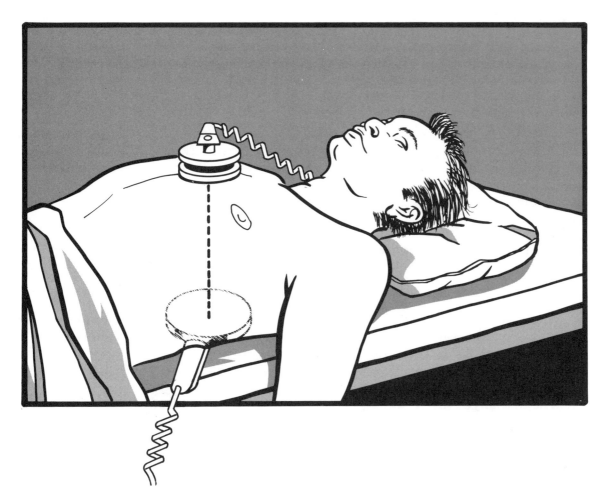

Figure 17.17. Alternative placement of paddles. A special flat paddle is placed under the left scapula, and another paddle is held directly over the upper sternum.

2. A thick layer of conducting jelly is placed on the face of the electrodes and distributed evenly. Additional electrode paste is applied to the chest wall where the paddles will be held. Unless there is an adequate amount of jelly at the electrode–skin interface, serious skin burns can occur.
3. One paddle is placed in the right sternal area and the other on the left lateral chest wall. The precise location of the paddles is not critical as long as the flow of current traverses the heart (Fig. 17.16). An alternative method of paddle placement is to position one electrode (a special flat paddle) under the left scapula and to hold the other paddle directly over the upper sternum (Fig. 17.17). In this way the flow of current passes directly through the heart in an anterior–posterior direction.
4. Before the energy is discharged it is important to ascertain that the conducting paste remains localized at the electrode sites and has not spread over the chest wall. Excess jelly should be wiped dry before proceeding, otherwise the current will flow across the skin surface (rather than through the heart), creating a large spark and perhaps causing a burn.
5. The paddles must be pressed firmly and evenly against the chest wall; failure to preserve good contact results in dissipation of energy. Furthermore, tilting of the paddles may cause skin burns.
6. Since there is a theoretical threat that the electrical force being delivered to the patient could pass through the bed and reach the operator or others, it is a wise practice to have all personnel stand clear of the bed at the moment of discharge.
7. The discharge switch is pressed, and the effect is immediately evident by a sud-

den generalized contraction of the patient's muscles. Observation of the oscilloscope will confirm whether normal rhythm has been restored.

8. In some instances premature ventricular contractions are noted following cardioversion, and lidocaine should be administered promptly to combat this cardiac irritability.

9. In the extremely unlikely event that the cardioversion attempt causes ventricular fibrillation, the synchronizer switch must be turned *off*, the energy increased to 400 watt-seconds, and a second shock delivered instantly to defibrillate the patient. Remember that defibrillation cannot be accomplished if the synchronizer is *on*!

Technique of Emergency Defibrillation

Although the method for defibrillation has been described in the discussion of ventricular fibrillation, it is important to review this procedure with particular emphasis on the differences between defibrillation and elective cardioversion.

1. Defibrillation is a lifesaving technique and must be accomplished within a minute or so to be successful. This means that precordial shock must always be the *initial* step in treatment (within the setting of a CCU), and that no time should be wasted with other measures such as the administration of oxygen or closed chest massage. The first person reaching the bedside, whether a physician or a nurse, should proceed to defibrillate the patient at once.

2. The discharge energy should be set at its maximum level: 400 watt-seconds; the use of lesser energies is pointless and should never be attempted.

3. It is absolutely essential that the synchronizer switch be in the *off* position for defibrillation so that the discharge will occur the instant the trigger is pressed.

4. Conductive jelly is applied to the electrode surfaces, and the paddles are held firmly against the chest wall in the same manner described for elective cardioversion.

5. If for some reason defibrillation is unsuccessful, precordial shock should be repeated immediately. With some equipment it is necessary to recharge the capacitor by pressing an appropriate button before a second discharge can be delivered.

18

Antiarrhythmic Drugs

From the foregoing chapters it is apparent that the successful management of arrhythmias depends not only on the recognition and diagnosis of the particular rhythm or conduction disturbance but also on the selection and proper use of appropriate antiarrhythmic therapy. The object of this chapter is to elucidate the actions and methods of administration of the main drugs used in treating arrhythmias associated with acute myocardial infarction. Before discussing the antiarrhythmic agents individually it is useful to consider the basic mechanisms by which this group of drugs affects the heart's electrical activity and controls arrhythmias.

MECHANISMS OF ANTIARRHYTHMIC ACTION

Antiarrhythmic drugs act by altering automaticity, excitability, or conductivity of cardiac cells.

Automaticity refers to the ability of certain cells within the heart to initiate electrical impulses spontaneously. An increase or a decrease in automaticity (spontaneous firing) produces certain types of arrhythmias. For example, increased automaticity of pacemaker cells within the atria, AV junctional tissue, the His-Purkinje network, or the ventricles results in ectopic beats or tachyarrhythmias. In contrast, sinus bradycardia is due to decreased automaticity of the cells comprising the SA node. One of the fundamental actions of antiarrhythmic drugs is to restore normal automaticity. Many agents—including lidocaine, quinidine, procainamide, and propranolol—serve to decrease spontaneous firing (particularly of ectopic pacemakers), while other drugs such as atropine and isoproterenol are used to increase automaticity.

Excitability refers to the ability of cardiac cells to respond to stimulation. As noted in the preceding chapter there is a critical (threshold) level at which the heart will respond completely or not at all to an electrical stimulus. If this threshold level for stimulation is reduced (because of low potassium levels, for example), the cells become more easily excitable and rapid-rate arrhythmias or repetitive firing may develop. On the other hand, if excitability is decreased (because of inadequate myocardial perfusion), a normal stimulus will not evoke a response (i.e., depolarization and contraction). The beneficial effects of antiarrhythmic drugs are often related to the control of excitability, either decreasing or increasing cellular responsiveness.

Conductivity refers to the velocity at which impulses are transmsitted through the specialized fibers of the conduction system. Certain arrhythmias are characterized by slow conduction velocities and others by accelerated propagation of impulses. Among the antiarrhythmic drugs, atropine and isoproterenol increase the velocity of conduction, while digitalis, quinidine, and procainamide decrease conduction velocity.

Antiarrhythmic drugs influence automaticity, excitability, and conductivity through two basic mechanisms: (1) a direct effect on cardiac cells, and (2) an indirect effect by way of the autonomic nervous system.

Direct Cellular Effect

When a cardiac cell is stimulated by an impulse, the cell membrane immediately responds by allowing sodium ions to enter the cell and potassium ions to leave the cell. This exchange and flow of ions creates an electrical current (depolarization). During repolarization potassium ions reenter the cell and sodium ions leave it. The effect of the movement of ions across the cell membrane on the electrical behavior of the heart has been demonstrated in the animal laboratory by recording the electrical events that occur after stimulation of a single cardiac muscle fiber. The recording (which in effect represents an electrocardiogram taken from one cell) is called a transmembrane action potential. A typical transmembrane action potential tracing is shown in Figure 18.1.

After the cell membrane is stimulated (Fig. 18.1, arrow) there is a sharp upstroke from the resting baseline (called phase 0), which represents depolarization of the cell. Unless the stimulus is strong enough to exceed the threshold level, the cell will not respond. After depolarization, repolarization occurs (phases 1, 2, and 3), and finally the potential returns to the baseline (phase 4). Critical to an understanding of antiarrhythmic drug action is the fact that the cell is insensitive (refractory) to another stimulus and cannot be reexcited until the repolarization curve has descended below the threshold level. In other words, if an impulse arrives at any time during the *effective refractory period* the myocardium will not respond to the stimulus.

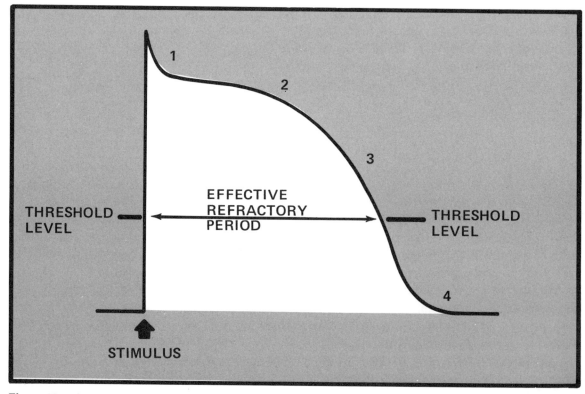

Figure 18.1.

Antiarrhythmic drugs that act directly on cardiac cells do so by altering the various phases of the transmembrane action potential and particularly by changing the duration of the effective refractory period. The control of automaticity, excitability, and conductivity is achieved in this way.

Autonomic Nervous System Effect

In addition to antiarrhythmic agents that act directly on the cell membrane, a second group of drugs controls arrhythmias indirectly by either stimulating or blocking sympathetic or parasympathetic nervous system activity.

As mentioned previously, the sympathetic and parasympathetic nervous systems have antagonistic actions on the heart. Stimulation of sympathetic nerves results in an increase in the rate of impulse formation (heart rate) and an increase in conduction velocity. In addition, sympathetic stimulation causes an increase in the force of contraction of the atria and ventricles (inotropic effect). The effects of parasympathetic (vagus) stimulation are just the opposite: The inherent heart rate slows, and the speed of conduction decreases. At the same time, the force of atrial contraction is diminished. (Ventricular contraction is not affected directly by parasympathetic stimulation because the ventricles do not contain vagal fibers.)

Drugs that alter the autonomic nervous system's control of heart rate, conduction velocity, and myocardial contractility can be classified into four groups: (1) agents that *stimulate* sympathetic nervous system activity; (2) agents that *block* sympathetic nervous system activity; (3) agents that *stimulate* vagal activity; and (4) agents that *block* vagal activity.

With this brief background the following antiarrhythmic agents are considered in this chapter:

Quinidine
Procainamide (Pronestyl)
Lidocaine
Digitalis (digoxin)
Diphenylhydantoin (Dilantin)
Potassium
Isoproterenol (Isuprel)
Atropine
Propranolol (Inderal)

QUINIDINE

Uses

1. To control or terminate atrial arrhythmias, particularly atrial fibrillation.
2. To suppress ventricular ectopic activity that has not responded to lidocaine or procainamide.
3. To prevent recurrent supraventricular tachycardia (prophylactic treatment).

Action

Quinidine acts directly at the cell membrane level and also inhibits vagal influences on the heart (vagolytic action).

The direct cellular action produces a decrease in spontaneous impulse formation (automaticity), a decrease in excitability (of atrial cells in particular), and a slowing of conduction (especially at the AV node). However, in achieving these antiarrhythmic effects, quinidine depresses myocardial cells and thereby reduces the strength of myocardial contractility; this results in a reduction in stroke volume and cardiac output.

Because quinidine has an inhibitory (blocking) effect on vagal impulses to the heart, the drug can cause the heart rate to increase and the conduction time to decrease. This vagolytic action may sometimes counteract the direct cellular effects.

Methods of Administration and Dosage

1. Although quinidine can be administered orally, intramuscularly, or intravenously, the oral route is by far the safest and is the method of choice (except perhaps in rare emergency situations).

2. When quinidine therapy is started it is advantageous to begin treatment with a loading dose. This usually consists of 300 mg quinidine orally every 3 hours for three doses.

3. The oral dose thereafter (the maintenance dose) is 200–600 mg every 6 hours; the average dose is 400 mg every 6 hours. The daily dosage should not exceed 1.6 grams unless serum quinidine levels can be measured regularly (to identify toxic levels).

4. The customary prophylactic dose for preventing recurrence of arrhythmias is 200–300 mg every 6 hours.

5. The drug usually acts within 2–4 hours after oral administration, when peak blood level concentrations are reached.

Contraindications

1. Quinidine should not be given to patients who have evidence of a ventricular conduction disturbance (manifested by widened QRS complexes), nor should it be administered in the presence of advanced AV heart block.

2. Patients with known sensitivity or adverse reactions to quinidine should not be treated with this drug.

3. The drug should be used cautiously in patients with elevated BUN levels.

Side Effects

Cardiac Effects

1. Quinidine may cause atrioventricular and intraventricular heart block.

2. It may produce excessive depression of myocardial contractility, predisposing to or exaggerating heart failure.

3. In *toxic* doses quinidine may lead to ventricular tachycardia or ventricular fibrillation (sudden death).

Systemic Effects

1. Gastrointestinal symptoms—nausea, vomiting, and especially diarrhea—may occur.

2. Visual and auditory symptoms—blurred vision, tinnitus, and deafness—may develop.

3. Allergic reactions—fever, skin rashes, thrombocytopenic purpura, and hemolytic anemia—are uncommon responses.

Nursing Implications

1. Careful electrocardiographic monitoring is essential to detect signs of cardiac toxicity. Progressive widening of the QRS complexes, the development of AV heart block,

and major increases or decreases in the heart rate are of great significance and should be reported to the physician promptly.

2. Manifestations of systemic reactions should always be considered before the next dose is administered. Diarrhea, nausea, or vomiting are the most frequent side effects.

3. When there is reason to suspect quinidine toxicity, serum quinidine levels should be measured. A serum quinidine level greater than 8 mg/liter is in the toxic range. (The desired serum level is 5–7 mg/liter.)

PROCAINAMIDE (PRONESTYL)

Uses

1. To suppress or terminate premature ventricular contractions or ventricular tachycardia.

2. To prevent recurrent ventricular arrhythmias.

3. To treat supraventricular tachyarrhythmias not controlled by quinidine (or when quinidine cannot be used because of hypersensitivity or side effects).

Actions

The electrophysiological effects of procainamide are very similar to those of quinidine. The drug, a myocardial depressant, decreases automaticity, excitability, conductivity, and myocardial contractility. In addition, procainamide inhibits vagal activity, but this action is usually not of sufficient magnitude to cause an increase in the heart rate.

Procainamide is now seldom used as a primary drug in the treatment of arrhythmias. It is less effective than lidocaine in terminating ventricular arrhythmias and less effective than quinidine in controlling supraventricular arrhythmias. The drug is employed most often to prevent the recurrence of ventricular arrhythmias.

Methods of Administration and Dosage

1. Procainamide can be given orally, intravenously, or intramuscularly. The parenteral routes are used to terminate or suppress arrhythmias, while oral administration is reserved mostly for prophylactic treatment.

2. When procainamide is used intravenously to terminate ventricular arrhythmias, 2 grams of the drug are diluted in 500 cc 5% dextrose in water and administered by continuous drip at a rate of 100 mg every 5 minutes (25 cc). (In this dilution each milliliter contains 4 milligrams of procainamide.) The total intravenous dosage should not exceed 1 gram in an hour (250 cc).

3. If the arrhythmia is successfully controlled, maintenance therapy is usually continued intravenously for the first 24 hours. In this circumstance the customary dosage is 2–3 mg of procainamide per minute (or a total of about 1 gram each 6 hours).

4. If for some reason an intravenous line has not been established (for example, while the patient is enroute to the hospital) procainamide may be injected intramuscularly. The usual intramuscular dose is 500 milligrams.

5. In less urgent situations the drug should be given orally. A loading dose of 1 gram procainamide produces effective blood levels in less than an hour (4–8 mg/liter). Because the action of the drug lasts only 3–6 hours, repeated doses of 500 mg are given every 4 hours. The total oral dosage in 24 hours should not be more than 3.0 grams.

6. When used for prophylactic purposes the recommended oral dose is 250–500 mg every 4 hours.

Contraindications

1. Procainamide should not be administered to patients with advanced atrioventricular heart block or intraventricular conduction defect (unless a demand pacemaker is functioning).

2. The drug is contraindicated in patients with known hypersensitivity to procaine and chemically related drugs.

Side Effects

Cardiac Effects

1. Procainamide may slow conduction velocity and produce atrioventricular or intraventricular heart block. Widening of the QRS complex by more than 50% of the pretreatment width, or the development of a prolonged PR interval, is reason to discontinue the drug temporarily.

2. The drug may precipitate or potentiate heart failure because of its depressant action on myocardial contractility.

3. Occasionally procainamide may cause an acceleration of the heart rate (as a result of its vagolytic action) and induce ventricular tachyarrhythmias.

Systemic Effects

1. A fall in blood pressure is often observed after parenteral administration of the drug (rarely after oral administration). In most instances the drop in pressure is less than 15 mm Hg. However, in some patients procainamide produces serious hypotension. As a general rule, if the blood pressure falls more than 20 mm Hg the drug should be discontinued.

2. Gastrointestinal symptoms develop in about 10% of patients. These side effects include anorexia, bitter taste, nausea, vomiting, abdominal pain, and diarrhea.

3. A syndrome resembling lupus erythematosus may develop during the course of prolonged procainamide therapy. This reaction usually consists of chills, fever, skin lesions, joint and muscle discomfort, and pleuritic pain.

4. In patients sensitive to procainamide, allergic reactions manifested by urticaria and chills and fever may be noted.

5. Agranulocytosis, leukopenia, and thrombocytopenia occur rarely after the administration of procainamide.

Nursing Implications

1. The nurse should examine the electrocardiogram (monitor strip) before each dose of procainamide is administered. Of particular importance is the development of intraventricular blocks (widening of the QRS complexes) or signs of atrioventricular block (particularly prolongation of the PR interval). These findings may represent cardiotoxicity and if present should be brought to the attention of the physician. The drug should be withheld if the QRS complex widens more than 50% of its original duration or if first- or second-degree AV block is observed. Also of concern is a significant reduction or acceleration of the heart rate. Again, a rate change may reflect a toxic effect.

2. The blood pressure should be carefully recorded before the drug is administered initially and then checked at regular intervals thereafter. A reduction in blood pressure of greater than 15 mm Hg should be reported to the physician.

3. Because of its myocardial depressant action, procainamide may cause, or worsen, heart failure. Careful assessment of the patient's clinical condition is essential in detecting early signs of this complication.

4. The nurse should be aware of the diverse systemic side effects of procainamide and if there is any suspicion of drug-induced reactions the physician should be notified before the next dose is given.

LIDOCAINE

Uses

1. To terminate premature ventricular contractions and ventricular tachycardia.
2. To suppress ventricular ectopic activity prophylactically and to prevent recurrent ventricular arrhythmias.

Actions

Lidocaine controls ventricular arrhythmias by depressing automaticity in the His-Purkinje network and by raising the excitability threshold of the ventricles. (The drug has little or no effect on the atria and therefore is not particularly useful in treating atrial tachyarrhythmia.)

Unlike quinidine and procainamide, lidocaine in customary doses does not affect conduction velocity; consequently it does not produce atrioventricular or intraventricular conduction disturbances. (In higher dosages conduction may be depressed.)

In usual doses lidocaine has only a minimal effect on myocardial contractility and peripheral vascular resistance. Therefore cardiac output and systemic blood pressure are not ordinarily decreased during drug administration.

The drug penetrates cardiac tissues very rapidly, and its onset of action occurs within 60 seconds following an intravenous bolus dose. Lidocaine is successful in abolishing ventricular arrhythmias in more than 75% of cases.

Methods of Administration and Dosage

1. Lidocaine is administered intravenously except in rare circumstances when an intramuscular route must be used.
2. For the initial treatment of ventricular arrhythmias, an intravenous bolus injection of lidocaine is given. The dosage is 50–100 mg (or 1 mg/kg of the patient's body weight). Effective blood levels are achieved at once. If the ventricular arrhythmia is not controlled with this injection the same dose may be repeated every 5 minutes until the arrhythmia is terminated or until a total dosage of 300 mg has been administered during a 1-hour period.
3. Because the effect of the bolus dose lasts no more than 15 minutes, it is necessary to start a continuous infusion of lidocaine to maintain effective blood levels and prevent the recurrence of ventricular ectopic activity. This infusion is prepared by diluting 3000 mg 2% lidocaine in 500 cc 5% dextrose solution. This dilution provides a solution containing 6 mg lidocaine per milliliter. The infusion is administered at a rate of 1–4 mg/minute (10–40 microdrops/minute) depending on the clinical response. Although maintenance doses of lidocaine can be continued for several days if necessary, it is desirable to discontinue therapy as soon as the cardiac rhythm appears to be stable in order to minimize toxic effects.
4. When an intravenous route is not immediately feasible, lidocaine may be administered intramuscularly. The intramuscular dose is 200 mg and may be repeated every 5–10 minutes. However, intravenous administration is always preferable.

Contraindications

1. Lidocaine should not be used in the presence of complete heart block since the drug may suppress or abolish the ventricular focus which is maintaining the heartbeat. The same principle applies wherever sinus node activity is depressed (e.g., sinoatrial block or marked sinus bradycardia) or when there is evidence of advanced atrioventricular or intraventricular block.

2. Because lidocaine is metabolized primarily in the liver, the drug must be administered with great caution if at all in patients with severe liver disease or congestive failure. In these conditions lidocaine may accumulate in the blood and produce toxic levels.

3. Although lidocaine does not depress myocardial function in usual doses, large doses may reduce myocardial contractility, especially when the heart is severely damaged. For this reason the drug may be hazardous in patients with cardiogenic shock or pulmonary edema.

4. Patients with known hypersensitivity to local anesthetics should not receive the drug.

Side Effects

Cardiac Effects

The toxic effects of lidocaine on the heart have been described in previous paragraphs.

Systemic Effects

1. The most serious side effects of lidocaine involve the central nervous system. Of particular importance is the occurrence of convulsions (grand mal seizures), which result most often after large doses of the drug are administered for prolonged periods.

2. Other common central nervous system manifestations of lidocaine toxicity are drowsiness, paresthesias, difficulty in hearing, and muscle twitching. Also, patients may become acutely disturbed, agitated, or disoriented when lidocaine is administered on a continuous basis.

3. Nausea and vomiting are less common side effects than those involving the central nervous system but are by no means rare.

Nursing Implications

1. The maintenance dosage of lidocaine must be adjusted according to the clinical response. A microdrip technique should be used for accurate titration. As a general rule the rate of infusion should not exceed 4 mg lidocaine per minute.

2. The nurse should be aware of the total dosage of lidocaine that has been administered in a given period (e.g., total mg in 8 hours).

3. Because of the high incidence of side effects involving the central nervous system, the nurse must seek manifestations of such reactions at frequent intervals. In the event of seizures the drug should be discontinued. If the convulsions persist, the physician may choose to administer a short-acting barbiturate. Less obvious central nervous system reactions (especially drowsiness or behavioral changes) can be recognized only by thoughtful repeated assessment of the patient's clinical state. The latter effects can often be controlled by reducing the rate of infusion.

4. Although lidocaine is a relatively safe drug and does not usually cause heart block or depression of myocardial function, the possibility of these cardiac side effects must

be kept in mind. Widening of QRS complexes, prolongation of the PR interval, a change in rate or rhythm, the development of hypotension, or left ventricular failure should be brought to the physician's attention at once.

DIGITALIS (DIGOXIN)*

Uses

1. To control atrial fibrillation associated with a rapid ventricular rate.
2. To terminate other rapid-rate supraventricular arrhythmias, particularly paroxysmal atrial tachycardia.

Actions

Digoxin exerts multiple and diverse effects on the electrophysical properties of the heart. Its main action is to increase the strength of myocardial contraction, but this effect is unrelated to its antiarrhythmic activity. Fundamentally, the drug controls arrhythmias by increasing vagal activity and slowing the rate of conduction in the AV node and in the bundle of His.

Methods of Administration and Dosage

1. Digoxin may be given intravenously or orally, the choice depending on the urgency of the clinical condition.
2. In patients with rapid ventricular rates due to supraventricular arrhythmias, it is customary to administer 0.5 mg digoxin intravenously as an initial dose. Slowing of the ventricular rate begins within 15 minutes, and a maximum effect is usually reached within 1 hour. Depending on the heart rate response, an additional dose of 0.25 mg digoxin can be given within 3 hours if necessary; however if the ventricular rate is adequately controlled by the initial dose, the second injection should be administered at 6 hours. Further doses of 0.25 mg, or 0.125 mg, digoxin may be given at 12 and 18 hours after the first injection. The total intravenous dose of digoxin in patients with acute myocardial infarction should not exceed 1.2 mg in 24 hours.
3. Oral administration of digoxin produces an effect within 2–6 hours and can be used in less critical situations. The oral dosage consists of 0.5 mg initially, followed by 0.25 mg every 6 hours for two additional doses or until a satisfactory rate control is achieved. Subsequent doses of 0.125 mg or 0.25 mg digoxin may be given at 6-hour intervals if needed until a total dose of 1.5 mg is reached.
4. After a supraventricular tachyarrhythmia is terminated (or controlled) by digoxin, oral doses of 0.125 mg or 0.25 mg digoxin are administered once a day for maintenance purposes.

Contraindications

1. Digoxin should not be used to treat any arrhythmia that may in itself be a manifestation of digitalis toxicity (for example, junctional tachycardia).

---

*This discussion considers digoxin only as an antiarrhythmic agent. (The use of digoxin in the treatment of heart failure has been discussed previously.) Although digoxin is but one of several cardiac glycosides used in the management of arrhythmias, it is by far the most popular digitalis preparation. Other agents such as digitalis leaf, digitoxin, deslanoside, and ouabain are not discussed here.

2. Because digoxin decreases conduction through the AV node it should be administered with great caution in patients with ECG evidence of first- or second-degree AV block.

3. The presence of frequent premature ventricular contractions may be a relative contraindication to the use of digoxin because the drug tends to increase automaticity and to stimulate ectopic pacemakers; this action may precipitate ventricular tachycardia.

4. Acidosis, alkalosis, hypokalemia, and other electrolyte disturbances are known to increase sensitivity to digoxin. Thus the risk of inducing digitalis toxicity in patients with these conditions must always be weighed before selecting digitalis as an antiarrhythmic agent.

Side Effects

Cardiac Effects

1. In toxic doses, digitalis may induce practically any type of rhythm disturbance. Premature ventricular contractions (particularly in the form of bigeminy), non-paroxysmal junctional tachycardia, and paroxysmal atrial tachycardia with block are the most frequent digitalis-induced arrhythmias.

2. Digitalis toxicity may also produce second-degree heart block and, less frequently, sinus arrest.

Systemic Effects

1. Gastrointestinal symptoms include anorexia, nausea, and vomiting.

2. Central nervous system manifestations of digoxin overdosage are mental depression, confusion, and lassitude.

3. Visual complaints, although mentioned frequently in textbooks, are not especially common. Abnormal color perception and blurred vision are sometimes noted.

Nursing Implications

1. It is important for the nurse to ascertain precisely which digitalis preparation is to be administered. The dosages of the various drugs in the digitalis group are distinctly different. For example, the oral maintenance dose of digitalis (leaf) is 100 mg, the maintenance dose of digoxin is 0.25 mg, and the maintenance dose of digitoxin is 0.1 mg. Administering the wrong digitalis preparation may have fatal consequences.

2. There is only a narrow margin between a therapeutic and a toxic dose. Consequently it is essential to constantly seek signs suggesting digitalis toxicity.

3. If ECG or systemic signs of digitalis toxicity are noted or suspected, the nurse should withhold the next dose of digoxin until the physician has been consulted.

4. If the heart rate decreases to below 60/minute, the physician should be advised before further doses of the drug are given.

5. Because hypokalemia is a common cause of digitalis toxicity the nurse should be aware of the serum potassium level before administering digoxin. This caution is particularly important in patients who are being treated concomitantly with diuretic therapy.

DIPHENYLHYDANTOIN (DILANTIN)

Uses

1. To terminate digitalis-induced tachyarrhythmias.

2. To control ventricular ectopic beats when lidocaine and procainamide have been ineffective.

3. To prevent or treat supraventricular tachyarrhythmias but only as a secondary choice to quinidine or other agents.

Actions

Dilantin, well known for its antiepileptic action, also has antiarrhythmic properties. These electrophysiologic actions are unlike those of other antiarrhythmic agents, and the drug is unique in this sense. The main effect of Dilantin is to accelerate conduction velocity through the atria (by increasing the rate of depolarization). As a result, the greatest use of the drug is in combating depressed AV conduction resulting from digitalis or other drug toxicity. In effect, diphenylhydantoin (DPH) reduces automaticity without decreasing conduction through the heart.

Clinically, Dilantin does not affect the QRS complex but may shorten the PR interval.

Methods of Administration and Dosage

1. When used in emergency situations, Dilantin is administered intravenously. In less critical circumstances or when used as maintenance therapy, oral dosages are employed.

2. The initial intravenous dose is 125–250 mg; this amount is injected *slowly* over a period of 3–5 minutes (about 50 mg/minute). The drug usually acts within 15 seconds, and its maximal effect is evident at 5 minutes. If not successful in controlling the arrhythmia, the same dose can be repeated every 15 minutes if necessary; however, the total dosage should not exceed 750 mg in 1 hour.

3. The drug should *not* be given by continuous intravenous infusion because a precipitate forms within most intravenous solutions.

4. Oral administration consists initially of 200 mg, followed by 100 mg every 6 hours.

5. Following termination of the arrhythmia, Dilantin may be continued for maintenance purposes in dosages of 100 mg three times a day.

Contraindications

1. Because Dilantin decreases automatic firing of the SA node and ectopic pacemakers, the drug probably should not be used in patients with marked sinus bradycardia or sinus arrest. Similarly, the drug should be avoided in patients with complete heart block in whom depression of the ventricular focus may lead to ventricular standstill.

2. Hypersensitivity to diphenylhydantoin, although rare, is a specific contraindication to the use of the drug in treating arrhythmias.

Side Effects

Cardiac Effects

1. Depression of automaticity may lead to excessively slow heart rates.

2. Atrioventricular heart block may develop during the course of Dilantin therapy; however AV conduction is only rarely affected.

Systemic Effects

1. When administered intravenously Dilantin may cause hypotension, particularly if the rate of injection is too rapid.

2. Drowsiness, ataxia, dizziness, incoordination, and nystagmus are central nervous system side effects. (It is believed that if these findings are allowed to persist they may become permanent.)

3. Nausea, vomiting, pruritus, urticaria, and skin rashes may occur; these effects are probably allergic manifestations of the drug.

4. Gingival hypertrophy is commonly observed in patients on long-term treatment with Dilantin. This effect, however, is seldom observed during acute therapy for arrhythmias.

Nursing Implications

1. Dilantin should not be given as a bolus injection intravenously. Rather, the drug should be injected slowly, at a rate of 50 mg/minute.

2. Continuous observation of the monitor is essential during intravenous administration, particularly since the drug may begin to act within seconds. Blood pressure monitoring during the postinjection period is also advisable.

3. Complaints of drowsiness, nervousness, and depression should alert the nurse to the possibility that these behavioral changes are toxic manifestations of the drug.

4. When the drug is given orally, it is good practice to have the patient drink at least a half glass of water to minimize gastric upset.

POTASSIUM

Uses

1. To abolish digitalis-induced tachyarrhythmias, for example, paroxysmal atrial tachycardia with block and junctional tachycardia.

2. To suppress premature ventricular contractions that may be caused by a deficiency of potassium in myocardial cells.

Actions

The basic effect of potassium is to decrease the threshold of excitability and to increase intraventricular conduction. These actions are related to alterations in the exchange of sodium and potassium across the myocardial cellular membrane.

Methods of Administration and Dosage

1. In patients with acute myocardial infarction in whom arrhythmia control must be achieved promptly, potassium is often administered intravenously. In less critical situations the drug is given orally.

2. For intravenous use, 40 mEq potassium chloride is diluted in 500 ml 5% dextrose solution and the infusion is administered by slow drip during a 2- to 3-hour period. *Potassium should never be injected directly into a vein without being diluted.*

3. Oral dosage consists of a total 40–80 mEq potassium per day. This amount is divided into two, three, or four doses depending on the concentration of potassium in the particular preparation being used. Oral potassium preparations should be given after meals with a full glass of water to minimize the saline laxative effect and gastrointestinal irritation.

4. The ultimate amount of potassium required to combat digitalis-induced arrhythmias is not constant; it depends on the severity of digitalis toxicity and the response to therapy.

Contraindications

1. Because of the threat of producing *hyperkalemia*, potassium should not be given to patients with evidence of renal insufficiency or failure (e.g., oliguria, elevated BUN) who are unable to excrete potassium loads.
2. A high serum potassium level is a definite contraindication for the use of potassium therapy. (Potassium should never be administered until the serum potassium level has been determined.)
3. Elevating the serum potassium level may increase atrioventricular block in patients with normal serum potassium levels. For this reason potassium should not be used in the presence of second-degree or complete heart block unless the serum potassium level is markedly low to begin with.

Side Effects

Cardiac Effects

Although the initial effect of potassium is to decrease excitability and increase intraventricular conduction, these desirable effects may be reversed with prolonged infusion of potassium. Ultimately, conduction slows and excitability diminishes so that bradycardia or heart block may develop.

Systemic Effects

1. Nausea, vomiting, diarrhea, and abdominal discomfort may occur with the use of oral potassium.
2. Overdosage of potassium may lead to toxicity. Common manifestations of potassium intoxication are weakness, a feeling of heaviness of the extremities, listlessness, mental confusion, and a fall in blood pressure.
3. With intravenous administration, patients may experience pain or a burning sensation at the infusion site and along the venous pathway.

Nursing Implications

1. Potassium must *never* be injected directly into an intravenous line; the drug should always be diluted in at least 500 cc of fluid and administered by slow drip. The flow rate should not be greater than 20 mEq/hour. If the patient experiences pain at the intravenous site the rate of infusion must be decreased.
2. Any change in heart rate, rhythm, or the duration of the QRS complexes occurring during potassium administration should be reported immediately to the physician.
3. The nurse should consider the possibility that continuous potassium infusion may produce hyperkalemia and therefore should observe the patient for signs of toxicity. In addition the ECG should be examined carefully. Findings such as a narrowed peaked T wave, shortened QT interval, prolonged PR interval, and diminished P waves may reflect hyperkalemia.
4. Oral potassium preparations should be given with a full glass of water (for reasons explained previously).

5. Serum potassium levels should be monitored regularly in all patients receiving potassium. The normal serum potassium level is from 3.8–5.1 mEq. If the laboratory reports a serum level in excess of 5.1 mEq, the physician should be notified.

ISOPROTERENOL (ISUPREL)

Uses

1. To accelerate the heart rate in advanced heart block (especially complete heart block) until a temporary pacemaker can be inserted.
2. To control Stokes-Adams attacks due to marked bradycardia.
3. To treat symptomatic bradyarrhythmias that are not responsive to atropine (or when atropine cannot be used).
4. To restore heart action after the development of primary ventricular standstill.

(The use of isoproterenol in the treatment of cardiogenic shock has been discussed previously so this action is not included in the present discussion.)

Actions

The effect of isoproterenol is very similar to that of epinephrine. The drug is a sympathetic nervous system stimulant.

Isoproterenol increases automatic firing of both supraventricular and ventricular pacemakers, and produces an increase in the heart rate. In addition, the drug improves AV conduction. (Other than these antiarrhythmic properties, isoproterenol causes a marked increase in the force of myocardial contractility.)

Methods of Administration and Dosage

1. Isoproterenol can be given in any of the following ways: subcutaneously, intramuscularly, intravenously (directly or by continuous infusion), or sublingually. In addition, an intracardiac injection may be used in the emergency treatment of ventricular standstill. The route of administration depends on the arrhythmia being treated and urgency of the clinical situation, but the most common method of administration is by continuous intravenous infusion.
2. An intravenous infusion of isoproterenol is prepared by diluting 1 mg isoproterenol in 250 ml 5% dextrose in water (in this dilution each milliliter contains 4 micrograms). Microdrip administration and the use of "piggyback" technique is essential. The infusion rate initially is 2–4 micrograms per minute. If this dosage is ineffective in maintaining the heart rate at 60/minute or more, the infusion rate may be increased to 6–10 micrograms/minute.
3. When used to treat ventricular standstill or severe Stokes-Adams attacks, the customary intracardiac or direct intravenous dosage is 0.02 or 0.04 mg; however, 0.1 mg may sometimes be necessary.
4. The customary subcutaneous or intramuscular dosage is 0.1–0.4 mg isoproterenol every 2–4 hours as required.
5. Sublingual administration (the least common method of administration in a CCU) consists of 10–20 mg every 3 hours. The action begins within 15–30 minutes.

Contraindications

Because isoproterenol increases the heart's oxygen consumption, the drug must be used cautiously in patients with signs of acute coronary ischemia. For this reason the drug is reserved for emergency use until a temporary pacemaker can be inserted.

Side Effects

Cardiac Effects

1. The most serious effect of isoproterenol is that it may provoke ventricular tachycardia or ventricular fibrillation! This complication stems from the drug's ability to increase automatic firing of ectopic ventricular foci.

2. Angina may develop during isoproterenol therapy, reflecting the increased oxygen demand created by the drug.

Systemic Effects

1. Sweating, flushing of the skin, and a feeling of weakness are perhaps the most common side effects.

2. Nervousness, excitement, tremors, headaches, and dizziness also occur frequently.

3. Hypotension may develop because of the vasodilating effect of the drug on skeletal and mesenteric vessels.

Nursing Implications

1. During the course of continuous intravenous administration of isoproterenol the nurse should remain near the patient at all times. The threat of ventricular tachycardia or ventricular fibrillation is ever present, even when small doses are used.

2. In the event premature ventricular contractions develop with increasing frequency the rate of infusion should be reduced. A syringe filled with lidocaine should be available at the bedside.

3. Monitoring of the blood pressure and vital signs is essential.

4. Since most patients who are treated with isoproterenol are likely candidates for temporary pacemaker insertion, preparations should be made for this procedure.

ATROPINE

Uses

1. To accelerate the heart rate in sinus bradycardia, sinoatrial arrest, and slow junctional rhythms caused by parasympathetic (vagal) overactivity.

2. To increase the rate of conduction through the AV node in first- and second-degree AV block.

Actions

1. Atropine inhibits parasympathetic (vagal) activity on the SA node (and AV junctional area) and permits the sympathetic nervous system to gain control of the heart rate.

2. The increase in conduction velocity occurring after the administration of atropine is also related to vagal blockade. (Conduction disturbances due to organic damage to the SA or AV nodes are not benefited by atropine.)

3. Atropine may produce an increase in blood pressure and cardiac output. This effect is particularly apparent in patients with bradycardia and hypotension.

Methods of Administration and Dosage

1. Although atropine can be given subcutaneously and intramuscularly, intravenous administration is preferable in the treatment of arrhythmias. The initial intravenous dose may range from 0.3 mg to 1 mg; the average dose is 0.5 mg. The drug is

injected as a bolus. The onset of action is rapid, usually within 1–3 minutes.

2. If the heart rate does not increase to a satisfactory level with this initial dose, a similar dosage may be given in 5 minutes.

3. The drug is usually active for 4 hours, at which time an additional dose may be required. The cumulative dosage, however, should not exceed 4 mg.

4. When used intramuscularly, a 2-mg dose of atropine is generally used.

Contraindications

1. Patients with known glaucoma should not receive atropine because of the risk of increasing intraocular pressure to dangerous levels.

2. Because atropine has an antispasmodic effect and decreases urinary bladder tone, caution must be exercised in using the drug in patients with symptoms of urinary obstruction. The danger of causing urinary retention is particularly high in men with prostatic hypertrophy.

Side Effects

Cardiac Effects

1. The heart rate response to atropine is not wholly predictable, and certain patients may develop excessively rapid heart rates after receiving only small amounts of atropine.

2. The drug can produce atrioventricular dissociation because the atrial rate may be accelerated more than the ventricular rate.

3. Ventricular tachycardia and ventricular fibrillation have been reported to occur following the administration of atropine; however this arrhythmic complication is rare.

4. A *decrease* in the heart rate may occasionally develop before the rate increases. This paradoxical effect usually develops if atropine is injected too slowly or if the dosage is too small (less than 0.3 mg).

Systemic Effects

1. Atropine inhibits glandular secretions and therefore produces dryness of the mouth and diminished sweating.

2. Dilation of the pupils and blurred vision are common side effects. As noted, atropine may cause an exacerbation of glaucoma.

3. Atropine sometimes has a stimulating effect on the central nervous system and causes euphoria, excitability, and mental confusion.

Nursing Implications

1. For a period of at least 5 minutes after atropine is administered intravenously, the monitor should be observed continuously to determine the effect of the drug on the heart rate. The possibility of inducing an overly rapid rate must be considered. Also, paradoxical rate slowing may be noted immediately after the injection.

2. The duration of action of atropine, as manifested by the maintenance of an adequate heart rate should be carefully observed. If bradycardia returns within a short time, temporary pacing may be required.

3. The nurse should ask the patient if he has a known history of glaucoma or of difficulty in voiding. (Normally the physician would have determined these facts prior to ordering atropine, but for safety's sake it is a wise practice to recheck this possibility.)

4. Because a dry mouth and blurred vision are common side effects of atropine, the nurse should advise the patient that these symptoms may occur but are only transient in nature.

5. If the patient does not void for several hours after receiving atropine, urinary retention should be suspected and the physician notified.

PROPRANOLOL (INDERAL)

Uses

1. To control supraventricular tachyarrhythmias associated with rapid ventricular rates.

2. To terminate tachyarrhythmias due to digitalis toxicity.

3. To suppress ventricular ectopic beats not controlled by other antiarrhythmic drugs.

Actions

The primary effect of propranolol is to reduce sympathetic stimulation of the heart. This is accomplished by blocking beta receptor cells in the heart, thus inhibiting the secretion of catecholamines (norepinephrine) at the receptor sites.

Propranolol also has a direct action on the electrophysiological properties of cardiac tissue. Specifically, the drug decreases automaticity in the SA node, atria, the AV junction, and the His-Purkinje system. Furthermore, propranolol slows electrical conduction through the atria and bundle of His.

At the same time propranolol seriously decreases the strength of ventricular contraction and in turn reduces cardiac output.

Methods of Administration and Dosage

1. When used in the emergency treatment of arrhythmias, propranolol is given intravenously. The drug is injected slowly at a rate of 1–2 mg/minute. If necessary, the same dose may be repeated after 5 minutes. Further intravenous doses are not advisable for at least 4 hours. Following intravenous administration the drug acts within minutes, and the effect persists for at least 3 hours.

2. In noncritical situations (e.g., to suppress premature ventricular contractions), propranolol is administered orally in doses of 10–30 mg every 4–6 hours.

Contraindications

1. Because propranolol decreases the heart rate and prolongs AV conduction time, it should not be used in patients with marked sinus bradycardia, sinus arrest (or block), or second- or third-degree heart block.

2. As the result of its adverse effect on myocardial contractility, propranolol is extremely dangerous in the presence of heart failure or cardiogenic shock. The reduction in cardiac output induced by the drug can only exaggerate or intensify the pumping failure of the heart.

3. Propranolol should not be given to patients with a known history of bronchial asthma or bronchospasm because the blocking of beta receptors in the lung may produce severe airway resistance.

Side Effects

Cardiac Effects

1. Excessive slowing of the heart rate may develop, even after small doses of propranolol. This bradycardia may be accompanied by syncope, hypotension, and angina pectoris.

2. In patients with acute myocardial infarction, propranolol may precipitate heart failure or cardiogenic shock.

3. The drug may decrease atrioventricular conduction sufficiently to cause complete heart block, particularly in patients with preexisting conduction disorders.

Systemic Effects

1. Gastrointestinal symptoms including nausea, vomiting, or constipation may occur during propranolol therapy.

2. Weakness, fatigue, and lassitude are common side effects.

3. Confusion, insomnia, hallucinations, and mental depression are sometimes observed.

4. Allergic reactions including skin rashes, fever, and paresthesias of the hands are rare toxic manifestations.

Nursing Implications

1. Intravenous propranolol should be injected slowly (1 mg/minute) and not as a bolus.

2. Continuous observation of the monitor is essential during and following intravenous administration of the drug. Particular attention must be given to the heart rate. If severe bradycardia (a rate less than 50/minute) develops, the physician may order 1 mg atropine intravenously to combat this complication.

3. The possibility of second- and third-degree AV block developing in patients receiving propranolol should be considered.

4. The nurse should examine the patient at regular intervals for signs or symptoms of heart failure or hypotension. Any evidence of this untoward effect should be reported to the physician promptly.

5. If patients develop wheezing or other signs of bronchospasm, the drug should be discontinued and the physician notified.

6. Behavioral changes, particularly lassitude and depression, resulting from propranolol treatment should be considered in the nursing assessment of the patient.

Appendix

Exercises in the Interpretation of Arrhythmias

On the following pages 30 electrocardiographic (ECG) rhythm strips are presented for the reader's interpretation. This exercise is meant to serve three purposes:

1. To permit self-testing of the ability to identify common arrhythmias
2. To demonstrate variations in the ECG patterns of certain arrhythmias (particularly with different monitoring leads)
3. To introduce a few less common arrhythmias that were not described in previous chapters

In interpreting these arrhythmias the nurse should examine the ECG in an orderly way, never making a snap decision. It is important to point out that despite careful analysis of a tracing, many arrhythmias cannot be identified precisely from a single monitoring lead; multiple leads are often required to reach a definite conclusion. Whenever there is uncertainity about a particular ECG finding (e.g., are P waves actually present?), it is a wise practice simply to state that more than one possibility exists in interpretation (e.g., the arrhythmia may be *either* sinus tachycardia *or* atrial tachycardia).

The authors' interpretation of the 30 ECGs along with pertinent comments are found on the back of each page.

ECG 1

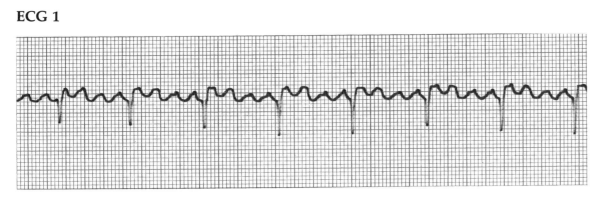

Interpretation:

_____

_____

_____

_____

ECG 2

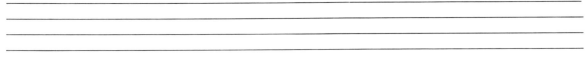
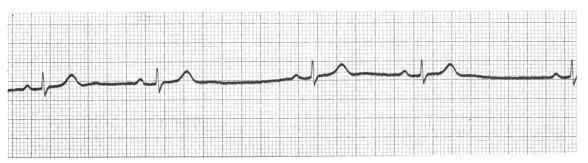

Interpretation:

_____

_____

_____

_____

ECG 3

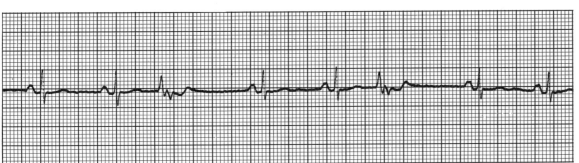

Interpretation:

_____

_____

_____

_____

ECG 1

Atrial Flutter with 4:1 Block

The atrial rate is 320/minute while the ventricular rate 80/minute. This indicates that only one out of every four atrial impulses is conducted to the ventricles (4:1 block). The P waves are replaced by typical flutter waves (F waves), creating the classic "sawtooth" configuration of atrial flutter. The regularity of the ventricular complexes excludes the possibility that the arrhythmia is atrial fibrillation.

ECG 2

Sinus Arrhythmia with Bradycardia

The cardiac rhythm is distinctly irregular. Because each QRS complex is preceded by a normal P wave, it can be concluded that the irregular rhythm is the result of unevenness in the rate of impulse formation at the SA node. This variation in automaticity is due to vagal influences on the SA node, as is the slow heart rate (50/minute).

ECG 3

Premature Junctional Contractions

The third and sixth beats are premature junctional contractions. The P waves of these ectopic beats are inverted and occur just *after* the QRS complexes, indicating their origin in the junctional tissue rather than in the atria. That these beats are not premature ventricular contractions is apparent from the normal width of the QRS complexes (0.08 second).

ECG 4

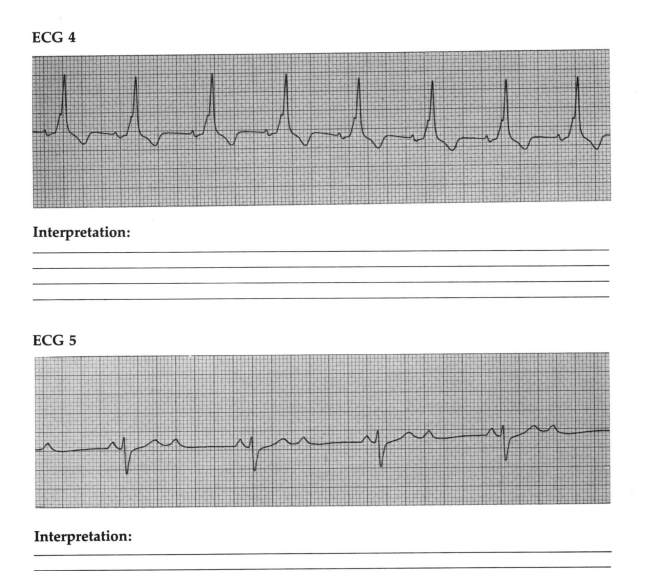

Interpretation:

_____
_____
_____
_____

ECG 5

Interpretation:

_____
_____
_____
_____

ECG 6

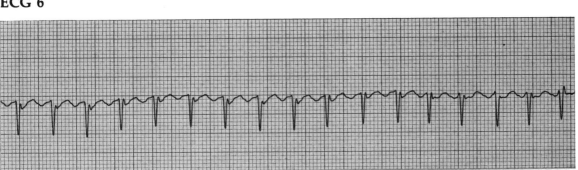

Interpretation:

_____
_____
_____
_____

ECG 4

Intraventricular Conduction Disturbance (Bundle Branch Block)

The QRS complexes are 0.16 second and have a slurred configuration. We know that these abnormal QRS complexes are not premature ventricular contractions because each is preceded by a P wave. The widening of the QRS complexes reflects a disturbance in conduction *below* the AV junctional area (bundle branch block). From this single monitoring lead, it is not possible to determine whether the left or the right bundle branch is involved.

ECG 5

Second-Degree AV Heart Block (with Constant PR Interval)

Every other P wave is blocked, producing a 2:1 second-degree heart block. The PR interval of the conducted beat is constant, unlike Wenckebach-type second-degree block in which the PR interval lengthens progressively with successive beats until a QRS complex is dropped. The normal width of the QRS complexes (about 0.10 second) suggests that the block is junctional rather than subjunctional in origin.

ECG 6

Supraventricular Tachycardia

From this single monitor lead recording, it is difficult to classify this arrhythmia in any more specific terms than "supraventricular tachycardia." The normal duration of the QRS complexes indicates that the tachycardia (170/minute) originates in either the atria or the junctional tissue (supraventricular) but not in the ventricles. Because of the inability to identify P waves specifically in this tracing, it cannot be determined if the arrhythmia is paroxysmal atrial tachycardia, paroxysmal junctional tachycardia, or atrial flutter with 2:1 block. Only by using additional leads can a definite interpretation be made.

ECG 7

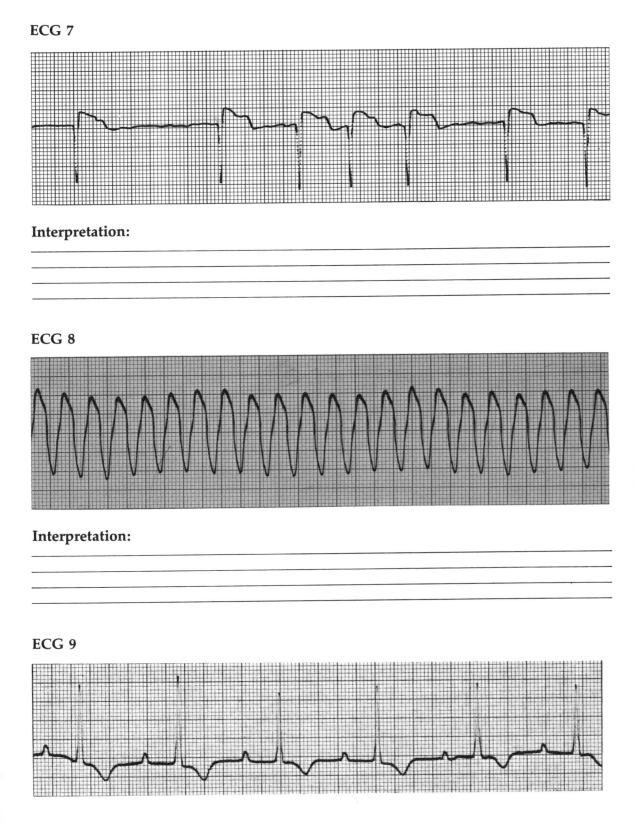

Interpretation:

_____

_____

_____

_____

_____

ECG 8

Interpretation:

_____

_____

_____

_____

_____

ECG 9

Interpretation:

_____

_____

_____

_____

ECG 7

Atrial Fibrillation

The totally irregular rhythm immediately suggests the probability of atrial fibrillation. This diagnosis is confirmed by the absence of P waves and the presence of fibrillatory (f waves). The elevated ST segments reflect acute myocardial injury.

ECG 8

Ventricular Tachycardia

This very rapid series of consecutive premature ventricular contractions (220/minute), typical of ventricular tachycardia, is an extremely dangerous arrhythmia. Sustained ventricular tachycardia of this type may progress to ventricular fibrillation at any time; the arrhythmia must be terminated at once.

ECG 9

First-Degree AV Block

The PR interval measures 0.36 second. This prolongation (greater than 0.20 second) is diagnostic of first-degree AV heart block. The inverted T waves reflect myocardial ischemia.

ECG 10

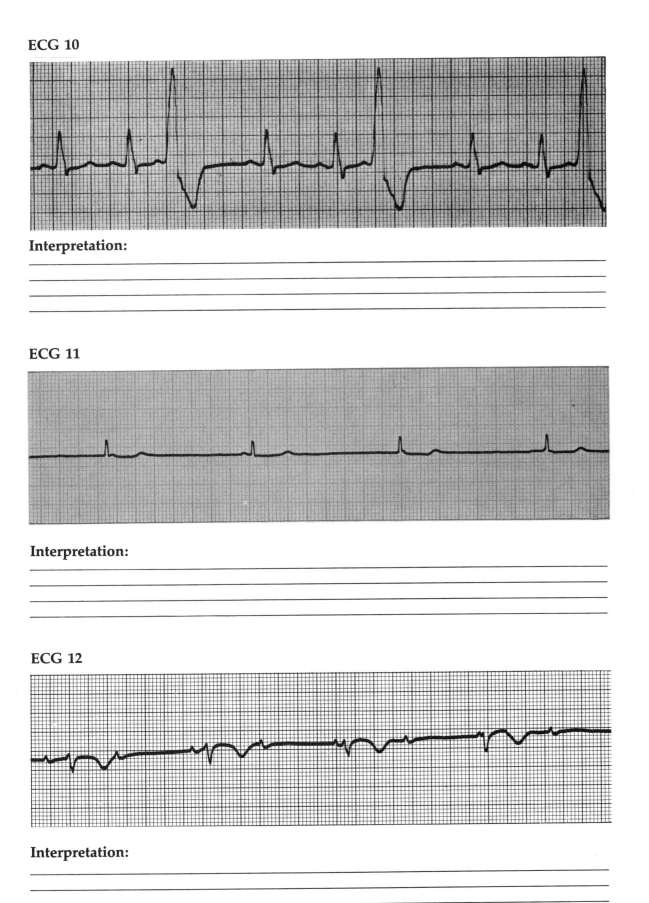

Interpretation:

_____

_____

_____

_____

_____

ECG 11

Interpretation:

_____

_____

_____

_____

ECG 12

Interpretation:

_____

_____

_____

_____

ECG 10

Frequent Premature Ventricular Contractions (Trigeminy)

Every *third* complex is a premature ventricular contraction. This sequence of two normal beats and then one premature ventricular contraction is described as *trigeminy*. (When every *second* beat is a premature ventricular contraction the pattern is termed *bigeminy*.) Because all of the premature ventricular contractions have the same configuration, it can be assumed that they arose from one irritable focus within the ventricles (unifocal rather than multifocal PVCs).

ECG 11

Junctional Rhythm

The pacemaker is in the AV junctional area, as is evident from the abnormal position of the P waves and the slow heart rate. In the first, third, and fourth beats, the P waves occur immediately after the QRS complexes; in the second beat the P wave precedes the QRS complex. With a passive junctional pacemaker the expected heart rate would be 40–60/minute, as is the case here (40/minute).

ECG 12

Complete (Third-Degree) Heart Block

The P waves bear no relationship to the QRS complexes since the atrial and ventricular pacemakers are wholly independent of each other (atrioventricular dissociation). All of the impulses originating in the SA node are blocked. That the QRS complexes are of normal width (0.08 second) suggests that the block is probably in the junctional area. (Subjunctional blocks are usually associated with wide QRS complexes.) The very slow ventricular rate (40/minute) is characteristic of complete heart block.

ECG 13

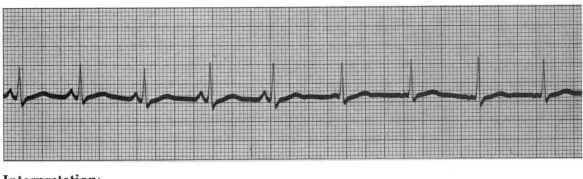

Interpretation:

_____

_____

_____

_____

ECG 14

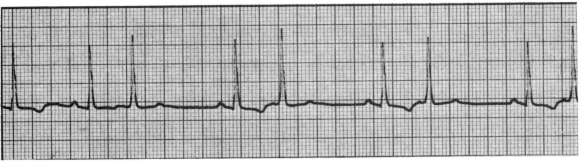

Interpretation:

_____

_____

_____

_____

ECG 15

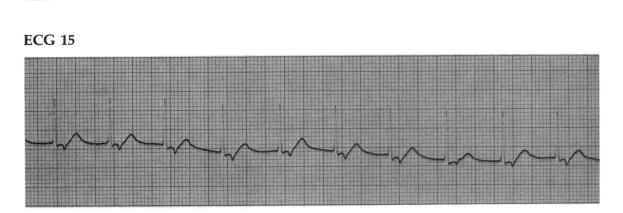

Interpretation:

_____

_____

_____

_____

ECG 13

Wandering Pacemaker

The pacemaker wanders from the SA node to the AV junctional area, as is apparent from the change in P wave configuration after the fifth complex. When the pacemaker is in the junctional area there is slight slowing of the heart rate.

ECG 14

Premature Atrial Contractions

A premature atrial contraction occurs after each normal beat (except the first beat). This pattern is described as atrial bigeminy. Note that the P waves of the ectopic beats are distinctly different from the P waves associated with the normal beats arising in the SA node.

ECG 15

Nonparoxysmal Junctional Tachycardia

The P waves are inverted and occur immediately after the QRS complexes, leaving no doubt about the junctional origin of the arrhythmia. The ventricular rate is about 100/minute. This rate excludes the possibility of a passive junctional rhythm (rate 40–60/minute) and paroxysmal junctional tachycardia (rate 140–220/minute). Although not evident on this short rhythm strip, the arrhythmia developed gradually rather than abruptly, typical of the onset of nonparoxysmal junctional tachycardia.

ECG 16

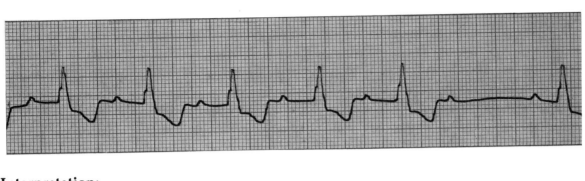

Interpretation:

_____

_____

_____

_____

ECG 17

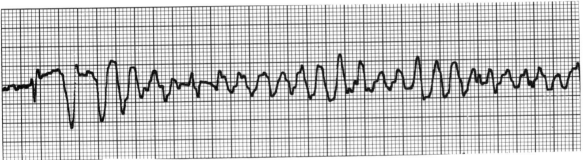

Interpretation:

_____

_____

_____

_____

ECG 18

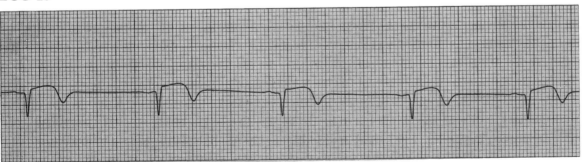

Interpretation:

_____

_____

_____

_____

ECG 16

Second-Degree Block (Wenckebach Type)

The PR interval lengthens gradually in each of the first five beats, after which the next P wave is not followed by a QRS complex. This sequence of progressive lengthening of the PR interval until a beat is dropped is the most characteristic feature of Wenckebach-type block. In most instances Wenckebach second-degree blocks are associated with QRS complexes of normal duration (because the block is usually in the AV nodal area). In this example, however, the QRS complexes are wider than 0.12 second, suggesting that the block is subjunctional in origin.

ECG 17

Ventricular Fibrillation

A premature ventricular contraction occurs at the time of the T wave (vulnerable period) of a normal beat and produces repetitive ventricular firing, which then degenerates almost immediately into ventricular fibrillation. This "R on T" pattern is one of the most common causes of ventricular fibrillation in patients with myocardial infarction.

ECG 18

Sinus Bradycardia

Because the P waves are not distinct and are difficult to identify in this particular monitoring lead, the possibility of a passive junctional rhythm cannot be excluded entirely. In order to identify the P waves more distinctly, a different monitoring lead was used (as shown below). The diagnosis of sinus bradycardia was then readily apparent.

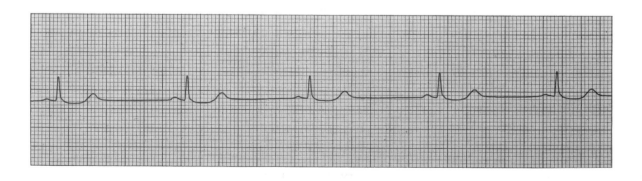

ECG 19

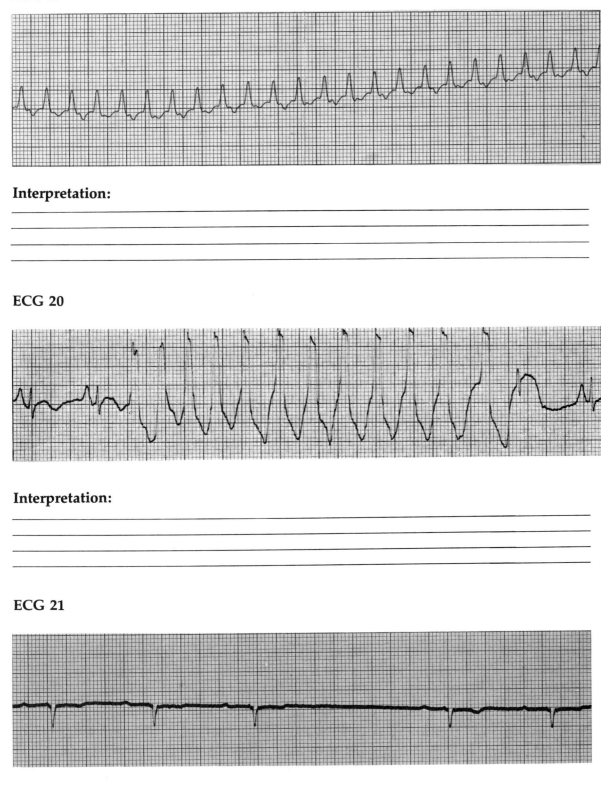

Interpretation:

_____

_____

_____

_____

ECG 20

Interpretation:

_____

_____

_____

_____

ECG 21

Interpretation:

_____

_____

_____

_____

ECG 19

Paroxysmal Junctional Tachycardia

The normal width of the QRS complexes (0.08 second) indicates that the tachycardia is atrial or junctional (supraventricular) in origin. The very rapid heart rate (about 240/ minute) is compatible with either paroxysmal atrial tachycardia or paroxysmal junctional tachycardia. However, since P waves appear to be present (just after the QRS complexes), the diagnosis of paroxysmal junctional tachycardia is reasonable.

ECG 20

Ventricular Tachycardia

After two normally conducted beats, there is a rapid series of 12 consecutive premature ventricular contractions. This sequence of four or more consecutive PVCs is, by definition, ventricular tachycardia. Because the repetitive ventricular firing stopped spontaneously after a few seconds, the episode is described as a short run of ventricular tachycardia. Despite the briefness of the episode and the return of normal sinus rhythm, lidocaine therapy should nevertheless be used to prevent further occurrences of ventricular tachycardia.

ECG 21

Sinus Arrest (or Block)

The absence of an entire PQRST complex (after the third beat) indicates that the SA node failed to initiate an impulse at the time (SA arrest) or that the impulse was blocked within the node (SA block). In addition, there is evidence of first-degree heart block (PR interval is 0.28 second). Both of these conditions may be the result of excessive vagal activity.

ECG 22

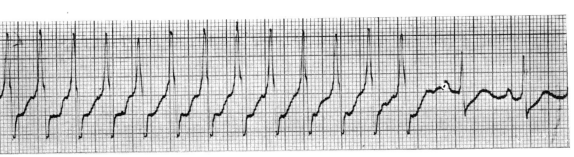

Interpretation:

_____

_____

_____

_____

_____

ECG 23

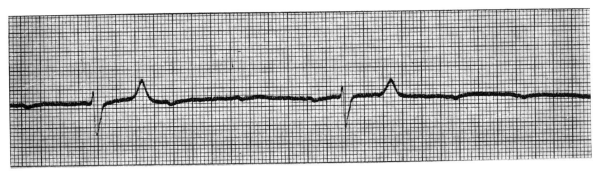

Interpretation:

_____

_____

_____

_____

_____

ECG 24

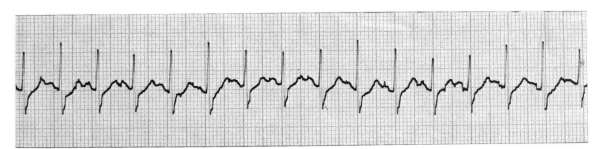

Interpretation:

_____

_____

_____

_____

_____

ECG 22

Paroxysmal Atrial Tachycardia with Aberrant Conduction

The occurrence of regular, very rapid QRS complexes (about 180/minute), each preceded by an abnormally shaped P wave, suggest that this arrhythmia is paroxysmal atrial tachycardia. The abrupt cessation of the tachycardia (note the last two complexes) is a characteristic feature of PAT. Because of the rapidity of atrial impulses, the ventricles are unable to recover (repolarize) fully before the next impulse arrives. As a result, conduction through the ventricles is abnormal (aberrant conduction), and the QRS complexes are distorted in shape. From this single lead the possibility that the arrhythmia is paroxysmal junctional tachycardia cannot be excluded. Therefore a more cautious interpretation would be either paroxysmal atrial tachycardia or paroxysmal junctional tachycardia.

ECG 23

Complete Heart Block Leading to Ventricular Standstill

Although atrial activity (P waves) persists, there are only two isolated ventricular complexes in 6 seconds, indicating that the inherent ventricular pacemaker has failed while the atria continue to beat. In effect, ventricular standstill has developed during the course of complete heart block. The patient died within minutes after this ECG was recorded.

ECG 24

Sinus Tachycardia

Although the heart rate during sinus tachycardia is 100–150 beats/minute in most instances, it is evident from this rhythm strip that sinus tachycardia may be associated with rates that exceed 150/minute. The diagnosis of sinus tachycardia is clear: each P wave is normal and is followed by a normal QRS complex.

ECG 25

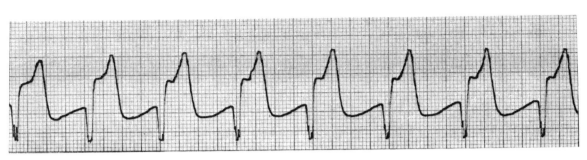

Interpretation:

_____

_____

_____

_____

_____

ECG 26

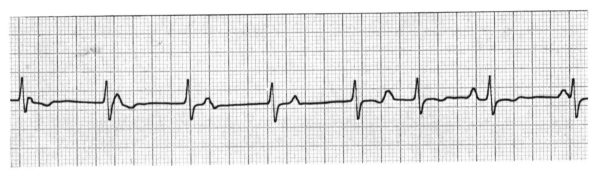

Interpretation:

_____

_____

_____

_____

ECG 27

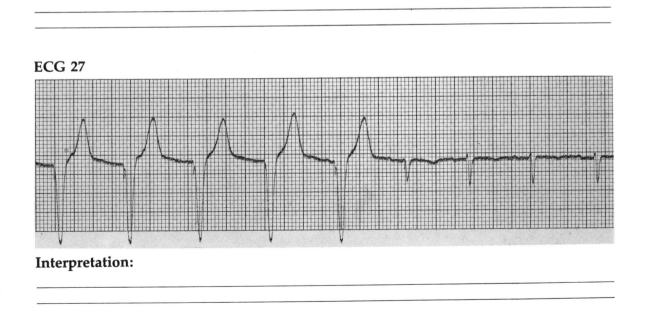

Interpretation:

_____

_____

_____

ECG 25

Accelerated Idioventricular Rhythm or "Slow" Ventricular Tachycardia

There is a series of eight consecutive premature ventricular contractions, which fulfills the diagnostic criterion for ventricular tachycardia. However, the ventricular rate is only 80/minute, and therefore the arrhythmia cannot be truly categorized as a tachycardia. Because of this latter fact, some clinicians classify this arrhythmia as "slow" ventricular tachycardia. A more appropriate term is accelerated idioventricular rhythm, which implies that the arrhythmia originates in the ventricles (idioventricular) but at a rate faster than the inherent rhythmicity of ventricular muscle (hence—accelerated idioventricular rhythm). This arrhythmia is considered to be less serious than true ventricular tachycardia.

ECG 26

A-V Dissociation

The P waves bear no relationship to the QRS complexes, as is apparent from the varying PR intervals. This indicates the atria and ventricles are beating independently; the SA node controls the atria, and a junctional pacemaker activates the ventricles. When the atria and ventricles beat independently, the condition is termed A-V dissociation. This arrhythmia differs from a complete heart block (which is also a form of A-V dissociation) in that the ventricular rate is equal to or greater than the atrial rate. (In complete heart block the ventricular rate is only 30–40/minute while the atria beat at a faster rate.)

ECG 27

Return of Normal Sinus Rhythm During Cardiac Pacing

The first five complexes on the rhythm strip are paced beats (as is evident from the pacing "spikes" and the bundle branch block configuration of the complexes). Then normal sinus rhythm returns, and the pacemaker instantly stops discharging impulses. This indicates that a demand pacemaker was being used and that the sensing mechanism recognized the naturally occurring beats and inhibited the discharge of further pacing impulses. With a set-rate pacemaker, pacing impulses would have continued despite the return of normal sinus rhythm.

ECG 28

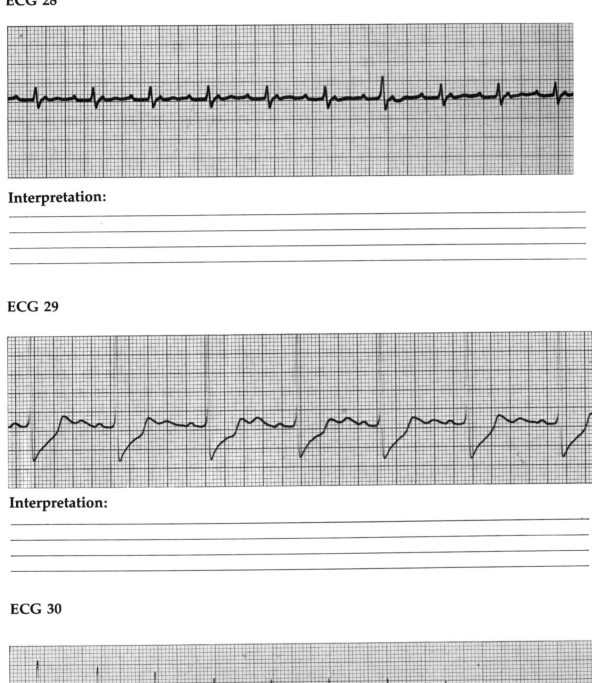

Interpretation:

_____

_____

_____

_____

ECG 29

Interpretation:

_____

_____

_____

_____

ECG 30

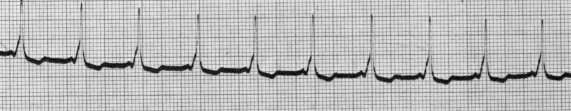

Interpretation:

_____

_____

_____

_____

ECG 28

Paroxysmal Atrial Tachycardia with Block

There are two evenly spaced P waves between each QRS complex. The atrial rate is 200/minute, typical of atrial tachycardia. The ventricular rate is 100/minute, indicating that every other atrial beat is blocked. This arrhythmia, called PAT with block, is one of the most common ECG manifestations of *digitalis toxicity*. The possibility of atrial flutter with 2:1 block can be excluded on the basis of the atrial rate (which would be 300 or more per minute with atrial flutter).

ECG 29

Normal Sinus Rhythm with Prominent U Waves

At first glance it might appear as if the arrhythmia is atrial flutter with 3:1 block. However, it is evident that the waves between each ventricular complex are different in shape and, more significantly, are not regularly spaced (as they would be in atrial flutter). The wave found between the T wave and P wave is called a U wave. It generally appears in the presence of low potassium levels.

ECG 30

Wolff-Parkinson-White Syndrome

Wolff-Parkinson-White syndrome is characterized by a short PR interval (0.06 second in this case) and slurring of the upstroke of the R wave (called a delta wave). It is believed that impulses from the SA node traverse a shorter-than-normal (an accessory) pathway in reaching the ventricles. This accelerated conduction accounts for the short PR interval and the slurred R wave.

Index

Index

A

Aberrant conduction, 155, 167, 270
Acidosis, lactic
  after ventricular fibrillation, 190
  after ventricular standstill, 211
  after ventricular tachycardia, 184
  with cardiogenic shock, 93, 98
Acute myocardial infarction, 13–22
  acute phase of illness, 18–20
  clinical course immediately after infarction, 14
  convalesence, 21–22
  definition and etiology, 10
  diagnosis, 16–18
  emotional disturbances, 20, 69–73
  extent of, 11–12
  fever, 19
  heart failure, 75–90
  location of, 11–12
  major complications, 15, 26, 31
  mechanism, 10–12
  mortality, 25, 30–31
  onset of the attack, 13
  physical examination, 18
  prehospital care, 34
  subacute phase of illness, 20–21
  types of, 11–12
  zones of damage, 12
Acute pulmonary edema, 79–80
  see also Left ventricular failure
  treatment of, 81–83, 89
Aldosterone, 84, 87
Angina pectoris, 8–9
Antiarrhythmic drugs, 235–252
  atropine, 249–251
  digitalis, 243–244
  diphenylhydantoin, 244–246
  isoproterenol, 248–249
  lidocaine, 241–243
  mechanisms of action, 235–237
  potassium, 246–248
  procainamide, 239–241
  propranolol, 251–252
  quinidine, 237–239
Anticoagulant therapy, 105, 106
Arrhythmias
  aggressive management of, 30
  atrial fibrillation, 158–161
  atrial flutter, 156–157
  atrial standstill, 162–163
  bundle branch block, 206–207
  classification of, 132–134
  disorders of conduction, 133, 193–195
  disturbances of impulse formation, 132–133
  ECG interpretation, 135–137
  first degree AV heart block, 196–197
  intraventricular subjunctional blocks, 193, 194–195, 198, 206–207
  junctional rhythm, 168–169
  nonparoxysmal junctional tachycardia, 172–173
  originating in the
    atria, 151
    AV junctional area, 165
    SA node, 139
    ventricles, 175
  paroxysmal atrial tachycardia, 154–155
  paroxysmal junctional tachycardia, 170–171
  premature atrial contractions, 152–153
  premature junctional contractions, 166–167
  premature ventricular contractions, 176–181
  SA arrest or block, 148–149
  second degree AV heart block, 198–201
  sinus arrhythmia, 144–145
  sinus bradycardia, 142–143
  sinus tachycardia, 140–141
  supraventricular, definition of, 175
  third degree AV heart block, 202–205
  ventricular fibrillation, 187–191
  ventricular flutter, 185
  ventricular standstill, 209–213
  ventricular tachycardia, 182–185
  wandering pacemaker, 146–147
  Wenckebach-type heart block, 198–200
Atrial fibrillation, 158–161
Atrial flutter, 156–157
Atrial standstill, 162–163
Atrioventricular junctional blocks, 194, 196, 205
Atropine, 249–251
  in treatment of
    first degree AV heart block, 196
    junctional rhythm, 168
    SA arrest or block, 148
    second degree AV heart block, 199
    sinus bradycardia, 142
    wandering pacemaker, 146
  method of administration and dosage, 249–250
Autonomic nervous system
  effect on arrhythmias, 237
  effect on impulse formation, 139
AV dissociation, 202–203, 272

B

Bigeminy, 176, 179
Blood gas studies, 38, 59, 94
Bronchodilators, 83
Bundle branch blocks, 206–207
  see also Intraventricular subjunctional blocks

C

Cardiac arrest, 187, 209
  see also Ventricular fibrillation, Ventricular standstill
Cardiac cycle, 122
Cardiac monitoring, 37–38, 109–120
  alarm system, 110, 116–117